Praise for

JABBED

"Two of my children—intelligent and caring individuals—have decided against careers in medicine. They have done so because they would be required to risk multiple and repeated vaccinations, just to get through medical school. How many more of Brett Wilcox's 'vaccine informed' have made or will make this same choice? All those, I suggest, that in a similar position to my children, read Wilcox's direct, informed, cut-to-the-chase narrative. A new documentary jumps out of every chapter."

—Andrew Wakefield, MB, BS
Director, *Vaxxed: From Cover-up to Catastrophe*
VaxxedTheMovie.com

"Brett Wilcox has done it again, this time taking on Big Pharma and the global vaccination program. This book is a must read especially if you still think vaccines are provably safe and effective! Toxic ingredients in vaccines work synergistically with glyphosate in food to damage children."

—Stephanie Seneff, PhD, Senior Research Scientist at the MIT Computer Science and Artificial Intelligence Laboratory

"A brilliant book on the sordid history of infectious disease and vaccines. It confirms my own conclusions on this subject, in that no vaccine prevents any infectious disease and that every vaccine poses serious dangers to public health. A must read for all ages."

—Shiv Chopra, DVM, PhD, Former Senior Scientific Advisor on Vaccinations for Health Canada, Author, *CORRUPT TO THE CORE: Memoirs of a Health Canada Whistleblower*, ShivChopra.com

"I used to be a vaccine believer but now consider myself vaccine informed. *Jabbed* is a valuable resource for those seeking to expand their knowledge about vaccines and break free of the deception of the profit-driven pharmaceutical industry. Brett's passionate exposé empowers you to make decisions for yourself and your family from a place of truth rather than fear. I see it as required reading for parents and health care professionals willing to have their eyes opened."

—Kathryn Azelia Hale, MD, MPH, FACOG, Holistic OB/GYN
AbundantHealthLife.com

"In 2000, my 12-month-old son was permanently vaccine injured by a lethal cocktail of vaccines. Reading Brett Wilcox's well-written summarization of the vaccine program in the United States reminded me of why I have chosen to live out the rest of my life as an advocate for informed consent and an activist for truth. *Jabbed* is a factual account of the indoctrinated fallacy that has created a sense of fear in societies all over the world and is a MUST READ for everyone no matter where you live on the planet."

—**Sheila Lewis Ealey MEd**, Featured in the documentary
Vaxxed: From Cover-Up to Catastrophe

"Brett Wilcox does an excellent job of revealing widespread dishonesty and corruption within the vaccine industry. Although peer-reviewed studies confirm numerous vaccine safety hazards, the pharmaceutical syndicate, FDA, CDC, World Health Organization, American Medical Association, American Academy of Pediatrics, and numerous other like-minded groups implement various ploys, scams, lies, and deception to hoodwink the public into believing that all vaccines are safe and effective. Parents and other concerned individuals must do their own research on this controversial issue or they may regret health consequences that could result from vaccine-related damage, including neurological and immunological disorders. I recommend this book to everyone wanting to learn about the unmitigated modern history of vaccine fraud, and to the beleaguered masses needing to disengage from a sacrosanct-like belief in the allopathic model of preventive medicine."

—**Neil Z. Miller**, medical research journalist and author of *Miller's Review of Critical Vaccine Studies* and *Vaccine Safety Manual for Concerned Families and Health Practitioners*

"*Jabbed* exposes extensive problems in the vaccine industry including conflicts of interests, corruption, the use of hyped-up fear campaigns, false historical narratives, and dangerous vaccine ingredients. Read it and you'll never look at vaccines the same way again!"

—**Dr. Nancy Tarlow**, Chiropractor, podcast and webinar host of *Healthy Alternatives to Vaccinations*, and owner of mBody Health and Wellness

"Cognitive dissonance regarding the vaccine program dies hard in this thorough and factual book. From polio to herd immunity, vaccine safety, and autism, *Jabbed* covers it all. If you value informed consent and if you're not afraid of the truth, then *Jabbed* is the book for you."

—**Michelle Rowton, MSN, RNC-NIC, C-NPT, NNP-BC,** Neonatal Nurse Practitioner and founding board member of Nurses Against Mandatory Vaccines

"*Jabbed* should be required reading for every new parent . . . and every adult. It exposes the unfortunate reality behind the US vaccine system, which is clearly driven by profit, not public health."

—**Brandy Vaughan**, Former Merck pharmaceutical rep & founder of the nonprofit, parent-driven Council for Vaccine Safety LearnTheRisk.org

"*Jabbed* is a comprehensive, well-referenced book providing the necessary answers for those with serious questions about vaccine safety and efficacy. This is a must-read for parents and parents-to-be especially!"

—**Robert Scott Bell, DA** Hom.

"In 1994, my daughter Lorrin was grievously injured by her one and only DPT vaccine, which was referred to as a 'hot' lot. This lot had reported injuries of seizures or worse to 30 other children and 10 surrounding deaths. The government immediately agreed that Lorrin was vaccine injured. Lorrin lived for 15 years as a quadriplegic, cortically blind and nonverbal; a young teen who was dependent on others for her every need. The same vaccine that was given to Lorrin was scattered throughout the US; this is just another way that our government protects the drug manufacturers, so no doctor will witness multiple injuries. I learned back in 1995 in my experience with The National Vaccine Injury Compensation Program that Lorrin's life was of no importance. It has been 22 years since that devastating time, and not much has changed. I encourage every single person to read this book and be part of the movement in taking our health freedom back. Thank you, Brett Wilcox, for bringing together the disturbing facts of vaccine history. A must-read for any person who considers jabbing a single vaccine into their body or the bodies of their precious children."

—**Karen Kain**, author, *A Unique Life Fully Lived: A Personal Journey of Love, Hope, and Courage*, vaccine safety advocate for informed consent, mother of a vaccine-injured child, KarenKain.com

"Despite the overwhelming scientific evidence that destroys 'the world's greatest scientific achievement,' there remain the vaxtremists whose faith in vaccines is stronger than science. Wilcox effectively pokes holes in the Religion of Vaccinology, where believers sacrifice Christian morality and God given freedom on the altar of Scientism. *Jabbed* provides fast-paced and well-researched insights into the hidden legacies of the vaccine program—insights that may leave readers righteously angry, prayerfully empowered and motivated to 'Speak out on behalf of the voiceless and for the rights of all who are vulnerable.'" - Proverbs 31:8

—**Lindey Hughes Magee**, codirector, Mississippi Parents for Vaccine Rights, MS state-portal codirector, National Vaccine Information Center

". . . for thy merchants were the great men of the earth; for by thy sorceries were all nations deceived." - Revelations 18:23

"Written in Greek originally, the word for 'sorcery' is 'pharmakeia,' from which our English word 'pharmacy' is derived. A look back through history shows that governments and empires come to an end for a number of reasons. Sometimes those reasons are due to external forces, but more often than not, the decline can be traced to internal forces; unemployment, inflation, urban decay, decline in morals and values, excessive military spending, political corruption, or declining public health. We are at a crossroads for the future of America, where political corruption has resulted in the biggest medical fraud in history coupled with the failure of journalists to remain objective and independent from the advertising dollars they rely upon to exist, and the combination is destroying the public health of the country. Brett Wilcox explores and exposes connections between a government influenced and corrupted by the pharmaceutical industry, and the resulting decline in the health of our citizens brought about through a vaccine program that is neither safe nor effective. Anyone who cares about the principles of liberty and freedom that were the foundation of the experiment in self-government that has become the American experience, and has a desire to understand and eliminate the powers that infringe upon those principles, ought to read this book."
—**Bob Snee, JD**, Director, Oregonians for Medical Freedom

"*Jabbed* is a historic and scientific chronicle that exposes the vaccine obsession of corporate rulers. I urge you to read it and to be brave, vigilant, and informed."
—**Camille Hayes, BSN**

"*Jabbed* tells a terrifying story of a government-vaccine industry partnership that kills, maims, and otherwise injures babies for money and of a medical system that callously turns a blind eye to the immense suffering vaccine-injured children endure. Brett Wilcox uses brilliant analogies to describe the endless abuse families like mine experience at the hands of arrogant doctors who took an oath to 'First do no harm.' As the parent of a 'Gardasil Girl,' I've spent countless hours in ERs and in the offices of doctors pleading for medical intervention and accountability. *Jabbed* unexpectedly brought out intense emotions as it paints a painfully vivid picture of this world we now live in, a world where parents make life and death decisions for their children based on the lies of sociopaths. The same government that profits from its collusion with industry is now maneuvering to gain free access to our children by stripping from parents our God-given right to choose what will and will not be injected into their bodies. *Jabbed* is the antidote to vaccine-related government propaganda and is essential reading for anyone who has ever loved a child."
—**Alicia Davis Boone**, Warrior mom fighting for my Gardasil-injured daughter, advocate for vaccine injury awareness, informed consent, and medical freedom

"Brett Wilcox expertly challenges the marketing maneuvers of the greedy vaccine manufacturers, supported by individuals at government agencies such as the 'vaccine sociopaths' at the CDC, some of whom attended the invitation-only criminal conference at Simpsonwood (2000) where 60 'vaccine industry insiders' concocted schemes to conceal the horrific dangers of thimerosal-containing vaccines, among other noxious ingredients. Their tactics were corroborated by the Institute of Medicine, theoretically an independent organization but one that is composed of people from medical schools, the drug industry, former FDA officials, and the Bill and Melinda Gates Foundation, founder (2000) of GAVI, the Vaccine Alliance whose objective is to vaccinate children in third-world countries. The FDA (largely funded by Big Pharma) does NOT test any vaccine or drug; it merely collects fees for the overhyped FDA approval. Wilcox observes that people are becoming more informed, which may have provoked the implementation of numerous mandatory vaccine programs for children as well as adults. He said, '[I]f sociopaths are denied voluntary access to our bodies, they will take them by force. The force of law.' Instead of mandatory jabs, this book should be mandatory reading!"

—**Deanna Spingola**, author, *The Ruling Elite Trilogy* and
Screening Sandy Hook, Causes and Consequences

"I came to the vaccine debate as a relative neophyte almost two years ago. Since then, I have spent many hours each week researching. Although I have gained a deep understanding of individual issues surrounding the debate, I have still felt I was missing some critical pieces of the overall picture. Brett Wilcox's book provides a comprehensive timeline, complete with those elusive puzzle pieces. Reading *Jabbed* will give you, in a matter of hours, a working understanding of this issue and an ability to advocate with confidence and authority."

—**Kristen S. Chevrier, MA**

"*Jabbed* is a beautifully thorough, accurately infuriating look at the vaccine industry. Brett Wilcox has done a masterful job of revealing with microscopic intensity the litany of insults, the trail of deception, the gall and guile of 'those at the very top,' as Dr. Archie put it, the fruits of whose labor are the stings of unavoidable immunological and neurological damage of every imaginable degree, in now-ongoing generations of kids, from the most intimate of environmental toxins: vaccines. A great read."

—**Shawn Siegel**, grandfather, vaccine researcher, author, and
Internet host of *The Vaccine Myth: An Issue of Trust*

Other Books by Brett Wilcox

We're Monsanto
Feeding the World, Lie After Lie
— Book One —

We're Monsanto
Still Feeding the World, Lie After Lie
— Book Two —

BRETT WILCOX

JABBED

How the Vaccine Industry,
Medical Establishment,
and Government
Stick It
to You and Your Family

SKYHORSE PUBLISHING

Skyhorse Publishing books may be purchased in bulk at special discounts for sales promotion, corporate gifts, fund-raising, or educational purposes. Special editions can also be created to specifications. For details, contact the Special Sales Department, Skyhorse Publishing, 307 West 36th Street, 11th Floor, New York, NY 10018 or info@skyhorsepublishing.com.

Skyhorse® and Skyhorse Publishing® are registered trademarks of Skyhorse Publishing, Inc.®, a Delaware corporation.

Visit our website at www.skyhorsepublishing.com.

10 9 8 7 6 5 4

Library of Congress Cataloging-in-Publication Data is available on file.

Cover design by Rain Saukas
Cover photo credit: iStockphoto

ISBN: 978-1-5107-5237-5
Ebook ISBN: 978-1-5107-2795-3

Printed in China

Disclaimer: This volume includes information from numerous sources. What you do with it is your business. Research. Consult. Inform yourself. Make up your own mind.

To our children.
May truth prevail.

"Our lives begin to end the day we become silent about things that matter."

— Martin Luther King, Jr.

CONTENTS

ACKNOWLEDGMENTS

I was about to become a grandparent when, in August 2014, Dr. William Thompson, a CDC scientist, announced that he and several of his colleagues had trashed the link between the MMR vaccine and autism. The timing of those events inspired me to study "the world's greatest medical invention," the result of which you're holding in your hand.

I stand in awe at the numerous people—mostly parents of vaccine-injured children—who have dedicated their lives to healing their children and protecting humanity from the rapacious pharmaceutical industry.

I was both humbled and honored when Kent Heckenlively, the coauthor of *Plague*, offered to write the foreword to this volume, and I was moved to tears when I first read his words. The spiritual connection he draws between his religious life and his advocacy for vaccine truth resonates with my own experience.

I was buoyed up by the people who read, critiqued, and endorsed this volume prior to publication.

Many thanks to Jim Catano for editing all three of my published books. May our collaboration continue for many books to come.

This volume includes numerous references to several books also published by the good people at Skyhorse Publishing. Their commitment to spreading the truth has blessed the lives of countless individuals, including my own.

I extend my deepest appreciation to Kris and our children. I could not have completed this labor of love without their support.

FOREWORD

Corruption always follows a similar pattern. It's just the players and the situation that change. Human nature remains the same.

I'm honored to write the foreword to Brett Wilcox's masterful and thoughtful book about vaccines and the devastating toll they are taking on our generation. Most people would be surprised to learn that in 1986, the United States removed vaccines from the traditional civil court system and placed them in a different judicial system. It was called the National Childhood Vaccine Injury Act. Even our own Justice Department recommended that President Reagan veto the bill. Reagan went ahead and signed the bill, but not before putting on the record his reservations about the constitutionality of the new court and a plea that changes be made before any such court came into existence. Sadly, these changes were never made, and we find ourselves today in a virtual civil war over vaccines. Even with all of these problems, this so-called "Vaccine Court" has already paid out more than three billion dollars in claims to vaccine-injured children, another fact of which most Americans are unaware.

When I say that corruption always follows a similar pattern, I mean that certain conditions must exist. The writers and thinkers of the Enlightenment, whose views on the nature of man found its greatest expression in our own US Constitution, believed a number of revolutionary things. They believed each of us were given certain rights and obligations by our Creator, and that in the exercise of our own judgment we would find our own best path. It followed that if our Creator gave each person the tools necessary to run their own lives, then any attempt to infringe upon the freedom of another person had to be closely examined.

Humanity will inevitably organize itself into political units, but each effort inevitably brings the danger of tyranny and injustice. That's why our Constitution has as part of its very soul an inherent distrust of any political organization and views the existence of any assembly as inherently suspect, unless there is a robust system of checks and balances. Any group of human beings that does not have strong oversight and is not periodically challenged as to their actions will inevitably fall into corruption.

Understanding this concept explains why I believe so strongly that the 1986 National Childhood Vaccine Injury Act set the stage for the litany of horrors described so thoroughly by Brett Wilcox in this book. Many writers have talked about the political uses of fear and how a perceived danger will often override the public's critical consideration of important issues. Shouldn't we as a society be asking whether it's a smart move to remove pharmaceutical companies from being required to provide all relevant safety data about vaccines? Isn't it valid to question the wisdom of removing pharmaceutical companies of any financial liability for harm caused by their vaccines? How is it that the media has been complicit in painting parents who ask for something as simple as a study of the health outcomes of vaccinated and nonvaccinated children as dangerous renegades who want children to die?

Corruption is the inevitable byproduct of powerful groups not being challenged. One need look no further than the clergy abuse scandals of the Catholic Church. Priests, Brothers, and Nuns were viewed by their congregations as doing God's work on Earth. For most of them this was true, but the lack of oversight was appalling. I was fortunate enough to go to a Catholic high school, De La Salle, which may be known to you for its football team, which had the longest winning streak of any sports team in history. This accomplishment is depicted in the movie *When the Game Stands Tall*, starring Jim Cazaviel and Laura Dern. The order that ran the high school and the college I attended is called the Christian Brothers, and I have rarely known a finer group of people. For many years, I considered whether I wanted to become a Christian Brother and dedicate my life to that mission. I wanted to serve God and humanity. Eventually, I opted not to join, as I wanted to have a family.

But De La Salle also had an abuse case, a Christian Brother who lived off-campus, gave drugs and alcohol to two of my friends, and sodomized them, eventually resulting in a six-million-dollar settlement. When this case came to light years later, I was appalled to read that many of the Christian Brothers I knew had personally taken measures to conceal these crimes or dismissed their importance. It is a betrayal at the most fundamental level, and it complicates my religious sentiments to this day.

Although I do not think I have completely resolved these feelings, I tell myself that these members of the clergy were simply human, doing things that humans inevitably do when they are not subject to proper oversight, which is to minimize the bad and focus on the perceived good. We need our critics, even the best of us.

I never expected that in my life I would become an adversary of the current vaccine program. But once my eyes were opened to the problem I could not turn away. The great scientist Albert Einstein once wrote, "Those who have the privilege to know, have a duty to act." Although I may have lost some measure of faith in the incorruptibility of the Catholic clergy, I still believe there will come a time when I will stand before my Creator and be asked to account for my life. In an infinite and loving voice, my Creator will ask me what I did for the weak and powerless, and those like my eighteen-year-old daughter, who still can't speak.

I will stand before my Creator in that moment and say that I tried to end the silence, both figurative and literal. I will not say these words with arrogant pride, because I know that all fall short in the eyes of God, but I will take some small measure of comfort that I did not remain silent. I encourage you to read this fine work by Brett Wilcox, use your own God-given powers of reasoning and deduction, and if you find his words to make sense, speak your truth. All of us have but a few, brief years in this world, and there is much work to be done.

Kent Heckenlively, JD
coauthor of *PLAGUE: One Scientist's Intrepid Search for the Truth about Human Retroviruses, Chronic Fatigue Syndrome (ME/CFS), Autism, and Other Diseases*
July 15, 2016

INTRODUCTION

"I have great shame now when I meet families with kids with autism because I have been part of the problem."[1]

These are the words Dr. William Thompson, a Senior Scientist employed by the US-based Centers for Disease Control (CDC), uttered in a phone conversation with Dr. Brian Hooker, a longtime researcher, advocate, and parent of an autistic child. Thompson was referring to his part in hiding various health conditions associated with the MMR vaccine, associations he and other CDC scientists had identified in their research. On August 27, 2014, Thompson issued a public statement, accepting responsibility for his misconduct.

I was no stranger to industry corruption when I read his apology. My son and I had just finished a run across the USA the previous month. We had run to educate people about the corruption in the biotech industry with a strong focus on one of the most corrupt companies in modern history: Monsanto. During our transcontinental adventure we shared my book *We're Monsanto: Feeding the World, Lie After Lie*, and we passed out some 3,000 organic seed packets labeled GMO Free USA to the people we met. Some were parents of autistic children. Yes, most of them said, the vaccines really were to blame. No matter what the government said, they had no doubt.

Initially, I was angry at Thompson and angry that I had been deceived by the endemic corruption that characterizes the most powerful vaccine-related regulatory body on Earth, angry that I had consented to the vaccination of our children, all of whom were born between 1991 and 2001, a period of time when children were injected with more thimerosal than ever in history.

Thompson's whistleblowing was big news. Very big news. Unless you follow the mainstream media, where it got little mention. This blackout piqued my interest. How deep did the corruption run? Was the vaccine industry no better than the biotech industry complete with a government-pharmaceutical revolving door, fraudulent science, bribes, threats against and intimidation of dissenting scientists, tainted educational curricula, industry PR machines pretending to be media, etc.?

I needed to know the answers. I was about to become a grandparent, and I was concerned. No, not concerned. I was scared—scared of yet another industry willing to lie and willing to hurt my posterity for economic gain.

Since that historic day when Thompson stepped out of the shadow of the CDC, I've immersed myself in the study of vaccines, which means, of course, I've immersed myself yet again in the study of corruption.

During the past few years of in-depth research, my anger has ebbed and flowed with every revelation of industry fraud, greed, and collusion. But I've also sensed a bit of Thompson's shame growing within me. He knew the truth, yet he remained silent for over a decade.

I was coming to know the truth as well. Like Dr. Thompson had done prior to his conversations with Dr. Hooker, would I remain silent? Would I hide my knowledge of the planned and purposeful choice by the pharmaceutical industry and the federal government to lie about the myriad problems associated with vaccines? Would I do as many privileged vaccine-informed people do—abstain from further participation in the corrupt vaccine industry—while watching other people hurry their children off to be jabbed with yet another round of vaccines that were brought to market through shady means? Would I shy away from conversations with dogmatic vaccine believers and misinformed physicians? Would I remain silent as the media continued to vilify men such as British doctor and researcher Andrew Wakefield?

No, I refuse to be silent. Silence is complicity. And I refuse to be complicit with corporations and governments that injure and kill children for the greater good of corporate profits. Quoting investigative journalist, Sharyl Attkisson, "I don't care if I piss off the entire government-pharmaceutical complex."[2]

And for those who charge that I am biased: you're absolutely right. In the words of researcher Andrew Gavin Marshall, "I am biased in favour of people over power, in favour of the oppressed over the oppressors, and in favour of freedom over domination."[3]

I extend my deepest thanks to Dr. Andrew Wakefield and to so many others who continue to stand against corrupt and powerful forces in industry, medicine, and government. Wakefield and others like him provide some of the loftiest examples of what it means to be human.

Just as I look forward to the day when biotech conspirators are held accountable, I look forward to the day when vaccine industry sociopaths—those who knowingly cash in on global human misery and death—are also brought to justice.

If we are to survive as a species, we must evolve in the way we treat one another. I look forward to a day when the lust for power, control, and wealth is eclipsed by our love for one another and for this ever-shrinking planet we call home.

CAST OF CHARACTERS

In the vaccine drama, there are three kinds of actors:

1. Vaccine Believers
2. the Vaccine Informed
3. and Vaccine Sociopaths

VACCINE BELIEVERS

Vaccine believers believe in the commercialized vaccine paradigm (a religious-based belief system), the vaccine program (the delivery system from manufacturer to the public), and the vaccine schedule (past, present, and future) with a black-and-white kind of devotion. Vaccines are safe and effective. Period. Vaccines save lives. Period. Disease is bad, vaccines are good. Period. Believers adhere to these beliefs just as surely as cultists believe that only they possess the truth.

Because vaccines are safe and effective, vaccine injury is nonexistent or vanishingly rare and of little importance. The good vaccines do for society is of infinitely greater value than the occasional ill effect vaccines might produce in a rare and peculiar case.

Vaccine believers are certain that vaccines protect them from infectious disease . . . except when they are exposed to unvaccinated individuals. The unvaccinated are tainted and should not be allowed to roam the streets or attend public schools spreading disease in their wake.

Vaccine believers see themselves as enlightened, progressive, and scientifically minded. Most people today are vaccine believers, including most medical professionals: primary care physicians, pediatricians, nurses, etc. Of these professionals, Paul Thomas, MD, coauthor of *The Vaccine-Friendly Plan*, writes, ". . . most of my MD doctor colleagues somehow have lost the ability to think independently on the vaccine issue. If you read the journals they read on a daily basis, it could happen to you too. These are not bad people, like 'weapons of mass destruction.' It is just a case of when you hear something enough and you don't have anywhere to get the other side of the story, the hidden truths, then you base your decisions on the information you have."[4]

THE VACCINE INFORMED

The vaccine informed are in some stage of knowing that no pharmacological intervention is completely safe. They have become aware that vaccines contain various toxic compounds that are, by definition, toxic. Therefore, they can see that all vaccines result in harm to a greater or lesser extent based on a host of variables in vaccine recipients as well as a host of variables in vaccines, the number and mixture of vaccines given at the same time, variables in vaccine schedules, etc.

They sense that no vaccine-believing doctor would consider it safe to orally ingest the contents of a vaccine. Many realize that federal law requires spilled vaccine contents to be cleaned up according to HAZMAT protocol. They understand that vaccines are created and marketed by the pharmaceutical industry—an industry that has paid $30 billion in fines for repeated fraud.[5]

They've learned that the industry has infiltrated national and state governing bodies, including but not limited to the White House, the Judiciary, Congress, and regulatory agencies. They've witnessed the control the industry holds over media. They're aware that the medical education curriculum is heavily influenced by the pharmaceutical industry, which results in a never-ending supply of doctors willing to scare and intimidate parents to vaccinate their children yet are blind to the negative outcomes of many vaccinations. The vaccine informed understand how little is known about the interactions between cells, tissues, systems, bodies, species, ecosystems, and the Earth we share.

Most vaccine-informed people are former vaccine believers who once recited the dogma, scorned the unvaccinated, and participated in the ritual of vaccination with devotion and faith. For many, the transition from vaccine believer to vaccine informed began with the injury or death of their own child or one close to them.

For many vaccine-informed medical professionals, their journey started at the other end of the needle. As painful as it was to acknowledge their role in vaccine injury or death among their patients, these professionals opened their hearts to the sting and their minds to the truth. Others simply opened their eyes and began to recognize the problems with vaccines and the vaccine paradigm.

Even certain members of Congress, after repeated exposures to the endemic corruption in the Centers for Disease Control, Food and Drug Administration, Department of Defense, American Medical Association, American Academy of Pediatrics, etc., couldn't help but join the ranks of the vaccine informed.

The vaccine informed may or may not self-identity as anti-vaccine, but they all recognize that there is a vast chasm between the theory and the practice of vaccination. Most, if not all, self-identify as pro-science, pro-safety, pro-informed consent, pro-vaccine choice, pro-individual rights, and pro-freedom. And most, if not all, are anti-corruption, anti-fraud, anti-cover-up and lies, anti-greed, anti-propaganda, anti-fear mongering, and anti-fascist. In short, vaccine informed people are anti-hogwash.

Being vaccine informed is a journey, not a destination. It happens in degrees. Once a mother realizes that vaccinating her newborn with the Hepatitis B vaccine provides considerable and proven risk with zero benefit, she is informed on that point. Once a father realizes that injecting his healthy pregnant wife with a thimerosal-containing flu vaccine is a medical atrocity, he is informed on that point. Once a couple realizes that mandated vaccinations are nothing more than medical tyranny, they are informed on that point. Once they know, they know. There is no going back.

It doesn't take long for newly vaccine-informed individuals to realize what all vaccine-informed people eventually come to know: the vaccine paradigm is a grand illusion created and maintained by people who personify the classic definition of a sociopath: "a person with a psychopathic personality whose behavior is antisocial, often criminal, and who lacks a sense of moral responsibility or social conscience."[6]

VACCINE SOCIOPATHS

There are two types of vaccine sociopaths: believers and the informed. The first are true believers. These are good people with good intentions whose belief in vaccines is so strong that they are able to justify the commission of sociopathic acts. Kevin Barry, Esq., the author of *Vaccine Whistleblower*, includes William Thompson and his colleagues in this group:

> The CDC personnel protecting the vaccine program are true believers in the "greater good" theory. And because of their unshakeable "vaccines save lives" belief, the CDC inflates the benefits and minimizes the risks of vaccination to benefit the greater good.[7]

Believing sociopaths—good people who commit sociopathic acts—are found throughout the medical profession; however, they make a mockery of its professed ethic of informed consent by pushing the CDC schedule using CDC propaganda. They believe it's their right and responsibility to minimize the risks associated with vaccines. It's their responsibility to report nonvaccinating parents to child protective services. It's their responsibility to sponsor and advance pro-industry legislation resulting in coercive vaccination legislation. Such people may treat parents of vaccine-injured children—the children whom they have injured—with contempt and hostility. They might deny injury or accuse mothers of being hysterical. Some demonstrate their closed minds by refusing contact with nonvaccinating parents.

Vaccine-informed sociopaths, on the other hand, are not good people. Their motivation lies more in personal profit or advancement than public health. They are aware of the problems with the vaccine paradigm, the program, the schedule, and vaccine ingredients. They know about the tainted science, crooked policies, and contaminated vaccines. That knowledge is important to them only in how they strategize to spin it or hide it from the public.

Vaccine-informed sociopaths work side by side with vaccine believers in the government, the medical establishment, and industry. Their loyalty to personal gain trumps their loyalty to law, ethics, and decency. Much of this book exposes the dealings of vaccine-informed sociopaths.

In the end, it doesn't really matter whether individuals are dealing with believing sociopaths or informed ones. Their motives and their values may be different, but both are dangerous.

A vaccine-informed citizenry represents the biggest enemy to vaccine sociopaths. Corporate and personal profits from the burgeoning vaccine pie depend upon the larger-than-life, myth-based vaccine paradigm. Sociopaths inject this paradigm into medical journals, medical curricula, congressional hearings, regulatory policies, White House statements, executive orders, and finally into the minds of vaccine believers.

Million-dollar sociopathic propaganda campaigns ensure that vaccine believers unleash their wrath against the vaccine informed, effectively keeping The Herd immune to the truth and ready and willing to roll up their sleeves to any and all vaccines currently on the schedule and to those yet to come down the vaccine pipeline.

In spite of and in part because of the propaganda, the number of vaccine-informed individuals is increasing. The day is soon coming when consumer distrust of vaccine sociopaths will gut the vaccine industry. Don't expect the sociopaths to roll over, play dead, and sacrifice their multibillion-dollar generating machine, however. Human bodies are, after all, their ATMs. The waves of coercive and mandatory vaccination laws that are rolling out across the USA and beyond demonstrate that if sociopaths are denied voluntary access to our bodies, they will take them by force. The force of law.

A vaccine-informed public is the only thing that will have the power to stop them and to hold them accountable for their crimes.

Chapter One

PHARMA, MEDICINE, GOVERNMENT, AND THE RELIGION OF VACCINOLOGY

Once you understand Modern Medicine as a religion, you can fight it and defend yourself much more effectively than when you think you're fighting an art or a science.[1]
—Robert S. Mendelsohn, MD

If the entities responsible for the modern vaccine empire—the pharmaceutical industry, the medical establishment, and the government—had their way, their machinations, deceptions, and frauds would remain unknown and unconsidered. Their tyranny would remain hidden behind the façade of public health. Their empire would continue to expand with each addition to the vaccine schedule. And the public would remain ignorant of what is certainly one of the greatest frauds in the history of medical science.

This book and many others like it are proof that the days of public ignorance are coming to an end. Mothers and fathers are finding out too much to be intimidated by medical professionals who are unable or unwilling to provide informed consent. Growing numbers of vaccine-informed people realize that the vaccine program, schedule, and paradigm are not based upon principles of sound scientific methodology. They're based instead on mystical claims of miraculous benefits over the ever-present evil of viruses and bacteria.

In short, they see that the dangerous practice of vaccination has morphed from a filthy experiment into a pagan ritual in the religion of Vaccinology, complete with its unique false history, false dogma, false priests, and the false promise of salvation from infectious disease. They understand that the pharmaceutical industry has seized control of medicine and government. Big Pharma, Big Medicine, and Big Government function as three seemingly separate but deeply entangled entities that advance a common agenda. Such a relationship is like a bastardized version of the Holy Trinity. There is nothing holy about the enmeshment and rank conflicts of interest in the pharmaceutical industry, medicine, and government.

Framing government, medicine, and Pharma in a religious context may rankle those who have abandoned the confusion and chaos of religion for the perceived certainty of science, but science—as practiced in the modern profit- and power-driven vaccine paradigm—is no less of a salvation-offering religion than is Christianity, Judaism, or Islam. Pure science, on the other hand, is merely a method for uncovering facts and their interrelationship, but hardly worthy of worship. People of business have co-opted science and turned it into Scientism, the religion for the masses. Scientific bodies have displaced religious bodies just as scientific journals have displaced holy writ. The phrases "All scientists agree" and "The science is settled" have displaced phrases such as "God says" or "The Bible says."

For thousands of years, corrupt individuals have claimed the authority of God to justify atrocities. Today, the authority of science is used to justify atroci- ties. Many "moderns" who are proud to be free of rituals and superstitions have instead surrendered their minds and souls to popes and priests of the modern "church": scientists and doctors who are responsible for both advancements in civilization and health as well as atrocities committed against civilization and health. As will be explained further in this book, surrendering one's critical thinking skills to "science" has proven to be more destructive than surrendering one's critical thinking skills to religion. Robert S. Mendelsohn, MD, a devout Jew, advanced the medicine-as-religion concept in his 1979 book, *Confessions of a Medical Heretic*. He devotes his book to dissuading readers from belief in "The Church of Modern Medicine." His "Non Credo" begins: "I do not believe in Modern Medicine. I am a medical heretic. My aim in this book is to persuade you to become a heretic, too."[2] Later Mendelsohn writes, "Modern medicine can't survive without our faith, because Modern Medicine is neither an art nor a science. It's a religion."[3]

Mendelsohn refers to flu shots as a "farce" and the 1976 Swine Flu epidemic as a "fiasco." Following are his introductory remarks in a grand diatribe against the sacrament of vaccination:

> If you follow the sounds of medical-governmental drum-beating in favor of a "preventive" procedure, you'll more often than not find yourself in the midst of one of the Church's least safe and effective sacraments. For instance, with some immunizations the danger in taking the shot may outweigh that of not taking it![4]

Richard Moskowitz, MD, author of *Vaccines: A Reappraisal*, referred to vaccina- tion as a kind of involuntary Communion, a sacrament of our participation in the unrestricted growth of scientific and industrial technology, utterly heedless of the long-term consequences to the health of our own species, let alone to the balance of Nature as a whole.[5]

French journalist Olivier Clerc asserts that "medicine is actually ruled by a set of beliefs, myths, and rites of Christianity it has never freed itself from." In his book *The New World Religion: How Beliefs Secretly Influence Medical Dogmas and Practices*, he states:

> . . . physicians have taken the place of priests; vaccination plays the same role as baptism; the search for health has replaced the quest for salvation; the fight against disease has replaced the fight against sin; eradication of viruses has taken the place of exorcising demons; [and] the hope of physical immortality (cloning, genetic engineering) takes priority over eternal life. . . .[6]

Clerc argues that "the medical establishment has become the government's ally, as the Catholic Church has in the past. 'Charlatans' are prosecuted today, as 'heretics' were in the past, and dogmatism rules out promising medical theories."[7] The opening paragraph in Clerc's book reads:

> We traditionally associate the birth of modern medicine with the publication of the work of French biologist Louis Pasteur (1822-1895), the father of vaccines. This choice fits perfectly with my thesis, as it was with Pasteur that the progressive and systematic transference of Christian symbolism to medicine began.[8]

Pharmaceuticals play a major role in The Church of Modern Medicine, but they are not infallible. Drugs and their accompanying adverse effects, injuries, deaths, and the lawsuits that result come and go. Manufacturers claim their billions in profits, pay nominal fines not covered by liability insurance when their hidden dealings are made public, and then they move on their next blockbuster.

Vaccines, on the other hand, *are* infallible in the sect practiced by vaccine believers and sociopaths. Their infallibility is proclaimed in the primary vaccine creed: "Vaccines are safe and effective." Questioning the creed is verboten as is legal redress against vaccine manufacturers. The creed is an essential part of the vaccine paradigm because, unlike other pharmaceuticals, vaccines are administered to healthy individuals. Parents wouldn't let medical professionals jab their healthy kids if they didn't have faith in the creed. Vaccines—the sacred cow of public health—are a golden calf to the sociopaths who manufacture and manipulate the faith of the human herd. And with over 250 vaccines in development, that calf is growing ever more golden. By 2020, profits from the global vaccine market are expected to swell from nearly $24 billion to $61 billion.[9]

Referring to vaccines as a sacred cow and a golden calf is apropos from both religious and etymological perspectives. "Vacc" in the word "vaccine" is from the Latin word *vacca* ("cow"). The original "vaccine" was a preparation of the cowpox virus taken from infected cows and inoculated in humans with the belief that it would provide immunity to smallpox. In 1895, Arthur Wollaston Hutton, the author of *The Vaccination Question*, described in shocking details the treatment calves experienced in the process:

> . . . a realistic presentation at the Royal Academy of one of the wretched calves at the Vaccine Institute, with its stomach shaved clean of hair and punctured in some sixty places for the production of cow-pox lymph, might shock the British public into a sense of the disgusting folly of the situation. . . . There has, in truth, been no such calf-worship since the days when the children of Israel encamped beneath Mount Sinai; though on that occasion, if the records are to be trusted, the representative of the Law was not on the side of the superstition.[10]

The process of removing oneself from a fundamentalist religion can be a difficult and sometimes dangerous task. If social pressure against the heretic proves insufficient, the threat of eternal damnation may suffice. In some respects, removing oneself from the religion of Modern Medicine and more specifically from the subsect of Vaccinology is even more perilous. The Unholy Trinity—the pharmaceutical industry, the medical establishment, and government—has successfully convinced the faithful that abstaining from vaccinations puts the entire flock at risk of damnation in the form of lethal disease outbreaks. Under the bonds of such indoctrination, people who otherwise respect legal and religious freedom heartily endorse the use of scorn, shame, hostility, name calling, discrimination, loss of the right of public education, loss of parental rights, fines, and even imprisonment for those who refuse to inject any and all vaccines the indoctrinated impose upon the rest of the flock. Former pharmaceutical representative Brandy Vaughan, now an industry whistleblower, relates the following: "I've being called a murderer, told that I should be in jail, burned at the stake, that my child will kill other children on the playground, that he should be taken away from me."[11]

Such accusations protect believers against the uncomfortable realization that the sanctuary in which they worship may not be what it claims to be, that the data supporting their beliefs are more smoke and mirrors than they are science. Leaving the Church is not for the faint of heart.

Just as churches often hide, falsify, or erase faith-destroying information from their congregants, the sociopaths who run The Church of Vaccinology routinely hide, falsify, or erase faith-destroying information from the public. Thus, the spotlight of truth must not only shine on vaccines, it must also shine on the people who profit from the deliberate spread of vaccine-related propaganda and misinformation.

This book is dedicated to that purpose.

Chapter Two

THE VACCINE PARADIGM: INVISIBLE AND OMNIPRESENT

*Orthodoxy means not thinking—not needing to think.
Orthodoxy is unconsciousness.*

—George Orwell

The vaccine paradigm is a story or belief system used by vaccine believers and sociopaths to convert The Herd to the Vaccine religion. If the paradigm were a stock traded on the stock market, its value could be charted fairly accurately by averaging the stock values of all of the corporate contributors to the paradigm. If the value of the paradigm were charted from the 1850s to the present day, its growth would be astounding. The paradigm may not be a tangible thing, but without it there would be no vaccine program.

This vision creates the mental constructs and assumptions necessary to achieve public acceptance of the state-sponsored vaccine program. The vaccine paradigm provides the belief system common to all who worship the sacred vaccine cow. Like members of traditional churches, members of The Vaccinology Church enjoy benefits and approbation, social communion, and perceived protection from evil—in this case, evil from viruses and bacteria.

The phenomenal success of the paradigm's creators is measured by the fact that few people are even aware of its existence. Whether living in 1885 England or in the current day, vaccine-informed people, however, see evidence of the paradigm all about them and recognize that it rests upon "Fraud, Force and Folly."[1]

Glimpses of the paradigm create such cognitive dissonance within believers that unconscious defense mechanisms are aroused and vanquish any troubling thoughts and feelings, returning the indoctrinated to their comfortable state of ignorance. Those who have the most to lose through awareness—those with vaccine-related careers, for example—often have the strongest defense mechanisms in place.

For those who view themselves as too sophisticated to fall victim to religious or social manipulation, another illustration may be of value. Many young people who grow up in a predominantly white community in the USA are unaware of the societal culture that shapes their beliefs, attitudes, values, diets, lifestyles, etc. Beyond being "American," many such people are unable to identify specific aspects of their own culture. But if a young woman, for example, leaves her home and takes up residence in a foreign country, she will, in short order, become aware that cultural differences abound, and, for the first time ever, she will become consciously aware of her own culture. She may experience "culture shock" in the early stages of this process, accompanied by thoughts like: "These people are crazy."

Similarly, she may be surprised to learn that the pregnant women with whom she is now associating would never consider receiving a single vaccine, nor would they allow anyone to inject their newborns with vaccines. One of her new friends might inform her while nursing a newborn child that she's glad she had the measles when she was younger because her lifelong immunity also protects her baby through her breast milk. That might explain why no one seems concerned when some children in the neighborhood contract measles and when she sees a child with chickenpox playing in the park with friends.

Her new awareness leads to numerous questions: Why is there a big difference between her home and guest nations' vaccine schedules? Why is there a difference in the way people perceive risks associated with infectious diseases? Is it true that contracting measles is in many ways an advantage? If she pursues her questioning, she will almost inevitably become aware of the cracked foundation upon which her own society's vaccine paradigm is constructed.

Many expatriates reside in foreign countries long enough that when they say, "These people are crazy," they're referring to the citizens of their own countries. Likewise, most former vaccine believers who devote enough time and energy to the study of the vaccine paradigm come to realize that the paradigm itself is "crazy" and that those who believe in it are also "crazy," understandably so, but "crazy" nonetheless. Perhaps the individuals who best understand crazy are those who have both experienced it in themselves and have escaped from it.

Most people do not initially choose to venture away from the security of the vaccine paradigm. Rather, their journey toward vaccine awareness begins when a vaccine injury slams a child they love right up against that paradigm.

Comparing vaccines to religion and culture is a way by which vaccine awareness can be initiated and strengthened. Comparing the word "drugs" to "vaccines" accomplishes the same. If anyone were silly enough to say publicly that "all drugs are safe and effective," such a claim would not go unchallenged. Ironically, vaccine believers—the people who argue that vaccines are safe and effective—would be among the crowd shouting down the fool who believes all drugs are categorically safe and effective. Alcoholics use the same twisted logic when, in drunken states of bliss, they proclaim, "I would never use drugs," failing to realize that alcohol is a drug. Likewise, vaccine believers who are drunk on the paradigm fail to see the obvious: vaccines are drugs. Period.

The cultural distinction between the word "drug" and the words "vaccine," "vaccination," and "immunization" is not a chance phenomenon. It's a crucial component of the vaccine paradigm. Vaccine engineers, marketers, and profiteers have successfully imbued these words with the power to safely protect, regardless of the fact that vaccination (the act of injecting humans or other creatures with antigens, adjuvants, heavy metals, contaminants, and other toxins) and immunization (the body's natural response to infectious disease) bear few if any similarities.

The US Food and Drug Administration classifies vaccines as biologics, not as drugs. Without any scientific basis, the FDA allows vaccine manufacturers to compare the safety and efficacy of a new vaccine against other vaccines or against vaccine components, without comparing it to an inert placebo or to vaccine-free subjects.[2]

Needless to say, the process is a sham. But the sham is essential to the maintenance of the vaccine paradigm. It allows manufacturers to claim that experimental vaccines are safe because they are no more harmful than toxic "placebos" or toxic vaccines already on the market.

From laboratory, to licensing, to the schedule, and then into the bodies of patients, vaccines are granted separate treatment, separate terminology, and separate means of compensation following injury. Risks and dangers are denied throughout the process as evidenced by Dr. Richard Pan's absurd claim that water is the most dangerous substance in vaccines and Dr. Paul Offit's even more absurd claim that babies can safely be vaccinated with 100,000 vaccines.[3,4]

The paradigm ensures that indoctrinated believers respond with hostility to vaccine-informed individuals. The paradigm ensures that young parents fear benign childhood diseases more than they fear a life sentence of learning disabilities and vaccine-induced medical problems. The paradigm ensures that health care workers and others surrender their freedom to medical tyranny. The paradigm also ensures that critical thinking skills shut down in otherwise intelligent individuals anytime the subject of vaccination comes up. The words of Carl Sagan aptly describe the mindset of the indoctrinated:

> If we've been bamboozled long enough, we tend to reject any evidence of the bamboozle. We're no longer interested in finding out the truth. The bamboozle has captured us. It's simply too painful to acknowledge, even to ourselves, that we've been taken. Once you give a charlatan power over you, you almost never get it back.[5]

When the charlatan is as large as the Unholy Trinity, and "the bamboozle" is as powerful at the vaccine paradigm, leaving the fold is too frightening for the indoctrinated to bear. But for the parents of vaccine-injured children, remaining in the fold elicits far greater fear.

Fear is an essential component of the vaccine paradigm. Without it, the vaccine program would cease to exist. To prevent such an occurrence, vaccine manufacturers must not only manufacture vaccines, they must also manufacture fear.

How they create such emotional terror is the subject of the next chapter.

Chapter Three

BANKING ON FEAR

You've got to be taught
To hate and fear,
You've got to be taught
From year to year,
It's got to be drummed
In your dear little ear
You've got to be carefully taught.[1]
—Rogers and Hammerstein, "You've Got to Be Carefully Taught,"
South Pacific

You can't hate someone until you make them an enemy. You can't make them an
enemy until you fear them. Americans are being taught to fear CHILDREN. Your
children. My children. Healthy, disease free CHILDREN. By the United States
government. By Presidential candidates. By Senators. Congressmen.
CDC leadership. And the pharma-directed US mainstream media.
It's FRIGHTENING.[2]

—Age of Autism

To create fear among parents to strengthen their motivation to vaccinate is an
important part of the publicity used to promote vaccinations. A whole branch of
research is examining the question: What level of fear needs to be created to appear
as convincing as possible?[3]
—Dr. Gerhard Buchwald, MD

Fear is the very cornerstone of the vaccine ideology.[4]
—Roman Bystrianyk

Vaccine profiteers know how to keep the cash register ringing. They've had over a century to perfect the formula that results in public acceptance of vaccines and billions of dollars in profits. The formula is not rocket science, and it's certainly not vaccine science. It's the science of fear-based marketing; the science of trauma-based mind control. Here's the simple equation:

Irrational fear of infectious disease + Irrational belief that vaccines safely prevent infectious disease = Vaccine compliance

In reality, the irrational fear necessary to produce vaccine compliance has little if anything to do with legitimate fear of infectious diseases. When vaccine sociopaths display images of individuals covered with smallpox lesions or victims of polio lying in iron lungs to scare people into getting the chickenpox vaccine, they are appealing to irrational fear and not to fact or science. When doctors in developed countries tell mothers of newborns frightening stories about hepatitis B—a disease common to prostitutes and IV drug users, something that fewer than 1 in 50,000 young children per year would be exposed to—they are appealing to irrational fear.[5]

The same is true of the meningococcal vaccine—a jab that resulted in "serious adverse events" in up to 2.1% of study participants for a disease that affects less than 0.0003% of the population.[6,7] Referring to the meningococcal vaccine, Dr. Lance Rodewald, director of the immunization services division of the National Immunization Program, states, "Frightening parents about the consequences of failing to vaccinate their children will most likely be part of the campaign."[8]

After traumatizing society with the specter of suffering and death, vaccine marketers introduce vaccines as the antidote to public fear. They create the problem and then solve the problem while laughing all the way to the bank. The greater the public fear, the higher the profits.

Kelly Brogan, MD, author of the 2016 book *A Mind of Your Own*, explains the concept as follows:

> We must look at the beliefs—the fantasies—underpinning the creation of the vaccine, the simple play on the vulnerable human psyche, and those who stand to accrue power and wealth at the expense of the pawns in the game.
>
> **The belief, at its core, is that germs are bad, they kill us if they get near, in, or on us, and we have the know-how to not only defeat them, but to annihilate them forever**.
>
> We are acculturated to this belief through corporations and enmeshed government agencies. They tell us that we cannot trust ourselves, the wisdom of our bodies, or our collective experience, to tell us how to be safe and well. The companies that stand to profit from this distrust, are the very ones who have convinced you that you are in danger. The fox is feasting in the hen house. [emphasis in original][9]

Glen Nowak, PhD, is one of the foxes Brogan refers to. As the Acting Director of Media Relations at the CDC, Nowak uses a slide show presentation to teach media outlets exactly which words to use to scare people into getting an annual flu shot, a strategy he refers to as the "'Recipe' for Fostering Public Interest and High Vaccine Demand." Among other things, media talking heads are instructed to tell the public that the dominant strain of this year's "immunization 'season'" is "very severe," "more severe than last or past years," and "deadly." They are to emphasize the risk of "severe complications" and "predict dire outcomes." Nowak tells them to use such words because

> [f]ostering demand, particularly among people who don't routinely receive an annual influenza vaccination, requires creating concern, anxiety, and worry. For example:
> * A perception or sense that many people are falling ill;
> * A perception or sense that many people are experiencing bad illness;
> * A perception or sense of vulnerability to contracting and experiencing bad illness.[10]

Nowak's "recipe" explains why newscasters sound like they're reading from the same script. Pour the CDC recipe into viewers' minds, then mix, stir, shake, bake, and presto, the government has created irrational fear leading to the equally irrational perception that the flu shot is the silver stake that will protect the human race from evil flu vampires.

The *British Medical Journal* published a paper in 2005 on some of the problems associated with the influenza vaccine including the CDC's "marketing of fear." The article reads:

> US data on influenza deaths are a mess. There are significant statistical incompatibilities between official estimates and national vital statistics data. Compounding these problems is a marketing of fear—a CDC communications strategy in which medical experts "predict dire outcomes" during flu seasons.[11]

Vaccine profiteers learned long ago that nothing sells vaccines as well as epidemics or pandemics. Even today, they invoke the specter of smallpox and polio to frighten people into submitting to vaccines for benign and, yes, beneficial illnesses such as chickenpox. But the fear derived from such tactics tends to diminish among younger people who have no personal experience with smallpox or polio or the false narratives that profiteers pass off as history.

In the absence of serious disease outbreaks, vaccine sociopaths have mastered the art of hyping predicted disease outbreaks that turn out to be epidemic busts and Pharma profit boons. In 2009, industry and global governments teamed up under the pretext of protecting their citizens against the predicted H1N1 swine flu pandemic. Governments spent billions stockpiling H1N1 flu vaccines for a pandemic that failed to meet the World Health Organization's original definition of the word. According to several sources, the real pandemic was the corrupting influence of Pharma on the WHO. The cable news network RT presented evidence "that vaccine manufacturers pressured the World Health Organization into declaring a swine flu pandemic seeking to increase profits."[12]

A translated version from the Danish newspaper *Information* suggests that vaccine manufacturers didn't pressure the WHO as much as they colluded with their paid consultants who are also members of WHO committees.[13]

One of the experts in the WHO H1N1-specific advisory group, Dr. Albert Osterhaus, is known in Holland as "Dr. Flu" because he promotes vaccines as solutions to epidemics. Osterhaus also has financial interests in several pharmaceutical companies.

Dr. Frederick Hayden is an outside expert in the WHO's Strategic Advisory Group of Experts on Immunization (SAGE), which advises the WHO on vaccines. He is listed in official papers as a flu-research coordinator from the benign-sounding Wellcome Trust in London. Unlisted are his financial relationships with Big Pharma giants Roche, RW Johnson, SmithKline Beecham, and Glaxo Wellcome.

Dr. Arnold Monto is another SAGE member. The WHO lists Monto as the head of a department at the University of Michigan. Unlisted is his job as a paid consultant to Glaxo Wellcome, ViroPharma, and MedImmune, which produces an inhalable flu vaccine.

Not only do major vaccine manufacturers like GlaxoSmithKline, Novartis, and Baxter pay consultants who influence WHO policy, they even attend SAGE meetings as "observers."[14]

The Council of Europe castigated the World Health Organization's handling of the "H1N1 influenza pandemic" for

> the consequences of decisions taken and advice given leading to distortion of priorities of public health services across Europe, waste of large sums of public money, and also unjustified scares and fears about health risks faced by the European public at large.

According to the Council, the problem started when the WHO changed its definition of "pandemic":

> A number of members of the scientific community became concerned when WHO rapidly moved towards pandemic level 6 at a time when the influenza presented relatively mild symptoms. This combined with the change in the definition of pandemic levels just before the declaration of the H1N1 pandemic heightened concerns. As Dr Wolfgang

Wodarg, German epidemiologist and former member of the Parliamentary Assembly, highlighted at the public hearing on 26 January 2010, the declaration of the current pandemic was only made possible by changing the definition of a pandemic and by lowering the threshold for its declaration.

. . . The definition before 4 May 2009 was worded as follows: "An influenza pandemic occurs when a new influenza virus appears against which the human population has no immunity, resulting in epidemics worldwide with enormous numbers of deaths and illness. With the increase in global transport, as well as urbanization and overcrowded conditions, epidemics due [to] the new influenza virus are likely to quickly take hold around the world", whilst the same definition became the following on WHO's website after this date: "A disease epidemic occurs when there are more cases of that disease than normal. A pandemic is a worldwide epidemic of a disease. An influenza pandemic may occur when a new influenza virus appears against which the human population has no immunity. . . . Pandemics can be either mild or severe in the illness and death they cause, and the severity of a pandemic can change over the course of that pandemic".[15]

Paul Flynn, the Vice Chairman of the Council of Europe Health Committee, stated,

Britain has spent a fortune on preparations. We've caused a great deal of stress to the population; people are very anxious about it, and we've distorted the priorities of our health service. . . . The world has been subjected to a stunt for their own greedy interests of the pharmaceutical companies.

RT reporter Laura Emmett said,

Governments all over Europe are now saddled with billions of dollars worth of unnecessary swine flu vaccine. They are trying to sell it, but supply now far exceeds demand.

RT titled their coverage of the H1N1 scandal "H1N1 'false pandemic' biggest pharma-fraud of century?"[16]

The H1N1 fraud was certainly big, but how does one declare one instance of fraud to be the biggest when the industry's standard operating procedure is fraud?

Capitalizing on the swine flu fraud, drug company Roche sold 40 million doses of Tamiflu to Britain's Department of Health at a cost of £424 million (about $675 million) based on the claim that the drug would halt the spread of influenza. The *Telegraph* reported on a major study authored by Oxford University that declared, "the drug's Swiss manufacturer, gave a 'false impression' of its effectiveness and accuses the company of 'sloppy science'."[17] How sloppy? A paper published in The *International Journal of Risk & Safety in Medicine* concluded that

> Tamiflu use could induce sudden deterioration leading to death especially within 12 hours of prescription. These findings are consistent with sudden deaths observed in a series of animal toxicity studies, several reported case series and the results of prospective cohort studies. From "the precautionary principle" the potential harm of Tamiflu should be taken into account and further detailed studies should be conducted.[18]

The real "swine" in the 2009 swine flu fiasco may be the marketers at GlaxoSmithKline who "refused to supply governments" with vaccines "unless it was indemnified against any claim for damage caused." According to the UK's *International Business Times*, GSK's Pandemrix vaccine left hundreds of European children permanently disabled while leaving the British government paying the damages.[19]

Richard Bergström, the director-general of the European Federation of Pharmaceutical Industries and Associations, said,

> The worst nightmare of both the industry and the health authorities is an illness that turns out to be mild, while the vaccine that was supposed to prevent a dangerous epidemic causes a severe side effect that was previously unknown.[20]

As far as the final outcome, 60% of Swedes received the H1N1 vaccine compared to 8% of Germans. The death rate in both countries was identical with only 1 death per 300,000 people, which means millions of Europeans were put at risk for no reason other than to line the pockets of the pharmaceutical industry.[21]

The swine flu debacle takes its place on the dishonor role of hyped-up public relations campaigns designed to increase irrational fears, vaccine compliance, and industry profits. Others on the list include SARS, bird flu, Ebola, and the Zika virus.

The most ludicrous so-called epidemic in recent years was the 2015 Disneyland measles outbreak. News reporters around the world spoke of it as an apocalyptic event. Many laid the blame on the unvaccinated. So what befell the few dozen hapless measles victims? Death? Disability? Disfigurement? No, they gained lifelong immunity against measles along with a protective effect against heart disease, cancer, malaria, allergic diseases, juvenile rheumatoid arthritis, Infantile Hodgkin's Disease, atopy, and psoriasis.[22]

Dr. William Thompson, the man now known as the CDC whistleblower, discussed the topic of fear mongering with Brian Hooker in a legally recorded telephone conversation:

. . . I also have to say these drug companies and their promoters, they're making such a big deal of these measles outbreaks and they are now, they're making a big deal that polio is coming back and polio comes back all the time in third world countries. It's like a never-ending thing where the press loves to hype it and it scares people. It scares the crap out of people when they hype those two types of outbreaks.[23]

In 1961, Alexander Langmuir, MD, the "father of epidemiology," described measles as a "self-limiting infection of short duration, moderate severity, and low fatality."[24] During the same time period, mothers read the following passage from a 1958 children's book titled *Have a Happy Measle, a Merry Mumps, and a Cheery Chickenpox*:

And just about *everybody* gets measles, mumps, and chickenpox, some-time or other. They don't always come at the handiest time. They might interfere with Christmas or birthdays or the circus, BUT once you have had them, you almost certainly will never have them again. SO have a happy measle, a merry mumps, and cheery chickenpox, and grin and bear whatever else comes along.[25] [emphasis in original]

Isn't it amazing how the "happy measle" of yesteryear has morphed into "one of the most contagious and most lethal of all human diseases"?[26]

The real outbreak that took place at Disneyland was an outbreak of hysteria and fear. The creators of the hysteria are also afraid. And unlike the irrational fear that drives parents to vaccinate their infants, the fear of vaccine sociopaths is anything but irrational. They fear that their cover story—the vaccine paradigm—is about to be blown. They fear that the public will recognize them for what they are: a global network of criminal organizations working in concert with corrupt governments intent on extracting as much profit as possible from the collective mindless Herd. They fear that The Herd's irrational fear will be replaced with justifiable outrage once awareness dawns. They fear that they'll be charged, tried, and convicted of crimes and spend the rest of their lives in prison forever separated from their ill-gotten gains.

Their fear is well founded.

Two important vaccine-related events happened in the 1990s. Both the vaccine schedule and public access to information exploded. The former was a boon to industry profits; the latter foreshadowed the demise of the vaccine paradigm. Vaccine sociopaths now enjoy the potential for nearly unlimited gains in wealth from a nearly unlimited ability to add to recommended vaccine schedules. However, they also must contend with a technology that has the power to bring to light their hidden deeds of darkness: the Internet.

The ancient church controlled the faithful by blocking member access to accurate information found in written texts. Prior to the Internet, The Church of Vaccinology controlled its adherents by blocking member access to accurate information about the fraudulent science and endemic corruption.

These are momentous times! Almost limitless information is available with a few keystrokes. Naturally, vaccine believers and sociopaths mock those who access and share accurate information from the Internet. The irony is that much of the information they mock comes directly from government and industry sources. No matter, both paid and unpaid industry propagandists also use the same Internet to "advance" the boneheaded concept that the public is better served by learning about the vaccine industry from industry-funded and -influenced news sources.

The public still knows only a minute portion of the shady practices carried out by the world's vaccine power brokers, but thanks to the Internet, the balance of information has shifted immensely in the public's favor. A growing number of vaccine-informed individuals know that the vaccine paradigm is a work of fiction. The Vaccine Church's administrators know that their flock is becoming more informed, and they're panicked. They know that an increasingly savvy public is becoming immune to industry fear-based marketing. Without public fear, the vaccine paradigm and the profits it generates will shrink.

However, vaccine sociopaths will continue to turn nonevents such as the Disneyland measles outbreak into an outbreak of fear. Then they'll infect the legislative processes with fear and bribery to pass laws that remove citizens' personal belief exemptions for vaccinations. In other words, what they can't do by persuasion, they will try to do by force.

Louis Conte, coauthor of *Vaccine Injuries*, and Wayne Rohde, author of *The Vaccine Court: The Dark Truth of America's Vaccine Injury Compensation Program*, addressed this phenomenon in an article titled "Paul Offit, Fear, Intimidation and Astroturf":

> The measles hysteria fueled by paid industry advocates like Paul Offit is designed to remove parental choice from the health care decisions involving their children. It is designed to terrorize the public into forfeiting the right to full disclosure and informed consent. It is designed to

force people to surrender their rights to the government for the purposes of fueling drug company profits. Paul Offit wants to use corrupted science to have public policy exclusively determined by men like him.[27]

Pediatrician and California State Assembly member Richard Pan capitalized on industry fearmongering following the measles outbreak to convince California legislators to pass the infamous SB 277 mandatory vaccination bill. Now exposed as a liar, Pan had testified on another vaccine-related bill he authored in 2012, saying it would not eliminate personal belief exemptions: "We are not taking away the parental rights to be able to make a decision." Later, speaking of the same bill, Pan testified,

> Parents who decide not to vaccinate their children will no longer be able to exempt them from legally required vaccinations when enrolling them into school attended by other children, but would instead have to homeschool them.

The Supreme Court ruled that vaccines are "unavoidably unsafe," a detail that didn't deter Pan from declaring, "SB 277 was heard in Health Committee where it was established that vaccines are safe and efficacious." When confronted by Carol Liu, the chair of the Senate Education Committee, and committee member Loni Hancock, Pan lied to their faces by telling them that California children didn't have a 92 to 95% measles vaccination rate, when in fact most do.[28]

In November 2015, Pan spoke at a seminar held at the University of California Berkeley's School of Public Health, where he told the audience, "thimerosal is not in childhood vaccines." Many pediatricians might ignorantly believe such nonsense, but as the SB 277 cosponsor, there is no way Pan could have been ignorant of the fact that the CDC added the flu vaccine to the pediatric schedule in 2003 and that most flu vaccines still contain "50 micrograms of thimerosal . . . or approximately 25 micrograms of mercury" per dose.[29]

Then Pan, apparently taking his cue from the vaccine industry's biggest proponent and vaccine profiteer, Paul Offit, as previously cited made the outrageous claim that water is the most dangerous component in vaccines.[30]

If there were any scientific basis for mandatory vaccinations due to the Disneyland hysteria outbreak, it would apply only to measles. Vaccine sociopaths are capitalizing on the hysteria to mandate any and all vaccines on the current or future schedules. Only sociopathy can explain a law that requires compulsory vaccination of a low birth-weight, premature infant for hepatitis B with a vaccine that's not medically indicated and has been shown to cause liver damage in those it's purported to protect.[31] Even according to a paper published in the *Journal of Viral Hepatitis*, it's a vaccine that simply doesn't work as advertised.[32]

Only sociopathy can explain a law that would turn a minor measles out-break into compulsory vaccination program featuring worthless and dangerous thimerosal-containing flu vaccines (more in coming chapters). Only sociopathy can explain a law that would turn a minor measles outbreak into compulsory vaccination for any and all vaccines. Only sociopathy can explain state-man-dated vaccines. Period.

Free and open access to accurate information is the biggest threat vaccine sociopaths have ever faced. Their golden calf is melting in the fire of truth and public awareness. Mandatory vaccines are industry's defense against public knowledge. Even if citizens one day revolt against compulsory vaccinations as they did in Great Britain in the 1880s, the sociopaths will still have managed to bilk a few more billion dollars out of the hands of taxpayers, insurance compa-nies, and governments before their reign of terror ends.

In summary, vaccine sociopaths fear losing their ill-gotten gains more than they fear injuring others. They've thrown out the Hippocratic Oath's "First do no harm" and replaced it with the hippocritical oath's "First do no harm to the vaccine paradigm, program, schedule, and profits."

Fear is a normal and healthy response to danger. But the criminal behavior of vaccine sociopaths is far more dangerous and frightening than measles, chick-enpox, or the nearly nonexistent threat of hepatitis B in newborns.

This chapter has dealt with the first half of the equation The Vaccine Church uses to ensure vaccine compliance: irrational fear. Ensuing chapters deal with the second half of the equation: the belief that vaccines safely protect against infectious disease.

Chapter Four

VACCINES ARE SAFE AND EFFECTIVE AND OTHER LIES

Anyone who acquired their information in a trance state tends to be more confident and sincere sounding . . . .[1]

—Carla Emery

The next time vaccine experts loudly proclaim that vaccine safety is unassailable, consider whether the researchers exhibited any genuine curiosity about adverse events to begin with. It's not possible to find what you don't look for.[2]

—Claire Dwoskin

Prepare to enter the Inner Sanctum of The Church of Vaccinology. Prepare to drink from the Holy Grail. Prepare to kiss the hand of the Patron Saint of The Church, the Reverend Doctor Paul Offit. One proclamation echoes within the sacred chambers far more than any other. It embodies the religion's central tenet, the core doctrine, the cosmic creed:

"Vaccines are safe and effective."

So it is, so it has ever been, and so it will ever be. Amen and amen.

The Unholy Trinity—Pharma, the medical establishment, and government—has uttered, published, and broadcast this statement with such repetition that merely thinking or hearing it induces society into a hypnotic response, effectively shutting down critical thought processes while turning on faith-based magical thinking.

"Vaccines are safe and effective."

In a religious context, this proclamation is a creed. In organizational terms, it's policy. In marketing, it's the hook. In social psychology, it's propaganda. In literary parlance, it's myth. In legal vernacular, it's fraud. In the art of mind control, it's described as conversational hypnosis or "sleight of mouth." Under oath, it's perjury. In short, it's bunk.

"Vaccines are safe and effective."

This irrational statement disregards an infinite combination of variables in vaccines (ingredients, manufacturers, country of origin, batch, or lot), vaccine administration (number or combination of jabs, time between jabs), and vaccine recipients (age, sex, weight, race, genetic vulnerabilities, health status, allergies, autoimmune issues, previous adverse reactions).

The power of the vaccine paradigm imbues the word "vaccine" with its two central characteristics: safety and efficacy. To suggest that a vaccine is not safe is to suggest that safety itself is not safe because the word vaccine is synonymous with safety. Likewise, to suggest that a vaccine is not effective is to suggest that efficacy is not effective because the word vaccine is synonymous with efficacy.

No other term in current medical lexicon holds the power that the word "vaccine" holds over the minds of otherwise intelligent and thinking people. Vaccine sociopaths have recently invoked the power of the word *vaccine* in California and other US states to persuade legislators to pass coercive and compulsory vaccination laws for any and all vaccines on both current and future schedules based on a minor outbreak of measles—a childhood disease that was once portrayed in TV sitcoms as a trivial nuisance.

If the word *anti-psychotic* held the same power as the word *vaccine* over the minds of the public, every outbreak of public madness would result in ever-more coercive anti-psychotic drug mandates forced upon the general population. But perhaps that is not impossible either, as the trend to drug the general public with mind-altering pharmaceuticals, especially children and adolescents, is, in fact, spreading across the USA at a maddening pace.[3]

Vaccine believers view vaccines as a concept, not as assortments of chemical compounds. Since the concept of a vaccine is safe, then it stands to reason that a vaccine is safe. Since a vaccine is safe, then two vaccines are equally safe. Since two are safe, then four are safe. As is written in The Gospel of Paul—Paul Offit, that is—as many as 100,000 simultaneous vaccinations are safe.[4]

Surely, St. Paul spoke figuratively, not literally. In the minds of true believers there is no distinction between figurative and literal. There is no difference between conceptual and actual. As a single example of literal acceptance in a nation of literal "thinkers," consider the "facts" presented in the short video titled "Reasons to Immunize" hosted on the Brigham Young University school of nursing YouTube channel.[5]

According to the video, the side effects of disease include pneumonia, deafness, brain infection, blindness, heart defects, and death. The sum total of all vaccine side effects ever experienced includes soreness, swelling, redness, fever, and rash.

Nurses who graduate from programs that teach such nonsense become the nurses who are unable to see what's obvious to thousands of parents: vaccines have injured their children. Parents and professionals report a host of symptoms to the US government's Vaccine Adverse Event Reporting System (VAERS). According to Jane Orient, MD, Executive Director of the Association of American Physicians and Surgeons, some of the most common symptoms include: "prolonged screaming, agitation, apnea, ataxia, visual disturbances, convulsions, tremors, twitches, an abnormal cry, hypotonia, hypertonia, abnormal sensations, stupor, somnolence, neck rigidity, paralysis, confusion, and oculogyric crisis."[6]

The US National Library of Medicine, "the world's largest biomedical library," catalogues studies linking vaccine reactions to hundreds of diseases and disorders. Following is a partial list:

- Acute Flaccid Paralysis
- Aging
- Allergic Rhinitis
- Allergies
- Alopecia
- Aluminum Toxicity
- Anaphylaxis
- Anemia
- Arthritis: Juvenile Chronic
- Arthritis: Juvenile Rheumatoid
- Asthma
- Atopic Disease
- Attention Deficit Disorder
- ADHD
- Autism
- Autism Spectrum Disorders
- Bell's Palsy
- Birth Defects
- Brain Inflammation
- Breast Augmentation Complications
- Cardiovascular Diseases
- Cervical Cancer
- Child Mortality
- Childhood Infections
- Cholera
- Chorioretinitis
- Chronic Fatigue Syndrome
- Cystic Fibrosis
- Dermatomyositis
- Diabetes Mellitus: Type 1
- Diabetes Mellitus: Type 2
- Diarrhea

- Dravet syndrome
- Ear Infection
- Elevated C-reactive protein
- Empyema
- Encephalitis
- Encephalitis: Japanese
- Encephalomyelitis
- Encephalopathies
- Endogenous avian retrovirus
- Epilepsy
- Epstein-Barr Virus Infections
- Erythema
- Erythematosus Arthritis
- Excitotoxicity
- Febrile Seizures
- Fever
- Gastroenteritis
- Gastrointestinal Diseases
- Glomerulonephritis
- Glyphosate Toxicity
- Guillain-Barre Syndrome
- Gulf War Syndrome
- Hearing Loss: Sudden
- Hemolytic Anemia
- Hepatitis C
- Herpes Zoster
- Herpes: Ocular
- Hydranencephaly
- Immune Dysregulation: TH1/TH2 imbalance
- Infant Infections
- Infant Neurological Development Inflammation

- Infertility
- Inflammatory Bowel Diseases
- Inflammatory Myopathy
- Influenza A
- Influenza B
- Intussusception
- Joint Diseases
- Leukemia Cutis
- Lipoatrophy
- Liver Damage
- Liver Disease
- Lupus Erythematosus
- Lyme disease
- Macrophagic myofasciitis
- Malaria
- Mental Retardation
- Mercury Poisoning
- Miller Fisher Syndrome
- Miscarriage
- Morphea profunda
- Multiple Sclerosis
- Myasthenia Gravis
- Mycoplasma Infections
- Myelitis
- Myocarditis
- Myopericarditis
- Narcolepsy
- Neuritis
- Neuromuscular Diseases
- Neuropathies
- Non-polio acute flaccid paralysis (NPAFP)
- Optic Neuritis
- Orchitis
- Ovarian Failure
- Oxidative Stress
- Pancytopenia
- Parapertussis
- Parapneumonic Empyema
- Parkinsonian Disorders
- Peripheral Neuropathies
- Pharyngeal Diseases
- Pneumonia
- Pneumonitis
  Polyradiculoneuropathy
- Polyarteritis Nodosa
- Porcine Circovirus Type 2
- Pre-Eclampsia
- Preterm Birth
- Prostate Cancer
- Pseudolymphoma
- Psychiatric Disorders
- Purpura
- Respiratory Diseases
- Rift Valley Fever
- Rotavirus Infections
- Sarcoma
- Shingles
- Shoulder Injuries
- Silicone Implant Toxicity
- Simian Immunodeficiency Virus
- Spontaneous Rheumatoid Arthritis
- Stroke
- Sudden Infant Death Syndrome (SIDS)
- Syncope Thromboembolism
- Systemic Lupus
- Systemic Seizures
- Thrombocytopenia
- Tuberculosis
- Transverse Myelitis
- Tumors
- Ulcerative Colitis
- Upper Respiratory Infections
- Urinary Tract Infections
- Uveitis
- Vaccine-Related Retroviruses
- Vasculitis
- Viremia[7]

The video continues: "There is no relationship between **any** immunization and autism [emphasis in original]." If that's really the case, then perhaps the nurses should instruct the National Vaccine Injury Compensation Program to stop compensating parents and children for vaccine-induced encephalopathy resulting in autism.[8] They might also do well to inform the CDC that there was no reason for government scientists to cover up and destroy their own figures demonstrating the link between thimerosal and autism, as well as the link between the MMR vaccine and autism (more in later chapters).

Perhaps they should also correct numerous researchers at numerous laboratories who have confirmed CDC findings, starting with their colleagues to the north at Utah State University who, in 2002, cited numerous studies regarding the ". . . faulty immune regulation in autistic children . . ." and the ". . . autoimmune mechanism of pathogenesis for autism. . . ." The USU researchers published their own findings on the subject in the *Journal of Biomedical Science* under the title "Abnormal Measles-Mumps-Rubella Antibodies and CNS [central nervous system] Autoimmunity in Children with Autism." Among other things, the researchers documented ". . . a strong association between MMR and CNS autoimmunity in autism." Their findings led them to ". . . suggest that an inappropriate antibody response to MMR, specifically the measles component thereof, might be related to pathogenesis of autism."[9]

According to the video, the only side effect a baby has ever experienced from the DTaP vaccine is irritability while the side effects from actually contracting diphtheria, tetanus, and pertussis include paralysis, brain infection, pneumonia, and death. The nurses might want to consider informing vaccine manufacturers, the CDC, numerous doctors, and thousands of parents that the DTaP vaccine didn't injure or kill their children. It merely made them irritable. On second thought, the nurses might not want to say such a thing to mourning parents.

The video also declares: "It's important to vaccinate **on time** [emphasis in original]." The parents whose children have autism *because* they vaccinated on time may disagree. According to Dr. William Thompson, African-American boys who receive the MMR vaccine "on time"—between 12 and 18 months old—are 2.36 times more likely to be diagnosed with autism compared to those who receive the vaccine after age three. In addition, CDC scientists found that the risk of "isolated autism"—healthy children who manifest no symptoms other than autism—increased 7 times for babies, regardless of race, following "on time" MMR vaccination.[10]

And last but definitely not least, the video trumpets, "Babies can be given multiple shots at once. An immunization is like a drop in the ocean of the immune system. The immune system can handle 100,000 immunizations simultaneously. Seriously, 100,000." Really? Then why not greet newborns with the whole schedule for maximum protection?

Not to cast doubts on the nurses' adherence to the Gospel of Paul, but most 10-year-olds could beat these medical professionals in math and critical thinking skills. Vaccine doses range from 0.5 ml to 2.0 ml. At the lowest dosage volume, 100,000 vaccines total 50 liters or 13.2 gallons of vaccine solution.

In 2012, Michael Belkin, father of a baby girl who died 15 hours after receiving the hepatitis B vaccine, posted an April Fool's news release on his website The Refusers. The release covered the story of Saint Paul's condition after his pediatrician wife injected him with 38 injections per square inch of his body or a 24-hour period.

> Dr. Offit . . . developed seizures and was admitted to Philadelphia Children's Hospital with severe cases of atypical measles, chickenpox, pertussis, pneumonia, rotavirus and encephalitis. This hospital issued a statement saying that Dr. Offit was probably faking his symptoms, because scientific studies show that vaccines have been proven to be 100% safe and effective and never cause adverse reactions.

> A spokesman for Merck (which made 99,999 of the 100,000 vaccines) said: "Sometimes neurological diseases occur in a random temporal association with vaccination. Correlation is not causation. No one should know this better than Dr. Offit and we refuse to take responsibility for his health problems. If he erroneously believes that vaccines have caused his illnesses, he should apply to the National Vaccine Injury Compensation Program (NVICP) for relief. The NVICP was created expressly to protect innocent vaccine manufacturers like us from frivolous lawsuits by so-called vaccine adverse reaction victims."

> The Chief Special Master of the NVICP kangaroo court issued a statement saying: "Unfortunately, Dr. Offit's symptoms are not covered under our program. There is absolutely no scientific evidence showing that vaccines can cause the diseases they were designed to prevent. Dr. Offit is mistaken if he believes that he can milk the system with his phony vaccine injury claims. Anyway, the money obtained through vaccine taxes in the NVICP program has already been spent by the US government as part of the general budget, so we couldn't pay Offit even if we wanted to. Why do you think we reject so many claims anyway?"[11]

Of course, had Offit really attempted to prove his point, or in this case, 100,000 points, his spirit would have, depending on one's perspective, ascended to vaccine heaven or descended to vaccine hell long before his wife had injected even a fraction of the 100,000 vaccines that he claims are safe for babies.

As pleasing as it might be to the parents of vaccine-injured children to ponder the final resting place of Saint Paul, ponder as well the final question asked in the BYU nursing video: "So now what?" The obvious answer is "Wake the (insert your favorite swear word) up! Seriously, wake up!" The fact that a nationally ranked nursing program would post such an unscientific video on YouTube demonstrates the power of the vaccine paradigm over the medical establishment and over much of the public.

Administering one vaccine to an infant is dangerous. Two is more dangerous. Three is still more dangerous. The *Journal of American Physicians and Surgeons* published a paper in its Summer 2016 edition titled "Combining Childhood Vaccines at One Visit Is Not Safe." The author of the paper, vaccine researcher Neil Z. Miller, reviewed data from the Vaccine Adverse Event Reporting System (VAERS) and found

> a dose-dependent association between the number of vaccines administered simultaneously and the likelihood of hospitalization or death for an adverse reaction. Additionally, younger age at the time of the adverse reaction is associated with a higher risk of hospitalization or death.

According to Miller, "The hospitalization rate [of adverse events reported to VAERS] increased linearly from 11.0% for two doses to 23.5% for eight doses."[12]

As common sense would dictate, infant mortality subsequent to vaccinations followed a similar pattern. "Of infants reported to VAERS," Miller wrote, "those who had received more vaccines had a statistically significant 50% higher mortality rate compared with those who had received fewer."[13]

Speaking of infant mortality, after the 5-in-1 pentavalent vaccine (DPT, hepatitis B, Haemophilus influenzae type b) was introduced in India, deaths attributed to SIDS in Kerala increased to "five times greater than the all-cause mortality rate in the state."[14]

According to a British-based website Child Health Safety, the World Health Organization dealt with the problem of increased vaccine-related child mortality by watering down its method of assessing "Adverse Events Following Immunization [AEFI]."[15]

The trade journal *Vaccine* published a paper in 2013 describing the changes in the WHO's assessment tool. Virtually all of the comments posted below the online version of the article condemned the changes that have resulted in more deaths being recorded as "Not an AEFI."[16]

The vaccine paradigm is unique among all other medical paradigms. Both its power and absurdity are symbolized in the conviction that babies can safely receive up to 100,000 vaccinations. In that conviction, the truth is made manifest: the vaccine paradigm is, at its core, madness.

No vaccine believer would claim that because one baby aspirin is safe then 100,000 baby aspirins administered on the same day would also be safe. But one need not compare vaccines with aspirin to dismantle the fragile web of lies woven by vaccine sociopaths. The most difficult obstacle to seeing the obvious is not a lack of evidence; it's a profound, irrational bias against and hostility toward any information that counters one's belief that vaccines are safe and effective, a phenomenon that represents the antithesis to the scientific method of learning. This bias prevents countless medical professionals from acknowledging the reality of vaccine injury. It even prevents parents from recognizing vaccine injury in their own children, turning them into unwitting accomplices to further injury.

If vaccines were as safe and as effective as they are proclaimed to be, then vaccine sociopaths would have no reason to rewrite history, doctor data, silence scientists, and bribe bureaucrats, topics that will soon be explored.

And now, a deeper look into the myths of vaccine safety and efficacy is in order.

Chapter Five

SAFE AND EFFECTIVE: NOT WHAT YOU THINK IT MEANS

They have sold you yet another string of tales. This time, that the vaccine science is settled, that they are perfectly safe and effective for everyone.[1]
—Kelly Brogan, MD

It's not just that we don't know some very basic things about the safety of the sacred program, we also cannot know and should not seek to know.
This stance should offend even the most skeptical scientists.
Still, the farce continues.[2]
—Mark Blaxill

How does the Unholy Trinity—the vaccine industry, medical establishment, and government—get away with calling vaccines "safe and effective" when the US Supreme Court has ruled that vaccines are "unavoidably unsafe?" The short answer is: it lies. The longer answer is the same, it just takes longer to decode the lies.

Before decoding, it's important to point out that for governmental employees, the "vaccines are safe and effective" statement is more than a marketing slogan, more than a policy, and more than dogma: it's an edict. Exactly when, where, and how the phrase became an edict is uncertain, but there's evidence that is has existed for over half a century. Several scientists have had their careers destroyed when they defied the edict.

Dr. Bernice Eddy was a pioneer in that unfortunate group. Eddy worked as a polio control officer in the 1950s. Her story came to the attention of Congress and the public in 1972. According to the congressional record, Eddy had "found live virus in supposedly killed polio vaccine; in 1955 she was relieved of her duties as polio control officer."[3]

Vaccine researcher Marco Cáceres, wrote that had her supervisors listened to, rather than reprimand, Dr. Eddy, "40,000 children would not have been infected with polio, 200 would not have been severely paralyzed and 10 of them would not have died."[4]

The live virus Eddy found was from the infamous Cutter factory, the company mainly responsible for including live poliovirus in its inactivated polio vaccine. Another scientist, Julius Younger, accepted an invitation to visit the Cutter manufacturing operation. "I was appalled," he said.

> Tanks containing live-virus pools and other tanks containing virus lots in various stages of formalin inactivation were kept in the same rooms. Conditions were not neat or esthetically appealing. There was a worrisome lack of attention to the most basic rules. . . . They never let me look at their data, but it was obvious to me that they were having serious trouble with their inactivation procedures.[5]

Younger reported his experience to his boss, who "agreed that it was a serious situation with terrible potential consequences." His boss said he would write a letter to the appropriate authorities. After American children were paralyzed from the Cutter vaccine, Younger "realized that [his boss] probably had done nothing."[6]

Congressman Percy Priest ordered and chaired a full investigation of the Cutter incident, but the public was not to be informed of the investigation. Priest stated that

> . . . in the previous year (1955) many responsible persons had felt that the public should be spared the ordeal of "knowledge about controversy." If word ever got out that the Public Health Service had actually done something damaging to the health of the American people, the consequences would be terrible. . . . We felt that no lasting good could come to science or the public if the Public Health Services were discredited.[7]

Although Dr. Eddy had been demoted following her discovery of live poliovirus in polio vaccines, that didn't stop her from getting into trouble again a few years later when she discovered that polio vaccines also contained a cancer causing simian virus derived from the monkey kidneys in which the vaccines were cultured. The congressional record reads: "After her discoveries concerning the SV40 virus, her staff and animal space were reduced and she was demoted from head of a section to head of a unit."[8] According to the *Encyclopedia of World Scientists*, Eddy

> [d]escribed her experiments with the mystery virus at a meeting of the New York Cancer Society in the fall of 1960. [Her boss, Joseph Smadel] heard about her speech and telephoned her in a fury. "I never saw any-

body so mad," Eddy said later. Smadel ordered her not to speak in public again without clearing the content of her speeches with him. . . .

During her remaining years at NIH Bernice Eddy was pushed into smaller and smaller laboratories and denied permission to attend professional meetings and publish papers.[9]

The congressional record documents that

. . . even when the contaminating virus was found to be oncogenic [cancer causing] in hamsters, the DBS [Division of Biologics Standards] and its expert advisory committee decided to leave existing stocks on the market rather than risk eroding public confidence by a recall.

. . . There has been a tendency on the part of certain higher government circles to play down any open discussion of problems associated with vaccines . . . .[10]

Downplaying the "problems associated with vaccines" is not a "tendency," it's policy. Doing otherwise would violate the edict that vaccines are safe and effective. The FDA officially stated that policy in 1984 when it submitted changes in the manufacturing standards for the live oral poliovirus vaccine. The Federal Register reads:

. . . although the continued availability of the vaccine may not be in immediate jeopardy, any possible doubts, whether or not well founded, about the safety of the vaccine cannot be allowed to exist in view of the need to assure that the vaccine will continue to be used to the maximum extent consistent with the nation's public health objectives. Accordingly, because of the importance of the vaccine and of maintaining public confidence in the immunization program that depends on it, good cause exists to issue these amendments as a final rule effective immediately.[11]

When doubts about vaccine safety "cannot be allowed to exist," neither can research that leads to doubts about vaccine safety be allowed to exist. If John Martin, professor of pathology at the University of Southern California, had been aware of the prohibition against doubt in the vaccine program, he probably wouldn't have wasted time petitioning the federal government for funding and for vaccine samples to investigate the potential risk that monkey viruses other than SV40 found in polio vaccines might pose to human health. According to a 1996 *Money Magazine* article,

. . . government officials rebuffed Martin's attempt to research those risks back in 1978 and again in 1995 when he was denied federal funding and vaccine samples he needed to investigate the effects of simian cytomegalovirus (SCMV), an organism that his studies indicate causes neurological disorders in the human brain.[12]

Commenting on his experience, Martin said, "The resistance of those in authority to face the issue of prior vaccine contamination is particularly unfortunate, because research establishing a viral cause for neurological disorders or cancers can lead to effective antiviral treatments." The government also gave Cecil H. Fox the brush-off on his proposal to examine polio vaccines for simian immunodeficiency virus (SIV).[13]

The FDA fired one of its own scientists, J. Anthony Morris, for insubordination because he revealed his intent to tell the public the truth about the 1976 Swine Flu scam (more in Chapter 8).

In 2009, Judy Mikovits, PhD, a 20-year veteran of the National Institutes of Health, informed 24 leading NIH scientists of her discovery of a xenotropic murine leukemia virus-related virus (XMRV) "linked to chronic fatigue syndrome (CFS), prostate cancer, lymphoma, and eventually neurodevelopmental disorders in children," including autism.[14] According to the CDC, "XMRV is closely related to a group of retroviruses called murine leukema [sic] viruses (MLVs), which are known to cause cancer in certain mice."[15] Mice brains are used as a vaccine culture media. Mikovits estimated that at least 30% of vaccines on the market were contaminated with the gammaretroviruses.[16] Authorities eventually responded by throwing the biochemist in jail and imposing a four-year gag order. After the order was lifted, Mikovits joined forces with Kent Heckenlively, former attorney and founding editor of Age of Autism, to chronicle the saga in the book *Plague: One Scientist's Intrepid Search for the Truth about Human Retroviruses and Chronic Fatigue Syndrome (ME/CFS), Autism, and Other Diseases*.[17]

Dubbed "the best scientist-in-jail story since Galileo," Hillary Johnson, author of *Osler's Web: Inside the Labyrinth of the Chronic Fatigue Syndrome Epidemic*, wrote a lengthy foreword for *Plague*. The following passage from the foreword reveals both the profound implications of the researcher's discovery and her disdain for the CDC:

[Dr. Mikovits] would call XMRV ". . . the biggest epidemic in United States history," one destined "to turn the US into the equivalent of HIV-riddled sub-Sahara Africa" if it continued unabated. She labeled the Centers for Disease Control "criminal" for what she saw as the agency's failure to control the spread of XMRV. Inside her lab, the Atlanta agency's acronym stood for "Can't, Don't Care." She and her staff derided the agency's method of selecting patients—by random telephone surveys— calling the government's cohort "Publisher's Clearinghouse" patients.

Scientists of integrity are not the only professionals to incur the wrath of the vaccine politburo. As will be explored later, vaccine-informed medical professionals are also at risk. In addition, the drug industry has little tolerance for sales representatives who blow the whistle on industry crimes, something Brandy Vaughan, a woman sometimes referred to as "the Merck whistleblower," learned the hard way. Now Vaughan regularly speaks out against the industry she used to represent saying she's

> . . . tired of all the lies. The chemical additives in vaccines have absolutely no place in the human body and are causing irreparable damage. And we are being lied to for profit— vaccines are NOT safe. There are too many, too soon and this entire generation of children is suffering because of it. People have the RIGHT to know the risks before they do something that may change their lives forever — or the life of their innocent, healthy child [emphasis in original].[18]

Vaughan created and heads up the nonprofit organization called LearnTheRisk.org. She takes her message to strategically placed billboards in which she shares key messages about vaccine risks. By doing so, she has placed herself at risk and has paid a high price: "They broke into my house (now selling it because of the PTSD), threatened my life, CPS threats, hacked into all my bank accounts, I have to live my life very differently than before I spoke out."[19]

When research emerges demonstrating the risks associated with vaccines and vaccine ingredients, the government often responds by conducting fraudulent studies to shore up the faith of vaccine believers. Dr. Gordon Douglas, director of strategic planning for vaccine research at the National Institutes of Health, explained as much in a 2001 presentation at Princeton University when he said,

> Four current studies are taking place to rule out the proposed link between autism and thimerosal. In order to undo the harmful effects of research claiming to link the [measles] vaccine to an elevated risk of autism, we need to conduct and publicize additional studies to assure parents of safety.[20]

Robert F. Kennedy, Jr. pointed out that when Douglas spoke at Princeton, he was also employed by Aventis, a company that manufactures thimerosal-containing vaccines. In addition, Douglas had formerly served as president of Merck's vaccination program.[21] While serving in that capacity in 1991—the beginning of the thimerosal generation and the autism epidemic—Kennedy asserts that:

> Dr. Maurice Hilleman, one of the fathers of Merck's vaccination programs, warned Dr. Gordon Douglas . . . that six-month-old children administered the shots on schedule would suffer mercury exposures 87 times the existing safety standards. He recommended that thimerosal use be discontinued, "especially where use in infants and young children is anticipated."[22]

No doubt, Douglas's associates appreciated the government spending taxpayer dollars on crooked research to absolve thimerosal—a potent neurotoxin— of the role it plays, and perhaps more important, the role the industry, medical establishment, and government play, in the brain damage and developmental disorders in children.

According to Dr. William Thompson, the man who would become known as the CDC whistleblower, he and his colleagues employed the garbage can method to maintain the faith of believers. Thompson stated that he, Frank DeStefano, Tanya Karapurkar Bhasin, Marshalyn Yeargin-Allsopp, and Coleen Boyle, used this method to destroy documents linking the MMR vaccine to autism. In 2004, the same names were listed as coauthors on the fraudulent study that dismissed the role of the MMR vaccine in autism. In July 2015, Representative Bill Posey quoted Thompson on the house floor as he described the CDC's garbage can party:

> . . . [W]e decided to exclude reporting any race effects. The coauthors scheduled a meeting to destroy documents related to the study. The remaining four coauthors all met and brought a big garbage can into the meeting room, and reviewed and went through all the hardcopy documents that we had thought we should discard, and put them into a huge garbage can. However, because I assumed it was illegal and would violate both FOIA and DOJ requests, I kept hardcopies of all documents in my office, and I retain all associated computer files.[23]

In 2004, Thompson's conscience got the best of him. He wrote a letter to CDC Director Julie Gerberding to tell her about the sham research he and his colleagues had presented to the world as truth. Thompson heard nothing from Gerberding, but apparently Robert Chen, then head of CDC's Immunization Safety Office and Thompson's direct boss, didn't think highly of Thompson's conscience or his letter. Chen met Thompson in an agency parking lot and threatened, "I would fire you if I could."[24]

In 2014, Thompson turned over thousands of documents to Representative Bill Posey exposing CDC fraud and cover-up. Thompson told scientist and father of an autistic child Dr. Brian Hooker how he and his colleagues had manipulated and destroyed the evidence linking vaccines to autism. Thompson told Hooker,

> I shoulder that the CDC has put the [autism/vaccine] research ten years behind. Because the CDC has not been transparent, we've missed ten years of research because the CDC is so paralyzed right now by anything related to autism. They're not doing what they should be doing because they're afraid to look for things that might be associated.[25]

If the CDC's going to uphold the Vaccines Are Safe And Effective edict, it's got to do a better job of screening out employees of conscience.

In 2013, Representatives Bill Posey and Carolyn Maloney introduced a bill known as the "Vaccine Safety Study Act." The act is intended

> [t]o direct the Secretary of Health and Human Services to conduct or support a comprehensive study comparing total health outcomes, including risk of autism, in vaccinated populations in the United States with such outcomes in unvaccinated populations in the United States, and for other purposes."[26]

Representative Maloney introduced a similar bill in 2007 and 2009. It failed to pass both times.[27]

One would expect that if Posey and Maloney's bill were passed and if "a comprehensive study comparing total health outcomes" of vaccinated versus unvaccinated populations were conducted and if the outcomes demonstrated the superior health of unvaccinated populations over vaccinated populations, the government might be free to amend current vaccine-related legislation or at least comment on potential changes in the US vaccine program. Such a conclusion, however, would be incorrect. The bill includes a "rule of construction" that reads: "Nothing in this Act shall be construed to authorize the conduct or support of any study in which an individual or population is encouraged or incentivized to remain unvaccinated."[28]

There it is, the edict stated clearly in print, proposed in the same bill that has the potential to finally demonstrate once and for all the superior health status of vaccine-free individuals. The rule would muzzle and bury the outcome just as surely as government officials have muzzled scientists and buried outcomes for over half a century. Thou shalt not say or do anything that would encourage or incentivize citizens to remain unvaccinated. Notice the unspoken yet deafening implication. Being unvaccinated is verboten, bad, evil, not an option, not happening, not a chance. True to the language of the vaccine paradigm, no mention is made of specific vaccines, specific combinations of vaccines, specific vaccine ingredients, genetic variables, or other differences in vaccine recipients. All vaccines, all schedules, all people, all the time. In such a repressive governmental culture, it's no wonder that fewer than 30% of members of Congress are willing to state whether they vaccinate their own children.[29]

Kudos to Representatives Posey and Maloney for proposing a vaccinated versus unvaccinated study, but charging the US government with the facilitation of such a study is as farcical as asking a cackle of hyenas to perform a grass versus meat taste test—a taste test that is quite unnecessary. Several vaxxed verses vax-free studies have already been conducted in various countries. The results demonstrate why the government refuses to conduct its own studies. German researchers have compiled statistics from various studies and have found that unvaccinated children suffer from far fewer disorders than their vaccinated peers:

Disorder	Vax Free (%)	Vaxxed (%)
Diabetes mellitus:	0.07	0.20
Autism:	0.44	1.10
Thyroid Disease	0.10	1.70
Migraine	1.09	2.50
Epilepsy/Seizures	0.33	3.60
Scoliosis	0.49	5.30
Autoimmune Disorders	0.37	7.00
Hyperactivity	2.04	7.90
Hay fever	3.00	10.70
Otitis Media	1.91	11.00
Herpes	0.27	12.80
Neurodermatitis	7.00	13.20
Sinusitis	0.75	15.00
Asthma / chronic bronchitis	2.32	18.00
Allergies	10.60	22.90[30]

A study out of Salzburger, Germany, reported similar results:

Disorder	Vax Free (%)	Vaxxed (%)
Asthma:	0	8-12
Atopic dermatitis	1.2	10-20
Allergies	3	25
ADHD	0.79	5-10[31]

In addition, a 1992 study out of New Zealand documented:

Disorder	Vax Free (%)	Vaxxed (%)
Asthma:	3	15
Eczema or allergic reactions	13	32
Chronic otitis	7	20
Recurrent tonsillitis	2	8
Shortness of breath and SIDS	2	7
Hyperactivity	1	8[32]

The *British Medical Journal* published a paper in 2000 titled "Routine vaccinations and child survival: follow up study in Guinea-Bissau, West Africa," where "[t]he children of 15,000 mothers were observed from 1990 to 1996 for 5 years." Among other things, the researchers found that "the death rate in vaccinated children against diphtheria, tetanus and whooping cough is twice as high as the unvaccinated children (10.5% versus 4.7%)."[33]

Dan Olmsted wrote an article for UPI in 2007 describing a privately funded telephone survey of US parents. "In one striking finding," wrote Olmsted, "vaccinated boys 11-17 were more than twice as likely to have autism as their never-vaccinated counterparts."[34]

In 2015, a panel of 120 Italian doctors "submitted an open letter to the Higher Institute of Health; the Italian equivalent of the CDC" stating that "[u]nvaccinated children are healthier." A rough translation of their conclusion follows:

Unvaccinated children will undoubtedly appear and healthier overall, less prone to infectious diseases, especially airway, less prone to intestinal disorders and chronic diseases, less prone to neurological and behavioral disorders. . . .[35]

A 2017 study of vaxxed vs. vaccine-free homeschoolers confirmed the indisputable fact that poison-free kids are healthier than kids poisoned with vaccines. Findings include the following:

- Vaccinated children were over fourfold more likely to be diagnosed on the Autism Spectrum (OR 4.3)
- Vaccinated children were 30 times more likely to be diagnosed with allergic rhinitis (hay fever) than nonvaccinated children
- Vaccinated children were 22 times more likely to require an allergy medication than unvaccinated children
- Vaccinated children were over fivefold more likely to be diagnosed with a learning disability than unvaccinated children (OR 5.2)
- Vaccinated children were 340 percent more likely to be diagnosed with Attention Deficit Hyperactivity Disorder than unvaccinated children (OR 4.3)
- Vaccinated children were 5.9 times more likely to have been diagnosed with pneumonia than unvaccinated children
- Vaccinated children were 3.8 times more likely to be diagnosed with middle ear infection (otitis media) than unvaccinated children (OR 3.8)
- Vaccinated children were 700 percent more likely to have had surgery to insert ear drainage tubes than unvaccinated children (OR 8.1)
- Vaccinated children were 2.4 times more likely to have been diagnosed with any chronic illness than unvaccinated children.[36]

Also in 2017, a study of vaxxed vs. unvaxxed premature infants concluded that:

No association was found between preterm birth and NDD [neurodevelopmental disorders] in the absence of vaccination, but vaccination was significantly associated with NDD in children born at term (OR 2.7, 95% CI: 1.2, 6.0). However, vaccination coupled with preterm birth was associated with increasing odds of NDD, ranging from 5.4 (95% CI: 2.5, 11.9) compared to vaccinated but nonpreterm children, to 14.5 (95% CI: 5.4, 38.7) compared to children who were neither preterm nor vaccinated.[37]

A team of researchers from Yale School of Medicine and Pennsylvania State School of Medicine published a 2017 paper titled "Temporal Association of Certain Neuropsychiatric Disorders Following Vaccination of Children and Adolescents: A Pilot Case–Control Study." The researchers found that compared to vaccine-free subjects, subjects vaccinated in the previous three months were more like to be newly diagnosed with anorexia nervosa.

> Influenza vaccinations during the prior 3, 6, and 12 months were also associated with incident diagnoses of AN [anorexia nervosa], OCD [obsessive compulsive disorder], and an anxiety disorder. Several other associations were also significant with HRs greater than 1.40 (hepatitis A with OCD and AN; hepatitis B with AN; and meningitis with AN and chronic tic disorder).

The researchers concluded, "This pilot epidemiologic analysis implies that the onset of some neuropsychiatric disorders may be temporally related to prior vaccinations in a subset of individuals."[38]

So, knowing that vaccines are "unavoidably unsafe," and knowing that numerous studies have demonstrated that vax-free kids are healthier than their jabbed counterparts, and knowing that government officials cannot reveal anything that would encourage or incentivize individuals to remain unvaccinated, it becomes clear that any reading of vaccine-related governmental resources must be read and scrutinized as marketing propaganda.

Norman Baylor, director of the FDA's Office of Vaccines Research and Review Center for Biologics Evaluation and Research, provides a classic example of such propaganda in his slide show presentation titled "FDA's Role in Protecting Your Child's Health Through Safe and Effective Vaccines."[39]

It's important to realize that the government would prefer not to define the words "safe" and "effective" because in the absence of a government definition, people are left to the standard definitions of those terms. An online dictionary defines "safe" as "free from hurt, injury, danger, or risk." "Effective" is defined as "adequate to accomplish a purpose; producing the intended or expected result."

Such definitions are on the minds of parents when their physicians proclaim that the vaccines they are about to inject into a three-pound premature infant are safe and effective. And that child will get the same dosage that a 300-pound adult would receive. All are assured, of course, that these concoctions will safely prevent disease. Period.

If the government is forced to define the words, it chooses various definitions based on the target audience. Parents and patients get one set of definitions, medical professionals get another, while industry gets yet another. Baylor's presentation is designed for parents, so the intent is to reassure and persuade them to vaccinate their children with any and all vaccines licensed by the FDA and recommended by the CDC. Slide number three reads: "FDA Serves as the Gatekeeper for Assuring the Safety and Effectiveness of Vaccines." This sentence effectively reinforces the illusion that the FDA exists to protect American citizens. Once that is accomplished, Baylor provides definitions for the words "safe," "pure," and "potent":

Safe: "Relative freedom from harmful effect . . . when prudently administered, taking into account the character of the product in relation to the condition of the recipient at the time."

Pure: "Relative freedom from extraneous matter in the finished product, . . ."

Potent: "Specific ability of the product . . . to effect a given result [emphasis in original]."[40]

The phrases "relative freedom from harm" and "relative freedom from extraneous matter" and "effect a given result" are reassuring to uncritical minds, but to those who are even remotely aware of the FDA's repeated failures to live up even to these nebulous criteria, they are anything but reassuring.

Slides five through eight provide a detailed description of the process of clinical testing before new vaccines are licensed and brought to market. Careful reading of the text reveals that manufacturers—not the FDA—conduct the clinical tests and submit the results to the FDA for review, then the "FDA determines whether the vaccine is safe, pure, potent (i.e., vaccine immunogenic or efficacious)." All in all, the typical parent would conclude that the approval process is thorough and conducted according to sound scientific procedures.

Louise Kuo Habakus, editor of *Vaccine Epidemic: How Corporate Greed, Biased Science, and Coercive Government Threaten Our Human Rights, Our Health, and Our Children*, is not the typical parent. Her assessment of vaccine safety research differs from Baylor's description. According to Habakus, "There is so little vaccine safety research, it boggles the mind. Equally distressing is the fact that we rely upon vaccine makers to do the research for product approval and licensure."[41]

Habakus points out that "the government-hired think tank, The Institute of Medicine," shares her perspective—not the FDA's—on vaccine testing procedures. The IOM notes

[M]any gaps and limitations in knowledge . . . inadequate understanding of the biological mechanisms . . . insufficient or inconsistent information . . . inadequate size of length of follow-up . . . limited capacity of existing surveillance systems . . . [and] few experimental studies. . . .

Clearly, if research capacity and accomplishment in these areas are not improved, future reviews of vaccine safety will be similarly handicapped.[42]

While vaccine safety testing is inadequate for single vaccines, it's virtually nonexistent for vaccines administered in combination or for the entire vaccine schedule. Dr. Brian Hooker, university professor, researcher, and father of a vaccine-injured son, takes a dim view of people who lie about vaccine safety, including Richard Pan, the pediatrician whose lies contributed to the passage of California's mandatory vaccination bill in 2015. Hooker told a Chicago audience,

> The vaccine schedule has not been studied. . . . When folks like Richard Pan out in California talk about the vaccine schedule being safe, it's the ultimate lie. These people are lying through their teeth because the entire vaccination schedule has never been studied for neurological effects on children.[43]

Baylor introduces slide number nine with the question "What Does 'Safe' Mean?" Then, rather than answer the question, he provides four statements meant to further convince parents that the FDA is on top of its game and that vaccines are safe and necessary.

FDA takes vaccine safety very seriously throughout the vaccine life cycle
- A vaccine is a medication. Like any medicine, vaccines have benefits and risks, and although highly effective, no vaccine is 100 percent effective in preventing disease or 100 percent safe in all individuals.
- Millions of vaccine doses are given per year in the US and the vast majority have few, if any, side effects.
- The benefits of vaccines clearly outweigh their potential risks.

Slide number 10 defines "Effective."[44]

- Vaccine <u>effectiveness</u> is the assessment of whether a vaccine prevents disease in the general population.
- Vaccine development proceeds from a study of immunogenicity to a randomized controlled trial that determines vaccine <u>efficacy</u> under ideal conditions.
  - vaccine <u>efficacy</u> is defined as the reduction in the incidence of a disease among individuals who have received a vaccine compared to the incidence in unvaccinated people.
  - efficacy of a new vaccine is measured in phase 2 or phase 3 clinical trials by giving one group a vaccine and comparing the incidence of disease in that group to another group who do not receive the vaccine.
  - vaccine <u>effectiveness</u> depends upon vaccine <u>efficacy</u>[45] [emphasis in original].

The FDA's claim that "vaccine efficacy is defined as the reduction in the incidence of a disease among individuals who have received a vaccine compared to the incidence in unvaccinated people" is false. Vaccinated-versus-vaccine-free studies are rarely conducted, and, when they are, their measure of efficacy is a change in serum or blood antibody levels, not a reduction in the incidence of disease. There are numerous problems associated with vaccine efficacy in general, the efficacy of combined vaccines, and the efficacy of specific vaccines (more in Chapter 9).

Slide number 13 is titled "Vaccine Ingredients," a subject of utmost importance, because vaccines are chemical concoctions produced by pharmaceutical companies, and the simple truth is that nature did not arrange for the ingredients in vaccines to be injected into the blood streams of humans or any other creature. So what exactly does the FDA have to say about vaccine ingredients?

> A vaccine is made up of various ingredients and each ingredient present in a vaccine is there for a specific reason. Different ingredients have different roles in a vaccine, and vaccines licensed for use in the United States are demonstrated to be safe and effective before they are used by the public.[46]

But enough said. The FDA has decreed that vaccines include "various ingredients" and each ingredient is there "for a specific reason" accomplishing "different roles." And, since the FDA pronounces vaccines "to be safe and effective," any sane parent or patient would be a fool not to conclude that all of those unnamed ingredients are also "safe and effective."

Let's test that theory using FDA's logic. Formaldehyde, ethylmercury, aluminum, 2-phenoxyethanol, MRC-5 cells, peanut oil, polysorbate 80, and potassium chloride are a few of the dozens of ingredients found in vaccines. Formaldehyde—embalming fluid—is defined as a carcinogen, but when placed in vaccines, it miraculously becomes safe and effective. Ethylmercury and aluminum are neurotoxins and are synergistically neurotoxic when ingested, but when injected they change into something that's "safe and effective." 2-phenoxyethanol is an insecticide. Humans are not insects, but somehow injecting humans with this insecticide is "safe and effective." Potassium chloride is used in lethal injections to shut down the heart and stop breathing, but when injected into babies it's "safe and effective." Of course, the dosage in vaccines is a small fraction of a lethal dosage, but less of a poison does not equal safe, it equals less toxic. MRC-5 cells are cells from aborted human fetuses. Foreign proteins—human or otherwise—can result in a host of medical problems including autoimmune disorders when ingested, but when injected, they're "safe and effective." According to Heather Fraser, author of *The Peanut Allergy*

Epidemic, the explosion of peanut and many other allergies in recent years is linked to the use of peanut oil in vaccines.[47]

Speaking of peanuts, Robyn Charron, an advocate for allergy awareness, wrote a review of Fraser's book commenting that "It is now known that the structure and weight of the Hib bacteria proteins are very similar to the structure and weight of the peanut protein, which leads to cross reactivity to peanuts and tree nuts." Charron concludes, "We are, essentially, creating anaphylactic babies in the same manner researchers create anaphylactic mice: administering a peanut-like protein fused to adjuvant bacterial toxin."[48]

Lest readers conclude that Fraser and Charron are nut cases, Janet Levatin, MD, Board Certified Pediatrician and Clinical Instructor in Pediatrics at Harvard Medical School, wrote the foreword for Fraser's book. Levatin's endorsement could not be stronger:

> *The Peanut Allergy Epidemic* is a vital, groundbreaking book, covering material that resides at intersection of medicine, history, and public policy. I believe it should be required reading for everyone who administers injections, everyone who receives injections, and everyone who authorizes injections for children.[49]

Hmmm. Baylor's pronouncement that vaccine ingredients ". . . are demonstrated to be safe and effective before they are used by the public" doesn't sound so safe anymore, does it? Surely, there are published studies that support the FDA scientist's position, right? Indeed there are, but there are also hundreds of studies that suggest otherwise. Vaccine researcher Neil Z. Miller compiled 400 such studies in his 2016 book *Miller's Review of Critical Vaccine Studies*.[50] Following are but a few samples of the papers highlighted in Miller's book:

- the CDC's "analysis suggests that high exposure to ethylmercury from thimerosal-containing vaccines in the first month of life increases the risk of subsequent development of neurologic development impairment."[51]
- "boys in the United States who were vaccinated with the triple series hepatitis B vaccine, during the time period in which vaccines were manufactured with thimerosal, were more susceptible to developmental disability than were unvaccinated boys."[52]
- ". . . the effects of thimerosal in humans indicates that it is a poison at minute levels with a plethora of deleterious consequences, even at the levels currently administered in vaccines."[53]
- "Hyperstimulation of the immune system by various [vaccine] adjuvants, including aluminum, carries an inherent risk for serious autoimmune disorders affecting the central nervous system."[54]

- researchers "conclude that the [macrophagic myofasciitis] lesion is secondary to intramuscular injection of aluminium-containing vaccines, shows both long-term persistence of aluminium hydroxide and an ongoing local immune reaction, and is detected in patients with systemic symptoms which appeared subsequently to vaccination."[55]
- "Vaccines designed to reduce pathogen growth rate and/or toxicity may result in the evolution of pathogens with higher levels of virulence. We propose that waning immunity and pathogen adaptation have contributed to the resurgence of pertussis."[56]
- "There is evidence from both prospective epidemiological surveillance and recent experiments in model organisms that immunization with the acellular vaccine may actually increase the host's susceptibility to infection by B. parapertussis."[57]
- "Haemophilus influenzae type b immunization contributed to an increase risk for Haemophilus influenza type a meningitis."[58]
- "Current worldwide HPV immunization practices with either of the two HPV vaccines appear to be neither justified by long-term health benefits nor economically viable, nor is there any evidence that HPV vaccination (even if proven effective against cervical cancer) would reduce the rate of cervical cancer beyond what Pap screening has already achieved."[59]
- "Under universal varicella vaccination, there has been a vaccine-induced decline in exogenous boosting. We estimate universal varicella vaccination has the impact of an additional 14.6 million herpes-zoster cases among adults aged under 50 years during a 50-year time span at a substantial cost burden of 4.1 billion US dollars or 80 million US dollars annually."[60]
- "Compared to the unexposed, patients with zoster vaccination had 2.2 and 2.7 times the odds of developing arthritis and alopecia, respectively."[61]
- ". . . the hypothesis that immunization with the recombinant hepatitis B vaccine is associated with an increased risk of multiple sclerosis."[62]

Papers such as these lead to the disturbing conclusion that vaccines are *not* safe and that granting licensure to such products is in direct violation of the government's own safety regulations. If that is true, then vaccines are really no more legal than illicit street drugs and the FDA and associates are really no different from any other drug dealers.

Drug dealers routinely kill for profit. Vaccine sociopaths have knowingly put at risk virtually every person on the planet to protect and increase their profits. The drug company Wyeth provided a disturbing example of sociopathy in 1979 following a spate of "SIDS" deaths in Tennessee after the administration of the DTP vaccine. Rather than issue an immediate recall of the lot or batch that was associated with the deaths, "senior management staff" agreed that future lots should be distributed more widely to hide the dangerous effects of "hot lots."[63]

If industry sociopaths are willing to kill babies for profit, it is not hard to believe that they would do the same to people of influence who get in their way. In fact, since William Thompson issued his public statement in August 2014, dozens of holistic medical professionals have died under suspicious circumstances. Prior to their deaths, many had condemned the practice of sacrificing children on the altar of Vaccinology.[64] Whether the industry is responsible for their deaths is yet unknown, but it *is* well known that CBS News reported in 2009 that

> Merck made a "hit list" of doctors who criticized Vioxx, according to tes-
> timony in a Vioxx class action case in Australia. The list, emailed between
> Merck employees, contained doctors' names with the labels "neutralise,"
> "neutralised" or "discredit" next to them. . . . One email said: "We may
> need to seek them out and destroy them where they live . . . ."[65]

But never mind that. The industry, the medical establishment, the CDC, FDA, HHS, NIH, DOD, and LMNOP are the good guys—the crusaders on a mission to protect against evil germs. So take a big breath, count to ten, and become one with FDA marketing propaganda. In one of the final slides in Baylor's presentation to parents on the "FDA's role in protecting your child's health through safe and effective vaccines," this reassuring call to the faithful is issued:

> FDA employees are parents, aunts, uncles, and grandparents and we
> have complete confidence in FDA-approved vaccines for our own fami-
> lies. The public can be assured that FDA is diligent in ensuring that the
> vaccines licensed for use in the United States are shown to be safe and
> effective."[66]

The government has fed its citizens such propaganda for nearly as long as vaccines have been in existence. And, by and large, the public has heeded the altar call.

Much of humanity's faith in the Vaccine religion lies in the apocryphal accounts of vaccine history—the legendary role of scientists and doctors who wielded vaccines to vanquish smallpox and polio. In order to pull back the curtain on the modern vaccine paradigm, it's necessary to first pull back the curtain on the false narrative the public has been fed for over a century starting with a discussion of smallpox and then moving on to polio.

Chapter Six

SMALLPOX VACCINE: LEGEND AND LIES

He who controls the past controls the future.
He who controls the present controls the past.

—George Orwell

Smallpox killed millions of people. The smallpox vaccine eradicated smallpox. Therefore, all vaccines eradicate disease, as well. Not vaccinating will result in disease epidemics, including a resurgence of smallpox. Those who question these facts are science deniers and they are to be blamed for any and all disease outbreaks.

Most vaccine believers believe the preceding paragraph with the same devotion that doctors once believed that their filthy hands had nothing to do with the spread of disease and the death of their pregnant and newborn patients. Such beliefs do not originate out of thin air, nor do they originate from science, unless one includes the science of agnotology: the study of culturally induced ignorance or doubt. Vaccine sociopaths spawned and fed public ignorance with the nonsense that the smallpox vaccine eradicated smallpox and the polio vaccine will soon do the same for polio.

As if to affirm their place as orthodox members in the Vaccine religion, researchers, scientists, doctors, and politicians frequently preface vaccine-related communications by bearing testimony to these false narratives.

If vaccines eradicated smallpox or polio, one would expect to find a general consensus in the records from those fortunate enough to have witnessed these miracles. Such is not the case. From the 1700s onward, numerous educated people from around the world bore witness to the fact that the smallpox vaccine resulted in an increase in both severity and prevalence of smallpox outbreaks. Frederick Cartwright commented on that point in his 1972 book, *Disease and History*:

> . . . [I]t has been reckoned that two or three persons died out of every hundred inoculated. Further, many people rightly suspected that inoculation,

even though it might protect the individual by a mild attack, spread the disease more widely by multiplying the foci of infection. For these reasons inoculation fell into general disrepute in Europe after 1728.[1]

In 1764, *The Gentleman's Magazine and Historical Chronicle* published an article titled "The Practice of Inoculation Truly Stated."[2]

The title suggests that a 1700s version of the vaccine paradigm had been instituted to decrease public resistance against a vaccine derived from the lymph of "a smallpox corpse, the ulcerated udder of a cow, . . . the running sores of a sick horse's heels, . . . rabbit-pox, ass-pox, or mule-pox."[3]

The "truly stated" article decimated the smallpox vaccine paradigm as seen in the following paragraph:

> It does not follow Inoculation is a practice favourable to life. . . . It is incontestably like the plague a contagious disease, what tends to stop the progress of the infection tends to lessen the danger that attends it; what tends to spread the contagion, tends to increase that danger, the practice of Inoculation manifestly tends to spread the contagion, for a contagious disease is produced by Inoculation where it would not otherwise have been produced; the place where it is thus produced becomes a center of contagion, whence it spreads not less fatally or widely than it would spread from a center where the disease should happen in a natural way; these centers of contagion are manifestly multiplied very greatly by Inoculation. . . .[4]

In England, portions of the general population recognized the vaccinators as the cause of the outbreaks as well as the cause of their children's suffering and death. Out of such suffering was born the anti-vaccination movement. Dr. W.J. Collins, MD, identified himself as an anti-vaccinationist in 1866 when he described his "Twenty Years' Experience of a Public Vaccinator" in material printed by the Anti-Compulsory Vaccination League. Wrote Collins,

> I have no faith in vaccination; nay, I look upon it with the greatest possible disgust, and firmly believe that it is often the medium of conveying many filthy and loathsome diseases from one child to another, and no protection whatever against small pox. Indeed, I consider we are now living in the Jennerian epoch for the slaughter of innocents, and the unthinking portion of the adult population.[5]

The British government was not impressed with the likes of Dr. Collins. Compulsory vaccination became law in 1853, and the provisions were made more stringent in 1867, 1871, and 1874. Several parents chose to be jailed or fined rather than subject themselves or their children to further risk of harm.[6]

Thus were the circumstances when the borough of Leicester rose up in defiance against the government. No, they declared, they would not comply with medical tyranny. J.T. Biggs, a member of the Leicester Board of Guardians and author of the 1912 book *Leicester: Sanitation versus Vaccination*, described the battle between science and the "financially-interested," a battle that is eerily familiar to modern vaccine informed individuals. Said Biggs,

> Notwithstanding the innumerable failures of, and the disasters attributable to vaccination, indubitably proven, the language of the professional, financially-interested, and official supporters and apologists, remains now much the same as ever. Like the Bourbons, these strange protagonists appear to have learned nothing and forgotten nothing.[7]

It is no small irony that modern vaccine profiteers cite smallpox epidemics as justification for today's burgeoning vaccine schedule, because the people who survived those epidemics cite them as proof that vaccine peddlers and their pustulants caused disease outbreaks far worse than outbreaks caused by natural smallpox. Biggs, a self-avowed anti-vaccinationist, wrote,

> The experience of the terrible smallpox epidemic of 1871-73, when many thousands of vaccinated persons contracted the disease, and several hundreds died as the result of the alleged "protection" (!) having lamentably failed in its hour of trial, produced in the minds of the thinking people of Leicester pronounced hostility against the blood-polluting quackery, which was found to be more baneful in its ultimate results than the disease it was supposed to prevent.[8]

Great tyranny always leads to great change. In Leicester that change was symbolized in what is likely the greatest anti-vaccination demonstration in the history of the world. Biggs described a few of the events leading up to the historic occasion:

> All honour to the parents, both men and women, who, rather than submit the health of their children to the risk of the blood poisoners lancet, preferred the prison cell. William Johnson, whose name heads the list, was the first in the Kingdom to be imprisoned under the Vaccination Acts. Also, Henry Matts, the fourth name on the list, suffered the longest term of imprisonment under the old barbarous penal regime—namely,

thirty days, being ten days for each of three children. These honours, therefore, belong to Leicester.

Thus was the small flame of resistance fanned by these harsh proceedings into a huge conflagration, which culminated in a demonstration in 1885, when copies of the Vaccination Acts were defiantly burned in public on that never-to-be forgotten occasion! The people of Leicester were thoroughly aroused. They organised what was described as the largest and most impressive demonstration that has ever been witnessed within its boundaries. It took the form of a national outburst against the cruelties attendant upon the enforcement of compulsory vaccination.[9]

The citizens of Leicester were far from alone in the demonstration. Some forty different anti-vaccination leagues, fifty neighboring towns, and representatives from both Ireland and Scotland gathered on the historic day of March 23, 1885. The *Hawera & Normanby Star* covered the event with a compelling and descriptive article titled "Anti-Compulsory Vaccination Demonstration at Leicester," much of which is quoted below:

The borough of Leicester, was on March 23, the scene of an extraordinary demonstration against the Vaccination Acts. The proceedings commenced with a procession. . . . The first detachment wore rosettes, and was made up solely of those who had suffered terms of imprisonment, varying from seven to thirty days, the second of parents who had had their goods seized for vaccination fines, the third of those who had paid conscience fines, the fourth of members of the Board of Guardians who had opposed the enforcement of the Acts, and the fifth of unvaccinated children, on ponies and carriages, with bannerets, [sp] &c. Then followed the delegates from various towns. Then followed detachments of anti-vaccinators . . . . The devices included one of Dr. Jenner suspended from a gibbet, and being repeatedly executed and inscribed "Child Slayer." Another consisted of a complete "funeral cortege of a victim of vaccination." a real coffin for a child, covered with wreaths, &c., being placed on a carriage bier, and followed by mourners. . . . The mottoes, on the other hand, included "Who would be free themselves must strike the blow." "The price of liberty is eternal vigilance," "They that are whole need not a physician," "Rachels are weeping all over the world because their children are not," "The Three Pillars of Vaccination—Fraud, Force, and Folly," "A Dead Swindle—the Vaccination Death Certificate," "We no longer beg but demand the control of our children," "Health without adulteration," &c. The procession marched through the principal streets and back to the Market Place, where about fifty thousand took part in a demonstration against the Acts. A resolution condemning the Acts as subversive of parental liberty, destructive of personal rights, and tyrannical and unjust, and ought to be resisted by every constitutional means, was adopted with enthusiasm; as was another petitioning for the abolition of the Acts. A copy of the Acts was then publicly burnt amid cheers, and proceedings terminated by the singing of an anti-vaccination song entitled "Cause that is True."[10]

After the demonstration, Councillor Butcher, one of the leading representatives of the movement, spoke to a cheering audience. He not only described the failure of the smallpox vaccine; he also described a solution to infectious disease that many educated people now agree accounts for the marked decline in the incidence and the severity of smallpox and every other infectious disease: modern sanitation, clean water, good food, and healthy living quarters. "If such details were attended to, there was no need to fear small pox, or any of its kindred; and if they were neglected, neither vaccination nor any other prescription by Act of Parliament could save them."[11] Following Councillor Butcher's comments, Mr. W. Stanyon recited the following resolution:

> That the Compulsory Vaccination Acts, which make loving and conscientious parents criminals, subjecting them to fines, loss of goods, and imprisonment, propagate disease and inflict death, and under which five thousand of our fellow-townsmen are now being prosecuted, are a disgrace to the Statute Book, and ought to be abolished forthwith.[12]

J.T. Biggs documented the proceedings of the meeting, which ended in the unanimous passage of the resolution. The speeches offered on that momentous occasion are as timely today as they were when first uttered. They are included below nearly in their entirety:

> In supporting the motion, Mr. Tebb remarked: "Schiller says only great questions arouse the profound depths of humanity, and I venture to say that the question which has called us together this evening belongs to that category. The Demonstration which we have witnessed today could only have been aroused by a deep conviction in the justice and righteousness of our cause; and, if I am not mistaken, it will help forward the work of emancipation wherever this odious and indefensible tyranny exists, and will leave a broad mark in the history of our time. . . . When our victory is won, we may rest assured that we shall have shaken the foundations of other tyrannies besides vaccination; for injustice and

cruelty are linked together in more ways than one, and in the downfall of this superstition we shall feel that we have become a freer, healthier, and happier people."

Mr. Alfred Milnes, M.A., also supporting the motion, said: "I can assure you it gives me very great pleasure to come here and take part in this splendid meeting. Not merely because one seems to breathe a purer atmosphere in coming to this, the head-centre of revolt against what I look on as in every aspect a wicked and intolerable law, but chiefly because here in Leicester a man gets rid at once of all the mass of sophistries with which this matter of compulsory vaccination has been overlaid. Here, at last, one comes face to face with the question in its plain, broad issues. . . . We are not met here tonight to ask for any man's toleration. For my own part, toleration is a word I detest; and I wish that some revised version would give us a reading, Who art thou, to tolerate thy brother? We ask for no man's toleration, and we plead for no man's pity; we are met to-night to demand the birthright of free citizens—equality before the law. [Cheers.] . . .

Mr. Enoch Robinson, M.R.C.S., in supporting the motion, said it seemed to him an outrage on common sense that, after all the efforts made to raise the people out of ignorance and superstition, there should be an Act of Parliament to keep their minds down on one point to the level occupied 160 years ago. . . . When the law is repealed we shall witness a marvellous transformation, not only in the disuse of vaccination by the people, but in its repudiation by the intelligence of the medical profession; for many know, as we do, that vaccination, as a defence against small-pox, is one of the grossest superstitions that ever afflicted the human mind. [Cheers.]

The resolution was carried unanimously. . . .

Biggs then described "a conference of delegates" held the following morning "with 70 to 80 individuals representing several towns and more than fifty anti-vaccination leagues." The body proposed and passed a resolution. The final paragraph follows:

We appeal to our fellow-countrymen and countrywomen everywhere to countenance and aid us in this righteous struggle for the disestablishment and disendowment of a practice which is not only no security against small-pox, but which, as many of us know by bitter experience, poisons the blood of our children, and implants in their constitution the fatal seeds of disease and death, and violates that right of self-control over the person which is one of the ancient rights of the English citizen.[13]

According to Biggs, 73-year-old Dr. Spencer T. Hall stood following the passage of the resolution and stated that

> [h]e had been vaccinated at two years of age, and very seriously injured; but at fourteen he had a severe attack of smallpox, which was followed by improved health. Far rather would he have smallpox than be vaccinated. He had paid fines for all his children. In his long and wide experience he had never seen such evil results from smallpox as he had seen from vaccination.[14]

If the aged Dr. Hall were wrong about his assessment of the "evil results . . . from vaccination," his error would have been manifest in ensuing plagues of smallpox falling upon the non-vaccinating citizens of Leicester and the surrounding villages. The vaccine sociopaths of the day were no doubt disappointed that such a scenario never played out. But of course it didn't because the people of Leicester had learned that resistance to smallpox did not come in a syringe filled with pus and other contaminants; it came from immune systems strengthened by clean water, nutritious food, and healthy environments and from quarantining people with active cases of smallpox.[15]

Eleanor McBean recounted smallpox related details in the USA and the Philippines in her 1957 book, *The Poisoned Needle,* saying that ". . . the gradual abandonment of vaccination laws . . ." resulted in a ". . . steady decline of smallpox. . . ." By contrast, compulsory vaccination in the Philippine Islands resulted in a death rate of 74%, the highest in history. McBean concludes:

> In spite of these cold facts and thousands of others like them, the promoters of vaccines insist that vaccination has been a blessing to the world and has reduced disease. This all goes to prove the old saying that figures can't lie but liars can figure.[16]

More recently, Vernon Coleman, MD, one of Britain's most prolific modern writers and a former professor of Holistic Medical Sciences at the International Open University in Sri Lanka, presented the indisputable fact that improvements in food, water, and lifestyle eclipse the role vaccines purportedly play in the reduction of infectious disease. The professor noted that smallpox vaccine resulted in so many deaths that the WHO abandoned "[m]ass vaccination programmes" and replaced them with "surveillance, isolation and quarantine." Coleman's opinion is unwavering: "The myth that smallpox was eradicated through a mass vaccination programme is just that—a myth."[17]

Seconding Coleman's conviction, pathologist and medical writer Glen Dettman, PhD, states, "It is pathetic and ludicrous to say we ever vanquished smallpox with vaccines, when only 10% of the population was ever vaccinated."[18]

If that is the case, then the CDC is made up of "pathetic and ludicrous" people, because they advance the one germ, one vaccine theory of the eradication of smallpox as if it were gospel truth.[19] And in doing so, they are building upon more than 100 years of lying about the multiple problems associated with the smallpox vaccine, including the fact that the vaccine often caused the disease it was alleged to protect against. And just as modern doctors sometimes intentionally refuse to acknowledge vaccine injury, their predecessors intentionally doctored medical records by claiming that vaccinated people who succumbed to smallpox were unvaccinated. Dr. Russell of the Glasgow Hospital stated, "Patients entered as unvaccinated showed excellent marks (vaccination scars) when detained for convalescence."[20]

Some of these shenanigans became well known outside of the club of medical corruption, as evidenced by George Bernard Shaw's statement:

> During the last epidemic at the turn of the century, I was a member of the Health Committee of London Borough Council. I learned how the credit of vaccination is kept up statistically by diagnosing all the re-vaccinated cases (of smallpox) as pustular eczema, varioloid or what not—except smallpox.[21]

The case for the smallpox vaccine would be stronger if smallpox were the only disease that has disappeared. But history tells a different story. The bubonic plague came and went without the assistance of a vaccine. Scarlet fever was well in decline in the latter part of the 1800s before the scarlet fever toxin vaccine was introduced. Suzanne Humphries, MD, coauthor of the seminal book *Dissolving Illusions: Disease, Vaccines, and the Forgotten History*, explained that the vaccine for scarlet fever was "never widely used because it had severe consequences to many of its recipients." And yet, even without a vaccine, a "marked decline in scarlet fever death occurred long before any antibiotic was used."[22]

In 1999, Dr. Viera Scheibner addressed a letter to The Subcommittee on Criminal Justice, Drug Policy, and Human Resources. After presenting evidence that "vaccination is the single biggest cause of SIDS," Dr. Scheibner informed elected officials that ". . . the largest epidemics occurred in the most highly vaccinated populations . . ." and that "better nutrition" did away with the bubonic plague and also reduced the incidence and severity of smallpox.[23]

The citizens of Leicester knew from experience that the smallpox vaccine spread smallpox. They also knew that improved public health conditions coupled with isolating contagious people contained the disease and resulted in a stronger, naturally immune population. The modern vaccine establishment dishonors the knowledge and experience the courageous people of Leicester demonstrated as they stood against the vaccine establishment of their day. The establishment can do no different because the story of the smallpox vaccine's victory over smallpox is not a story of medical science; it's a legend born and sustained by the "financially interested."

If the smallpox vaccine were truly safe and effective, it wouldn't have scarred and killed countless vaccine recipients. Parents wouldn't have gone to jail to prevent their children from further harm from the vaccine. The vaccine wouldn't have provided the catalyst for the anti-vaccination movement, nor would it have precipitated the world's largest anti-vaccine protest. And if the traditional story of the smallpox vaccine were based on truth, vaccine storytellers would have no objection to sharing these unflattering remnants from the past.

If the traditional smallpox narrative is symbolized by a sacred cow, then the history shared in this chapter reveals that the divine bovine worshipped by vaccine believers died long ago, diseased and forgotten in an unmarked grave. And when vaccine sociopaths promulgate the myth of the smallpox vaccine, they dishonor the memory of those who were injured and killed by that vaccine.

The truth is that each vaccine has its own story, its own safety record, its own level of efficacy, its own relative necessity, but vaccine profiteers can't stomach the truth. In the paradigm they've created, there is only one story: disease is bad and vaccines are safe, effective, and necessary. Inasmuch as various diseases have relative risks and benefits and inasmuch as no vaccine is entirely safe or effective, then all vaccines are implicated in the fraudulent paradigm. The question is not if fraud is present in the commercialization of a vaccine; the question, rather, is to what degree fraud is present.

It may be true that the greatest fraud is manifest in the greatest fear campaigns, because great fear generates great profits, not just for one vaccine, but also for the entire vaccine program. If that's the case, then the greatest vaccine-related fraud might well be associated with the most frightening and most well-known of all vaccine-targeted diseases: polio.

Chapter Seven

POLIO VACCINE: MORE LORE, MORE LIES

Had my mother and father known that the poliovirus vaccines of the 1950s were heavily contaminated with more than 26 monkey viruses, including the cancer virus SV40, I can say with certainty that they would not have allowed their children and themselves to take those vaccines. Both of my parents might not have developed cancers suspected of being vaccine-related, and might even be alive today.[1]

—Dr. Howard B. Urnovitz, PhD

Few words evoke as much fear as "polio," and it's felt the most among those who experienced the deadly polio outbreaks of the 1950s. The lingering message for the survivors of that generation and for their posterity remains firmly entrenched: the polio vaccine prevented a polio apocalypse, so only a fool would question the efficacy of polio vaccinations. Get ready for the shocker: many scientists, researchers, public health officials, and doctors not only question the efficacy, they question the entire polio vaccine narrative.

The 1950s was a heady time for scientists and researchers. They had identified what they believed to be the sole cause of poliomyelitis: three separate but related polioviruses. The race was on to create a vaccine that would—safely and effectively, of course—protect against the scourge of polio.

Whose name would be identified as the eventual savior of humanity against the dreaded illness? Two emerged: Dr. Jonas Salk and Dr. Albert Sabin, both American physicians and microbiologists. As the head of the Virus Research Laboratory at the University of Pittsburgh, Salk developed the "inactivated" polio vaccine by combining the three polioviruses in cultures made from monkey kidneys. Using formaldehyde, Sabin sought to kill or inactivate the viruses so a population injected with his vaccine would develop an antibody response without causing polio.

Sabin believed a stronger vaccine was necessary to achieve the equivalent of natural herd immunity. He developed a live virus vaccine from a weakened or attenuated "rare type of polio virus" that, in theory at least, would result in a more vigorous antibody response while still not causing the disease it was meant to prevent.

What could possibly go wrong? The answer to that question is voluminous and continues to balloon some 60 years later.

The initial problem was evident shortly after Salk's inactivated polio vaccine (IPV) was rushed to market in 1954 and hundreds of people contracted polio from the vaccine, and many died. Salk released a new and improved vaccine in 1955. By 1959, nearly 100 other countries were using Salk's vaccine.[2]

Perhaps Sabin learned from Salk that testing his live virus vaccine on American children made for poor public relations. That may explain why he conducted his initial human trials in the U.S.S.R., where his team vaccinated more than 6 million people in Latvia, Estonia, and Kazakhstan between 1958 and 1959.[3]

Sabin's "sugar-cube" vaccine made its way into the hearts of vaccine regulators and the bodies of American children by 1963. Most children responded to the vaccine without incident. However, some individuals with compromised immune systems contracted polio either as recipients of the vaccine or by coming into contact with recently vaccinated children. Such occurrences were rare because severely immunocompromised individuals are also rare due to the USA's relatively advanced standard of living.

Salk's oral polio vaccine (OPV) dominated the US market until the Advisory Committee on Immunization Practices (ACIP)—a body made up of 15 individuals with close ties to the pharmaceutical industry—recommended in 1999 that the CDC "update" its polio vaccine policy for the USA by reverting back to the killed-virus shot. The CDC described the process at follows:

> On June 17, 1999, the Advisory Committee for [sic] Immunization Practices (ACIP) voted to change the recommendation for routine childhood polio vaccination beginning in 2000 to a schedule using only the inactivated poliovirus vaccine (IPV) to eliminate the occurrence of vaccine-associated paralytic poliomyelitis (VAPP) in the United States. . . . The committee voted that oral polio vaccine will be acceptable only in special circumstances.
>
> Since 1979, the only cases of polio disease in the United States have been caused by the oral polio vaccine (OPV), which had been used routinely for childhood vaccination since 1965.[4]

Naturally, when parents in other countries learned that their children were being vaccinated with a vaccine the USA had banned because it caused polio in American children, they were not pleased. Kihura Nkuba, the Ugandan founder of Greater African Radio and president of the East African World Broadcasters Association and director of the Pan-African Center for Strategic and International Studies, gained access to an oral polio vaccine package insert and described the experience in a 2002 presentation he delivered to an American audience—a presentation televised by C-SPAN:

> . . . When I looked at the contraindications it stated that inactivated polio vaccine and not oral polio vaccine should be used in situations where families had HIV—where there was a history of HIV in the family. And when I got this information I was really shocked because since 1984 Uganda has had a very difficult HIV and AIDS problem. In fact it says that if a child is inadvertently given the oral polio vaccine, that that child should be quarantined for four to seven weeks because oral polio vaccine is "live" and they keep shedding it between that period, and they could contaminate other people.[5]

Nkuba goes on to explain more precisely how difficult the problem of HIV and AIDS is in many African countries:

> . . . HIV is very big in Uganda—very big in East Africa. I was born in a family of eleven, but from 1987 up to today I have lost eight members of my family through HIV.

> So when the manufacturer says "Do not give this vaccine to families that have a history of HIV" there are no families in Uganda that have no history of HIV. Everybody knows somebody who has died or has lost an uncle or a brother's wife or his children through HIV. And it's that relationship that people were able to put together saying "Maybe really the oral polio vaccine, when given . . . to a population that has HIV, it produces that reaction."[6]

The Ugandan government did not take kindly to Nkuba or to his radio program in which he exposed the dangers of the oral polio vaccine to immunocompromised people—his people. They initially told him that he could be charged with sedition and, if found guilty, put to death. But why fuss with due process when white men in pickup trucks can accomplish the same thing by running agitators like Nkuba off the road? Nkuba "knew that they were going to make their point and they were going to make it very well," after walking away from such an accident. But he "had passed the door of no return, and . . . could not take a step backwards."

In 2001, Nkuba traveled to Washington, DC, to give a lecture to the Voice of America. While there, he telephoned the Centers for Disease Control and recorded the conversation. He told the "expert" that he was living in the USA, was planning to take his family to Uganda, and that they had not received the oral polio vaccination. The CDC representative explained that they wouldn't be able to receive oral polio vaccination in the US. Nkuba asked, "Why not?" "Well," came the response, "you can get polio from oral polio vaccination." Nkuba followed up by asking, "What if I have a history of HIV and I receive oral polio?" The expert replied, "That would be really pretty dangerous. It could be a death sentence." After returning to Uganda, Nkuba played the conversation on the radio, saying,

> This is not me now. You can't arrest me. You have to arrest the Centers for Disease Control, because, I mean, it's them doing the talking. It's not me. I have just given them space on the radio![7]

Trust in the government eroded when Ugandan parents learned that a vaccine that was too dangerous for healthy American children was required for all children in developing countries, even though many of those children are immunocompromised from birth onward due to the effects of poverty, malnutrition, overcrowding, chronic exposure to pesticides and other chemicals, unsanitary living conditions, and diseases including HIV and AIDS. Sociopathy can be the only explanation for vaccinating such children at all, let alone vaccinating them with the oral polio vaccine. As Nkuba learned in conversations with numerous people, the results were catastrophic. As he said,

> So I was told by this preacher that when the government introduced the National Immunization Days in 1997, most of the children after vaccination started dying. The preacher told me that they had so much death that his cassock, that he wears to go and conduct the burial ceremony, got old. He said, "I buried the children and my cassock got old."
>
> . . . There was one mother who had four children, and she hid one and took three other children for vaccination, and three children died and that one survived. Now when I went to do my presentation and I asked most of the people who were there—about two, three thousand people—each person had the same story.[8]

Nkuba also learned that in the United States children receive vaccinations on a schedule and vaccinations are documented in medical records. In the rural regions of Uganda, public health officials drive into villages and vaccinate all children regardless of whether they already had the disease or were previously vaccinated. And, according to Nkuba, no vaccination records are kept.

Ugandan parents are no fonder of watching their children die than are American parents, so when the vaccinators approach their villages, they send their children "into the bush." In Uganda, when pharma-backed policies fail to achieve the desired results, gunpoint sometimes succeeds.

> . . . The government was ready for them—not really the government— the minister of health, the World Health Organization and the UNICEF. They mobilized the army, and the police and moved from house to house. They had asked the local authorities to do a list of people who had children, so they moved from house to house, grabbing children at gunpoint and vaccinating them.
>
> Now those that knew—as soon as the army got into the village— the rest of the people who had children would run into the bush, and they stayed there for a week. And there is the story of this child who was met on the road, and they grabbed him and asked him whether he was immunized, and he said "Yes." He lied to them—said "Yes"—He was running away, but he said "Yes" and they said "Well, we still have to immunize you anyway." So they got the (dose). They put it in his mouth and the child spit it out—first time. They put it a second time (spit)— third (spit)—fourth (spit) and then they hit the child and then the child ran away unvaccinated.[9]

The cruelest irony in administering the oral polio vaccine to African children with HIV or AIDS is that the first cases of HIV may have crossed the species barrier from chimpanzees to humans through experimental oral polio vaccines that were manufactured and administered to over one million Africans from 1957 to 1960. These experiments were led by Dr. Hilary Koprowski, director of the Wistar Institute in Philadelphia. Koprowski viewed himself as Dr. Sabin's competitor in the race to replace the Salk vaccine. Both Sabin's and Koprowski's vaccines were grown in monkey kidney tissue. No AIDS cases emerged following Sabin's human trials in the U.S.S.R. Koprowski conducted his trials in the Belgian Congo. "Between 1956 and 1960 more then 1 million African people were 'encouraged' to receive Koprowski's vaccine called CHAT."[10]

The OPV-HIV theory is not without its detractors, but dozens of articles, including some from prominent researchers, conclude that this theory is more plausible than any other. University professor and social scientist Brian Martin catalogues many of these articles on his webpage, which is part of the University of Wollongong Australia's website. Martin writes,

> One theory of the origin of AIDS is that it developed from contaminated vaccines used in the world's first mass immunisation for polio.

There are a number of reasons why this theory is plausible enough to be worthy of further investigation.

The location coincides dramatically. The earliest known cases of AIDS occurred in central Africa, in the same regions where Koprowski's polio vaccine was given to over a million people in 1957-1960.

The timing coincides. There is no documented case of HIV infection or AIDS before 1959. Centuries of the slave trade and European exploitation of Africa exposed Africans and others to all other diseases then known; it is implausible that HIV could have been present and spreading in Africa without being recognised.

Polio vaccines are grown (cultured) on monkey kidneys which could have been contaminated by SIVs. Polio vaccines could not be screened for SIV contamination before 1985.

Another monkey virus, SV-40, is known to have been passed to humans through polio vaccines. A specific pool of Koprowski's vaccine was later shown to have been contaminated by an unknown virus.

In order for a virus to infect a different species, it is helpful to reduce the resistance of the new host's immune system. Koprowski's polio vaccine was given to many children less than one month old, before their immune systems were fully developed. Indeed, in one trial, infants were given 15 times the standard dose in order to ensure effective immunisation.[11]

More well known than the probable link between OPV and HIV is the absolute link between OPV and SV40, or simian virus 40, the virus that Martin referred to in the quote above. SV40 was the 40th simian virus that researchers discovered in the vaccines grown in monkey kidney cultures. As mentioned previously, Bernice Eddy, a government scientist with the National Institutes of Health, discovered the oncogenic virus in 1959. Her superiors rewarded her good work by barring her from publicly revealing the news, removing her from her lab, and giving her a demotion.[12]

Vaccine researcher and author Neil Miller provided a detailed account of scientists' dealings with SV40 in his article titled "The polio vaccine: a critical assessment of its arcane history, efficacy, and long-term health-related consequences." Miller wrote,

In 1960, Drs. Ben Sweet and M.R. Hilleman, pharmaceutical researchers for the Merck Institute for Therapeutic Research, were credited with discovering this infectious agent—SV-40, a monkey virus that infected nearly all rhesus monkeys, whose kidneys were used to produce polio vaccines. Hilleman and Sweet found SV-40 in all three types of Albert Sabin's live oral polio vaccine, and noted the possibility that it might cause cancer, "especially when administered to human babies. . . ." According to Sweet, "It was a frightening discovery because, back then, it was not possible to detect the virus with the testing procedures we had. . . . We had no idea of what this virus would do. . . ." Sweet elaborated: "First, we knew that SV-40 had oncogenic (cancer-causing) properties in hamsters, which was bad news. Secondly, we found out that it hybridized with certain DNA viruses . . . such that [they] would then have SV-40 genes attached [to them] . . . . When we started growing the vaccines, we just couldn't get rid of the SV-40 contaminated virus. We tried to neutralize it, but couldn't . . . . Now, with the theoretical links to HIV and cancer, it just blows my mind. . . ."[13]

SV40 was bad news for the vaccine program, but apparently not bad enough to immediately remove from the market all vaccines potentially contaminated with the carcinogenic virus. The SV40 Cancer Foundation shares the following on its website:

Upon the discovery that SV40 was an animal carcinogen that had found its way into the polio vaccines, a new federal law was passed in 1961 that required that no vaccines contain this virus. However, this law did not require that SV40 contaminated vaccines be thrown away or that the contaminated seed material (used to make all polio vaccines for the next four decades) be discarded. As a result, known SV40 contaminated vaccines were injected into children up until 1963. In addition, it has been alleged that there have been SV40-contaminated batches of oral polio vaccine administered to some children until the end of the 1990's.[14]

Money Magazine published an article in 1996 titled "The Lethal Dangers of the Billion-Dollar Vaccine Business." The author of the article, Andrea Rock, wrote of Michele Carbone, a molecular pathologist at Chicago's Loyola University Medical Center, and his research on hamsters exposed to SV-40. According to Rock:

[Dr. Carbone] discovered SV-40 genes and proteins in 60% of patients with mesothelioma, a particularly deadly form of lung cancer, and in 38% of those with bone cancer. His most recent research . . . connects SV-40 and these cancers even more clearly by describing the mechanism through which SV-40 turns a cell cancerous. Carbone's research shows that SV-40 switches off a protein that protects cells from becoming malignant. Not everyone who is infected with SV-40 gets cancer for the same reason that not every smoker gets lung cancer: A variety of assaults on the immune system usually combine to trigger malignancy. But SV-40 could be a factor that predisposes some people to develop tumors of the brain, bone, and tissue that surrounds the lung.[15]

In 1999, the journal *Anticancer Research* published similar findings in an article titled "Cancer risk associated with simian virus 40 contaminated polio vaccine." Carbone's name is listed as one of three names on the paper. The circumspect tone of the authors fails to mute the horrifying results:

Our analysis indicates increased rates of ependymomas (37%), osteogenic sarcomas (26%), other bone tumors (34%) and mesothelioma (90%) among those in the exposed as compared to the unexposed birth cohort. . . .

These data suggest that there may be an increased incidence of certain cancers among the 98 million persons exposed to contaminated polio vaccine in the US; further investigations are clearly justified.[16]

In 2002, the National Academy of Science Institute of Medicine (IOM) Immunization Safety Committee published their findings in an article titled "SV40 Contamination of Polio Vaccine and Cancer." The committee concluded

. . . that the biological evidence is strong that SV40 is a transforming [i.e., cancer-causing] virus, . . . that the biological evidence is of moderate strength that SV40 exposure could lead to cancer in humans under natural conditions, [and] that the biological evidence is of moderate strength that SV40 exposure from the polio vaccine is related to SV40 infection in humans.[17]

The CDC tells a different story about SV40, and the language it uses to tell that story is not the language of science; it's that of religious dogma. The title of the webpage supposedly dedicated to the discussion of risks associated with vaccines is "Historical Vaccine Safety Concerns." SV40 is currently present in the bodies of millions of people throughout the world, and according to numerous respected scientists, the virus plays a part in the modern cancer epidemic. That's not history; it's a current and ongoing safety concern. The introductory paragraph to the CDC's rendition of "Historical Vaccine Safety Concerns" is as follows:

There is solid medical and scientific evidence that the benefits of vaccines far outweigh the risks. Despite this, there have been concerns about the safety of vaccines for as long as they have been available in the US. This page will explain past vaccine safety concerns, how they have been resolved, and what we have learned.[18]

Summary: Benefits far outweigh risks. Safety concerns have been resolved. No worries now. Go back to sleep. The single paragraph dedicated to the discussion of SV40 contains the same elements:

Some of the polio vaccine administered from 1955 to 1963 was contaminated with a virus called simian virus 40 (SV40). The virus came from the monkey kidney cells used to produce the vaccines. Once the contamination was discovered in the Salk inactivated polio vaccine in use at that time, the US government established requirements for vaccine testing to verify that all new batches of the polio vaccine were free of SV40. Because of research done with SV40 in animal models, there was some concern that the virus could cause cancer. However, evidence suggests that SV40 has not caused cancer in humans.[19]

End of discussion. The Herd must now lie down beside the still waters and be quiet.

For those who desire more information, the CDC provides a link to a PDF document titled "Vaccine Safety and Your Child: Separating Fact from Fiction." The link is dead, but the address indicates that the article was written by Paul Offit, the man made rich from his patented rotavirus vaccine and the man who said that babies can safely receive 100,000 vaccines. Very reassuring.

Less known than SV40 is the contamination of polio vaccines by the chimpanzee coryza virus, now known as respiratory syncytial virus (RSV). The *British Medical Journal* published a paper in 2012 authored by Dr. Viera Scheibner. According to the vaccine researcher and author,

RSV has spread via contaminated polio vaccines like a wildfire all over the world and continues causing serious lower respiratory tract infections in infants. . . .

Data from ten developing countries, with intense polio vaccination, showed RSV the most frequent cause of LRT infections (70% of all cases).

Polio vaccines are not only ineffective in preventing paralysis, they carry the risk of contamination with many harmful adventitious microorganisms, of which only some monkey viruses have been researched in more detail. Many other potentially dangerous microorganisms remain unaddressed.[20]

Returning to the discussion of the oral polio vaccine and the immunocompromised, it's worth noting that OPV is not the only vaccine recommended for individuals based on their country rather than their health status. The CDC follows the recommendations of the Advisory Committee on Immunization Practices (ACIP) made specifically for residents of the USA. ACIP provides a unique set of recommendations ". . . for persons with altered immunocompetence" as follows:

In general, persons known to be HIV infected should not receive live-virus or live-bacteria vaccines. . . .

MMR vaccine should not be administered to severely immunocompromised persons. . . .

OPV should not be used to immunize immunocompromised patients, their household contacts, or nursing personnel in close contact with such patients. . . . Immunocompromised patients may be unable to limit replication of vaccine virus effectively, and administration of OPV to children with congenital immunodeficiency has resulted in severe, progressive neurologic involvement. . . . If OPV is inadvertently administered to a household or intimate contact (regardless of prior immunization status) of an immunocompromised patient, close contact between the patient and the recipient of OPV should be avoided for approximately 1 month after vaccination, the period of maximum excretion of vaccine virus. Because of the possibility of immunodeficiency in other children born to a family in which there has been one such case, OPV should not be administered to a member of a household in which there is a history of inherited immunodeficiency until the immune status of the recipient and other children in the family is documented.[21]

The ACIP's recommendation also reads, "The degree to which an individual patient is immunocompromised should be determined by a physician."[22] It is unlikely that Ugandan doctors stand between vaccinators and gun-toting soldiers to prevent sick and malnourished children from receiving their latest round of undocumented live-virus vaccinations.

According to the World Health Organization, 158 member nations continue to receive the oral polio vaccine. Largely absent from the list are nations inhabited by "white" people. Numerous countries would be ranked among the poorest in the world, which means, of course, that their citizens are also living in a chronically immunocompromised state.[23]

Russell Blaylock, MD, comments on the bizarre policy of vaccinating sick children in developing countries with vaccines that are now banned in the USA:

> It . . . needs to be appreciated that children in developing countries are at a much greater risk of complications from vaccinations and from mercury toxicity than children in developed countries. This is because of poor nutrition, concomitant parasitic and bacterial infections and a high incidence of low birth weight in these children. We are now witnessing a disaster in African countries caused by the use of older live virus polio vaccines that has now produced an epidemic of vaccine related polio, that is, polio caused by the vaccine itself. In, fact, in some African countries, polio was not seen until the vaccine was introduced.
>
> The WHO and the "vaccinologist experts" from this country now justify a continued polio vaccination program with this dangerous vaccine on the basis that now that they have created the epidemic of polio, they cannot stop the program. In a recent article it was pointed out that this is the most deranged reasoning, since more vaccines will mean more vaccine-related cases of polio.[24]

India provides another example of the "deranged reasoning" that the WHO and other global vaccine architects use to justify the ongoing injuring and killing of millions of people already suffering from the effects of poverty. A 2010 Oxford analysis "concluded that there were more poor in India than in sub-Saharan Africa. Its 2014 analysis said the largest number of people classified as 'destitute' among developing countries was in India."[25]

The *Hindustan Times* reported in 2015 that more than 1,000 Indian children die every day from diarrhea, most caused by poor sanitation and hygiene and unsafe water. The article does not credit vaccines with childhood deaths, but endemic sickness, disease, and dying and dead children are proof that millions are living in a chronically immunocompromised state.[26]

In 2012, the *Indian Journal of Medical Ethics* published an article that documents the horrific consequences of India's ongoing use of the oral polio vaccine. The authors, Neetu Vashisht and Jacob Puliyel of the Department of Pediatrics at St Stephens Hospital, wrote,

> . . . While India has been polio-free for a year, there has been a huge increase in non-polio acute flaccid paralysis (NPAFP). In 2011, there were an extra 47,500 new cases of NPAFP. Clinically indistinguishable

from polio paralysis but twice as deadly, the incidence of NPAFP was directly proportional to doses of oral polio received. Though this data was collected within the polio surveillance system, it was not investigated. The principle of primum-non-nocere [first do no harm] was violated.[27]

To put this into historical context, the CDC reports, "Polio reached a peak in the United States in 1952, with more than 21,000 paralytic cases."[28]

Jagannath Chatterjee suffered an adverse reaction to vaccination in 1979, which may have sparked his interest in vaccine research and activism. In 2014, the Indian researcher published an article on his website titled "India's Polio-Free Status a Cruel Joke." Part of that joke was demonstrated in the response of health officials to the problem of viral shedding from recently vaccinated individuals and subsequent paralysis and disease outbreaks. Chatterjee commented,

> Because those vaccinated tend to shed the virus in their stool, it can mutate into a virulent form, causing paralytic polio in others, even leading to polio epidemics. When this phenomenon was noticed and reported by Indian doctors they were asked to increase the number of doses given to children![29]

The statistics Chatterjee cites below should be cause for great concern:

> The National Polio Surveillance Project data show that the polio eradication programme has increased paralysis among children—from 1,005 cases yearly in 1996 to 60,992 cases in 2012, most now being classified as NPAFP [Non-polio Acute Flaccid Paralysis] instead of polio. The government does not reveal how many of these cases are due to the vaccine. It was observed in 2005 that, against 66 cases of polio caused by the wild polio virus that year, 1,645 were caused by the vaccine. As the number of polio doses given to every child has increased exponentially over the years, the number of children affected by the vaccine has climbed new heights. Data reveals that those vaccinated are 6.26 times more likely to be paralysed. Doctors investigating the affected children have expressed anguish over how these children have been ignored by the government of India and have been left to fend for themselves. Deaths from the vaccine have also been reported.[30]

Merck's blockbuster drug Vioxx killed 60,000 people in the USA before the government pulled it from the market. Yet 60,000 Indian children contract a paralytic disease every year, and the leading cause of that disease not only remains on the market, it's given to every child again and again year after year regardless of individual health status. And India is only one country!

In 2015, the American Academy of Pediatrics published Vashisht, Puliyel, and Vishnubhatla Sreenivas's research documenting the "highly significant" correlation between the number of OPV doses with the rate of Non-polio Acute Flaccid Paralysis. They found no other positive correlation in their research.[31]

In 1988, the World Health Assembly—the governing body of the World Health Organization—declared a crusade to eradicate polio, presumably for humanitarian purposes. Sabin's oral polio vaccine was designated as the single weapon millions of vaccinators would use to achieve this goal.[32]

Modern scientists know full well that there are a host of potential negative consequences associated with the quixotic attempt to bring viruses to extinction. In the case of polio, one such consequence is paralyzing hundreds of thousands with the vaccine meant to prevent paralysis. But that's just the beginning. Like all living creatures, viruses evolve over time. Tinkering with viruses in laboratories results in novel life forms that have never existed in nature. So even if the global polio eradication initiative succeeds in eliminating the three viruses identified in the 1950s as the cause of polio, it will also result in novel viruses that may eclipse the pathogenicity of the original polioviruses.

According to Debabar Bannerjee, professor emeritus at Centre of Social Health and Medicine at Jawaharlal Nehru University, and other eminent doctors, "vaccine viruses had mutated into virulent strains and were circulating" in India since at least 2004, rendering polio eradication impossible.[33]

Chatterjee notes that the 1950s notion that polio is solely caused by three enteroviruses is false. Researchers in the USA have already documented more virulent strains that have the potential to replace the three viruses targeted by both the IPV and the OPV: "This phenomenon may soon become global as viruses change roles in response to misguided efforts that seek to eliminate them."[34]

In addition, scientists have mapped the genetic sequence of the polioviruses. The eradication of wild polio coupled with the existence of synthetic polio is the stuff of bioterrorists' dreams and the world's nightmare: polio in a non-immunized human population. Vashisht and Puliyel state, "The synthesis of polio virus in 2002, made eradication impossible. It is argued that getting poor countries to expend their scarce resources on an impossible dream over the last 10 years was unethical." They are not alone in their critique against the polio eradication plan. Critics include Richard Horton, editor of *The Lancet*, and Arthur L. Caplan, director of the University of Pennsylvania's bioethics center.[35]

According to Professor William Muraskin, author of *Polio Eradication and Its Discontents: A Historian's Journey Through an International Public Health (Un) Civil War*, the global polio eradication initiative has a political element to it that taints its supposed humanitarian purpose:

The literature on polio eradication is written by, and for, public health people, and it is massive. Unfortunately, much of that literature has been generated by the global polio eradication campaign itself. Even when it is being self-critical (which is not uncommon), it assumes the "natural-ness" and "inevitability" of polio eradication as a world goal, with the aim of supporting, justifying, and making the campaign more effective. In other words, it takes for granted the question that needs answering: Why polio eradication? In addition, many of the key articles dealing with polio policy questions show signs of being significantly affected by "political" considerations in the conclusions that they reach. . . . [T]he public health literature on polio eradication is less a "scientific" litera-ture than one would like or expect it to be. Especially disturbing is the discovery that conclusions of articles often do not follow the logic of the evidence presented in the heart of the text. When it comes to policy questions, the published literature is too often more a "hostile witness" than the objective resource it purports to be.[36]

Muraskin also noted in his book that from the first meetings in which the eradication of polio was discussed, scientists doubted the viability of such a plan.[37]

Meanwhile, decades later, the CDC is already referring to the "lasting legacy" of the eradication of polio as the only possible outcome:

When the spread of wild polio virus (WPV) is stopped, the interna-tional partners expect to plan and carry out a series of activities in vari-ous stages to certify the eradication of polio and minimize the possibility that the disease will return. . . .

The expansion of the national delivery systems that brought polio vac-cine to remote and medically underserved populations, paving the way for other preventive health services, will be a lasting legacy of the GPEI.[38]

According to a 1999 article published by the CDC, the failure to eradicate polio is not a public relations option: "A failure, especially in achieving polio-myelitis eradication, could as certainly call into question the credibility of the public health profession as did the collapse of the disastrous malaria eradication effort."[39]

This may well explain why the polio eradication initiative continues in spite of the fact that administering OPV to chronically immunocompromised children results in far more disability and death than it prevents. The initiative also continues in spite of the evidence that failure will be the real legacy and that success may be even worse than failure. Make no mistake: Sabin's oral polio vaccine is failing. If that were not the case, why would vaccinators subject Indian children to "30 to 50 doses of the vaccine" including children "who should be medically exempt" from the paralyzing vaccines?[40]

Vashisht and Puliyel conclude their article with a scathing rebuke:

> The polio eradication programme epitomises nearly everything that is wrong with donor funded 'disease specific' vertical projects, at the cost of investments in community-oriented primary health care (horizontal programmes). . . .

> With polio eradication there was a huge increase in non-polio AFP, in direct proportion to the number of doses of the vaccine used. Though all the data was collected within an excellent surveillance system, the increase was not investigated openly. Another question ethicists will ask, is why champions of the programme continued to exhort poor countries to spend scarce resources on a programme they should have known, in 2002, was never going to succeed.[41]

Chatterjee takes the rebuke up a level by calling for the legal prosecution against the perpetrators of India's modern epidemic of "non-polio" polio outbreaks:

> It is very important to find out exactly who have benefitted from the programme and take heed of calls by ethical doctors like Phadke that those guilty must be identified and punished. He says, "It is necessary that all these children who have lost their limbs be fully rehabilitated, and their parents adequately compensated. Criminal liability should be ascertained for those officials who have suppressed this information of breakup of follow-up of AFP cases, and those officials and policymakers who are responsible for continuing this policy of Polio Eradication Initiative."[42]

Those "who have benefitted from the programme" likely include members of the World Health Organization. Several doctors including Dr. Debabar Bannerjee, quoted previously, wrote a letter to WHO officials, charging them with inflating cases of wild polio "to justify the programme" and also repeatedly redefining polio "since the programme was launched, thus automatically leading to a drastic fall in the number of cases."[43]

As discussed earlier, the WHO is no stranger to redefining words to advance its purposes, having done so in 1998 with the H1N1 "pandemic," which resulted in billions of dollars of profits to the pharmaceutical industry—the same industry that influences and profits from WHO policy. And as also discussed, the WHO changed the classification scheme for recording child deaths from vaccines, which resulted in fewer deaths meeting the criteria for "Adverse event following immunization (AEFI) possibly due to vaccine" and more deaths declared "Not an AEFI."[44]

Redefining statistics to promote the safety and efficacy of vaccines that are neither safe nor effective is yet another legacy of the vaccine story.

Whether by accident or by design, the CDC mastered the art of redefinition from the onset of the polio vaccine program. When the vaccines first hit the market, virtually all cases of infantile paralysis were attributed to polio. By 1958, the polio pie had been divided into at least ten different conditions including: coxsackie or ECHO enteroviruses, congenital syphilis, arsenic and DDT toxicity, transverse myelitis, Guillain-Barré syndrome, hand, foot, and mouth disease, lead poisoning, and provocation of limb paralysis by intramuscular injections of many types, including a variety of vaccines.[45]

In the previous chapter, a portion of Dr. Viera Scheibner's letter to The Subcommittee on Criminal Justice, Drug Policy, and Human Resources was quoted, demonstrating the false narrative surrounding the smallpox vaccine. Following is the portion of her letter addressing polio:

> Polio has not been eradicated by vaccination, it is lurking behind a redefinition and new diagnostic names like viral or aseptic meningitis. When the first, injectable, polio vaccine was tested on some 1.8 million children in the United States in 1954, within 9 days there was huge epidemic of paralytic polio in the vaccinated and some of their parents and other contacts. The US Surgeon General discontinued the trial for 2 weeks. The vaccinators then put their heads together and came back with a new definition of poliomyelitis. The old, classical, definition: a disease with residual paralysis which resolves within 60 days has been changed to a disease with residual paralysis which persists for more than 60 days. Knowing the reality of polio disease, this nifty but dishonest administrative move excluded more than 90% of polio cases from the definition of polio. Ever since then, when a polio-vaccinated person gets polio, it will not be diagnosed as polio, it will be diagnosed as viral or aseptic meningitis. According to one of the 1997 issues of the MMWR [Morbidity and Mortality Weekly Report], there are some 30,000 to 50,000 cases of viral meningitis per year in the United States alone. That's where all those 30,000 - 50,000 cases of polio disappeared after the introduction of mass vaccination. One must also be aware that polio is a man-made disease since those well-publicized outbreaks are misrepresented that those huge outbreaks were causally linked to intensified diphtheria and other vaccinations at the relevant time. They even have a name for it: provocation poliomyelitis.[46]

It's interesting to note that India's problem with polio and "non-polio" polio may have more to do with its ongoing use of DDT and other toxic chemicals that are sprayed during summer months than with the polio virus. American doctors Morton S. Biskind and Irving Bierber were aware of that connection as early as 1949 when they published "DDT Poisoning—A New Symptom With Neuropsychiatric Manifestations" in the *American Journal of Psychotherapy*.[47] Biskind provided a statement to the Select Committee to Investigate the Use of Chemicals in Food Products, United States House of Representatives, where

> [h]e quoted another doctor that "wherever DDT had been used intensively against polio, not only was there an epidemic of the syndrome I have described but the incidence of polio continued to rise and in fact appeared where it had not been before.
>
> "This is not surprising since it is known that not only can DDT poisoning produce a condition that may easily be mistaken for polio in an epidemic but also being a nerve poison itself, may damage cells in the spinal cord and thus increase the susceptibility to the virus."
>
> "Facts are stubborn," Biskind concluded, "and refusal to accept them does not avoid their inexorable effects—the tragic consequences are now upon us."[48]

How might the state of public health be different today if it had modeled public health policy based on the disease-reducing policy instituted by the British town of Leicester's anti-vaccinators of the 1800s? How would the world be different if public health officials emphasized wholesome organic foods over toxic pharmaceutical formulations found in vaccines and other drugs? How might the world be different if public health officials studied to learn why 99% of the population experience polio much as they might experience a common cold? What do the 99% possess that protects them from experiencing the paralyzing effects of polio? What do the remaining 1% lack that makes them vulnerable to paralysis? What can be done to increase natural protective factors in immunocompromised individuals? How can the human race work with nature rather than fight against nature to increase mutual health and well-being? If public health had done more to promote healthy immune systems and done less to manipulate immune systems with vaccines, would the world be burdened with the ongoing cancer epidemic? Would the world know AIDS? Would the children in the USA and much of the rest of the world be suffering from a host of other chronic health problems and disabilities?

Well-meaning people in Western countries assume that vaccine recipients in developing countries are literally and figuratively dying for vaccines financed by the likes of Bill and Melinda Gates. It's long past time for a deeper look at the issues. Problems with a profit-based, one-sized-fits-all vaccination schedule in one country are multiplied when that profit-based schedule is exported around the world. Vaccinations with apparently good safety profiles in developed countries are death sentences in developing nations where immunocompromised individuals are the norm rather than the exception. People in developing countries are not dying from vaccine deficiencies, they are dying from their susceptibility to infectious diseases caused by chronic malnutrition, poor sanitation, dirty water, chronic exposure to pesticides, and yes, they are dying from their inability to deal with repeated vaccination assaults.

Dan Olmsted and Mark Blaxill, coauthors of the *The Age of Autism: Mercury, Medicine, and a Man-made Epidemic*, have researched and written about the numerous issues associated with the establishment's response to polio. The concluding paragraph of their 2014 series on the issue reads:

> The suffering of polio's victims is honored by learning all of its lessons, including the danger of environmental toxins and the perils of ignoring their role in modern disease; the risk of focusing all of our energy on vaccinations as magic bullets, and the fundamental ethical obligation to search for the truth without fear or favor. Only then can we work out the real nature of illnesses that confront us here and now, ranging from autism to Parkinson's to the persistence of poliomyelitis itself. Only then can we begin to prevent such disasters as The Age of Polio.[49]

Inasmuch as Africans may have suffered more harm from the devastating consequences of vaccinations than any other people, it is appropriate to conclude this chapter with a quote from Kihura Nkuba, who provides a poignant African perspective and asks a question that international public health officials should be required to answer:

> In Africa polio does not kill anybody and they say it's very rare to catch. It's really very rare to get paralytic polio. . . . So what is it that is killing people in Africa? Malaria. Every five seconds a child is dying of malaria in Africa. Now to get the dose of life-saving anti-malaria is about $5 but there is no government to give anti-malaria. When somebody gets malaria, if they have no money they even die.

So the question I was asking and many people were asking was "If you really want to help children, why begin with a disease that they don't have?"[50]

Well-meaning or not, people who support global vaccination initiatives are in fact party to policies that perpetrate ill-gotten pharmaceutical profits as well as institutional racism, classism, and genocide—policies that will certainly return home with ill will, hatred, and violence and may also return home in the form of plagues far greater than the diseases they hope to contain or eradicate.

Chapter Eight

VACCINE SAFETY: YESTERDAY AND TODAY

My own personal view is that vaccines are unsafe and worthless.
I will not allow myself to be vaccinated again.[1]
—Vernon Coleman, MD

The safety and efficacy of the smallpox and polio vaccines are illusions created and nurtured to strengthen the public's faith in all vaccines. Without faith the rational mind soon discovers the truth beyond the illusions: that each vaccine that the profiteers add to the schedule includes its own shady inception, development, and commercialization. It would be impossible for this book or any other single volume to explore all of the issues surrounding all vaccines; however, those discussed in the remainder of this book further illustrate the depths of industry corruption.

A quick review of vaccine history beyond smallpox and polio will shine more light on the dogmatic belief of vaccine safety, efficacy, and necessity—a belief that clouds the minds of millions of willing vaccinees.

Dr. Archie Kalokerinos was a vaccine believer when he first worked as a medical doctor among Australia's aboriginal people in the 1950s. Soon he noticed that the children he and others vaccinated did not respond as expected. In 1974, he described his moment of enlightenment as enthralling, beautiful, and horrifying in his provocative book *Every Second Child*:

> Then suddenly it clicked. "We have stepped up the immunisation campaigns," Ralph had said. My God! I had known for years that they could be dangerous, but had I underestimated this? Of course I had. There was no need to go to Alice Springs. I knew. A health team would sweep into an area, line up all the Aboriginal babies and infants and immunise them. There would be no examination, no taking of case histories, no checking on dietary deficiencies. Most infants would have colds. No wonder they died. Some would die within hours from acute vitamin C deficiency

precipitated by the immunisation. Others would suffer immunological insults and die later from "pneumonia", "gastroenteritis" or "malnutrition". If some babies and infants survived, they would be lined up again within a month for another immunisation. If some managed to survive even this, they would be lined up again. Then there would be booster shots, shots for measles, polio and even T.B. Little wonder they died. The wonder is that any survived. The excitement of this realisation is difficult to describe. On one hand, I was enthralled by the simplicity of it all, the "beautiful" way by which the pattern fitted everything I had been doing. On the other hand, I almost shook in horror at the thought of what had been, and still was going on. We were actually killing infants through lack of understanding.[2]

Every Second Child was so named because up to half of the vaccinated Aboriginal infants died following vaccination, which Kalokerinos attributed to an acute vitamin C deficiency. Kalokerinos learned independently what professionals had come to learn in Africa and India and what vaccine manufacturers had known all along: vaccines injure and sometimes kill immunocompromised children.

As is always the case when a priest apostatizes from the Vaccine Church, the medical establishment did not take kindly to the doctor's disclosures. The general bias white professionals of the era held against the dark-skinned Aborigines also played a part in the enmity Kalokerinos experienced. Professional bias against Aboriginal children is evident in the following passage:

> . . . I found that [the medical teams] were visiting the reservations, the outlying camps of Aborigines in the desert, and if for some reason a mother didn't want her child to be vaccinated they would simply grab the child and forcibly vaccinate it. I saw them chasing them on foot, and chasing them in Landrovers and grabbing the kids and vaccinating them. Now, a lot of these kids were terribly sick. They were malnourished and everything else. And if they survived the first vaccine, in a few weeks they would come back with booster shots. And then with more and more, and then they would come around with polio shots and so forth. . . .
>
> You cannot immunise sick children, malnourished children, and expect to get away with it. You'll kill far more children than would have died from the natural infection.[3]

In 1995, Dr. Kalokerinos granted an interview with the *International Vaccine Newsletter*. Speaking of the "extreme hostility" of his contemporaries, he said,

This forced me to look into the question of vaccination further, and the further I looked into it the more shocked I became. I found that the whole vaccine business was indeed a gigantic hoax. Most doctors are convinced that they are useful, but if you look at the proper statistics and study the instance of these diseases you will realise that this is not so.[4]

Numerous other doctors and scientists have come to the same conclusion. Emeritus professor of public health at the University of Glasgow, Gordon T. Stewart, MD, stated,

> There was a continuous decline [in disease] . . . from 1937 onward. [Whooping cough/pertussis] vaccination, beginning on a small scale in some places around 1948 and on a national scale in 1957, did not affect the rate of decline if it be assumed that one attack usually confers immunity, as in most major communicable diseases of childhood. . . . With this pattern well-established before 1957, there is no evidence that vaccination played a major role in the decline in incidence and mortality in the trend of events.[5]

Suzanne Humphries, MD, coauthor of the book *Dissolving Illusions*, wrote,

> All of the epidemics for which drug companies created vaccines were well into their decline or gone before the vaccine was introduced on a mass scale. The real reasons for the decline of the epidemics of smallpox, measles, polio, etc. were improvements in hygiene, sanitation, nutrition, working conditions and clean water delivery. The vaccines came in well after the fact. Then the vaccine makers/conventional medicine wrongly took credit for it.[6]

Robert S. Mendelsohn, MD, author of *How to Raise a Healthy Child in Spite of Your Doctor* and *Confessions of a Medical Heretic,* was an outspoken vaccine critic. Among other things, this "heretic" wrote,

> *There is no convincing scientific evidence that mass inoculations can be credited with eliminating any childhood disease.* While it is true that some once common childhood diseases have diminished or disappeared since inoculations were introduced, no one really knows why, although improved living conditions may be the reason. If immunizations were responsible for the disappearance of the these diseases in the United States, one must ask why they disappeared simultaneously in Europe, where mass immunizations did not take place [emphasis in original].[7]

E. Richard Brown wrote the following in his 1979 book, *Rockefeller Medicine Men: Medicine and Capitalism in America*:

In the great majority of cases the toll of the major killing diseases of the nineteenth century declined dramatically before the discovery of medical cures and even immunization. Tuberculosis, the Great White Plague, was one of the dread diseases of the nineteenth century, killing 500 people per 100,000 population at midcentury and 200 people per 100,000 in 1900. By 1967 the US rate had dropped to three deaths per 100,000. This tremendous decline was only slightly affected by the introduction of collapse therapy in the 1930s and chemotherapy in the 1950s. Similarly, for England and Wales John Powles shows that overall mortality declined over the last hundred years well in advance of specific immunizations and therapics.

Rene Dubos, the microbiologist formerly with the Rockefeller Institute, succinctly summed up the historical record. "The tide of infectious and nutritional diseases was rapidly receding when the laboratory scientist moved into action at the end of the past century," Dubos wrote in *Mirage of Health*. "In reality," he observed, "the monstrous specter of infection had become but an enfeebled shadow of its former self by the time serums, vaccines, and drugs became available to combat microbes." Improvements in general living and working conditions as well as sanitation, all brought about by labor struggles and social reform movements, are most responsible for improved health status. Improved housing, working conditions, and nutrition not medical science—reduced TB's fearsome death toll.[8]

Dr. Sherri Tenpenny, DO, has invested some 20,000 hours in vaccine research. Her position is clear:

It continually breaks my heart that people have to personally experience a severe vaccine injury—or observe a serious reaction in someone they love—before they wake up to the absolute truth: vaccines can and do cause harm. They have heard the arguments and the stories from others. They ignored the pleas about risks and poo-pooed the concerns about vaccine reactions put forth by concerned friends. Instead, they trusted their uninformed pediatrician or caved under the pressure of their badgering RN mother-in-law.

And now, they are left holding the bag, so to speak: a terrible tragedy and a lifetime of medical care and medical bills, as they watch their loved one's health deteriorate before their helpless, regretful, angry eyes. . . . The true cost of vaccination is more than the cost of buying and administering vaccines. The untold tens of millions spent on injuries are not included in the calculations.[9]

Dr. J. Anthony Morris, former Chief Vaccine Control Officer and Research Virologist at the FDA, testified before the Senate Committee on Ways and Means in 1987, saying, "There is a great deal of evidence to prove that immunization of children does more harm than good."[10]

James Howenstine, MD, wrote in his 2002 book, *A Physicians Guide to Natural Health Products*,

The use of multiple vaccines, which prevents natural immunity, promotes the development of allergies and asthma. *A New Zealand study disclosed that 23% of vaccinated children develop asthma compared to zero in unvaccinated children* [emphasis in original].[11]

The animal rights organization, In Defense of Animals, includes the following on its website:

Researchers from Harvard and Boston Universities concluded that medical measures (drugs and vaccines) accounted for between 1 and 3.5% of the total decline in mortality rates since 1900. Scores of animals were killed in the quest to find cures for tuberculosis, scarlet fever, smallpox and diphtheria, among others, but was their unwilling contribution important to the decline of these diseases? Dr. Edward Kass of Harvard Medical School, asserts that the "primary credit for the virtual eradication of these diseases must go to improvements in public health, sanitation and the general improvement in the standard of living."[12]

Vernon Coleman, MD, is one of Britain's most prolific authors. His titles include *The Medicine Men, Paper Doctors, The Good Medicine Guide, How to Stop Your Doctor Killing You, Health Secrets Doctors Share With Their Families*, and in 2011 *Anyone Who Tells You Vaccines Are Safe And Effective Is Lying. Here's The Proof*. Among other things, Coleman describes vaccines as "worthless":

Vaccination is widely respected by doctors and others in the health care industry because of the assumption that it is through vaccination that many of the world's most lethal infectious diseases have been eradicated.

But this simply isn't true. As I have shown in many of my books infectious diseases were conquered by the provision of cleaner drinking water and better sewage facilities. The introduction of vaccination programmes came along either just at the same time or later when the death rates from the major infectious diseases had already fallen. There really isn't any evidence to show that vaccination programmes have ever been of any real value—either to individuals or to communities.[13]

The preceding statements are but a small sample of statements made by vaccine-informed people. Speaking of small samples, the current vaccine schedule—as large as it is—represents only a small sample of vaccines ever brought to market. Many other vaccines were once in use but were withdrawn due to safety and efficacy concerns.

In 1972, US senators discussed these 32 "worthless vaccines" that were licensed and on the US market:

- Bacterial vaccine mixed respiratory
- Respiratory UBA
- Staphylococcus-streptococcus UBA
- Combined vaccine No. 4 with catarrhhalis
- Mixed vaccine No. 4 with H. Influenzae
- Staphylococcus vaccine
- Entoral
- Typhoid H antigen
- Vacagen tablets
- Brucellin antigen
- Staphylo-strepto serobacterin vaccine
- Catarrhalis serobacterin vaccine mixed
- Sensitized bacterial vaccine H. influenza
- Staphage lysate type I
- Staphage lysate type III
- Staphage lysate types I and III
- Catarrhalis combined vaccine
- Strepto-staphylo vatox
- Staphylococcus toxoid-vaccine vatox
- Respiratory vatox
- Respiratory B.A.C.
- Gram-negative B.A.C.
- Pooled stock B.A.C. No 1
- Pooled stock B.A.C. No 2
- Staphylococcal B.A.C.

- Pooled skin B.A.C.
- Mixed infection phylacogen
- Immunovac oral vaccine
- Immunovac respiratory vaccine (parenteral)
- Streptococcus immunogen arthritis
- N. catarrhalis vaccine (combined)
- No catarrhalis vaccine immunogen[14]

In a Senate Subcommittee meeting, Senator Charles Percy questioned Dr. Isacson, the Division of Biologics Standards (DBS) director, about the costs of the 32 "vaccines referred to as ineffective by the DBS director and their manufacturers":

> Doctor, right at the outset of your testimony, you make reference to the General Accounting Office report, that 32 vaccines of no known value, and some possible harm, have continued to be licensed. . . . I have never seen a figure as to what the total dollar value of those vaccines would be. What was the cost of the vaccines, which were either of little value or perhaps even harmful, and which were administered to people who felt they were being protected?[15]

Dr. Isacson replied, "Well, I think it must be astronomical. I do not think I could give you an actual figure. Since some of these appear from the investigation to have been on the market for 20 years, certainly it must add up."

Senator Abraham Ribicoff made these fiery comments on the senate floor:

> There are at least 32 vaccines currently on the market that are "generally regarded as ineffective by the medical profession," according to the DBS Director. I am releasing a list of these ineffective products. All of these drugs have been on the market for more than ten years, some of them for decades. Some [of] them can cause serious side effects. For example, one such drug, licensed in 1956 for the treatment of "upper respiratory infections, bronchitis, infectious asthma, sinusitis, and throat infections," contains six ineffective organisms. According to the circular on the package, there have been, associated with the use of the drug, "reports of children getting systemic reactions: fever, rash, abdominal cramps, and diarrhea four to eight hours after injection." All this from an ineffective drug.

> Or consider the possible side effects noted on a package circular for another ineffective vaccine used for treatment of infections and inflammations of the eye: "febrile reactions, preceded by chill, temperature

of 101-104. Fever subsides in a few hours and the patient may be left with muscular pains; chilly sensations and malaise may be expected. The patient should be kept under close observation through the period of increased temperature, and if excessive fever occurs, it should be combatted vigorously." There are many other examples.

And yet, in all these years, DBS never moved to take a single one of those ineffective drugs off the market, or even to inform the public or the medical profession of their ineffectiveness. In light of this kind of adverse reaction data, it is incredible that DBS could license such biologics as "safe." Since the agency believed that there was no corresponding benefit from the harm suffered by patients, it could have moved to take these drugs off the market under its undoubted authority and responsibility to withhold licenses for drugs which are unsafe. Instead, the DBS maintained that it had no authority to regulate biologics for effectiveness and simply washed its hands of the problem. . . .

For ten years, beginning in 1962, while memos were quietly exchanged within the bureaucracy, nothing was done to protect the public against drugs that were ineffective. The drugs stayed on the market; people continued to get adverse reactions from them. Those drugs are on the market today, ten years after HEW was given authority to do something about them.[16]

A mere four years after Senator Percy claimed to have closed the barn door on worthless vaccines, the American public fell victim to CDC shenanigans in the form of the Swine Flu vaccine—a vaccine that proved far more dangerous than the disease it was meant to protect against. The only pandemic experienced in the winter of 1976–77 was one of lies from top government sources beginning with US President Gerald Ford, when he announced on television: "This virus was the cause of a pandemic in 1918 and 1919 that resulted in over half a million deaths in the United States as well as twenty million deaths around the world." FDA scientist J. Anthony Morris had analyzed the virus and found that it was not the same as the 1918 virus, neither was it of particular importance. He felt the public had a right to know the truth. The FDA felt differently and made the point by firing Morris for insubordination. Authors Hilary and Peter Butler wrote of the unfolding fiasco in their book *Just a Little Prick*:

By October 1976, 33 people had died after receiving the Swine Flu vaccine, and by mid-December there were about 500 cases of Guillain-Barre. But even up to December all authorities were publicly stating that there was no relationship between any of the deaths or side-effects and the vaccine. In December of that year, at an urgent meeting, Dr Langmuir, one of the chief immunologists at the CDC said, "We cannot look at these data and not conclude that it was this influenza virus vaccine that precipitated Guillain-Barre in those who developed it, so we must consider stopping the programme." The round-the-table vote was 13 to 1 to stop the programme.

On 16 December 1976 after 46 million shots had been administered, three vaccine-associated deaths were officially admitted to, and the programme was stopped. But the main message continued to be denial, and more denial.[17]

Dr. David Sencer, the head of the CDC, protested the suspension of the program. According the *Washington Post*, "Dr. Sencer maintained there was no link between the vaccine and the deaths. . . ."[18] The unrepentant Dr. Morris told the *Washington Post*,

It's a medical rip-off . . . We should recognize that we don't know enough about the dangers associated with flu vaccine. I believe the public should have truthful information on the basis of which they can determine whether or not to take the vaccine.[19]

Then he added, "I believe that, given full information, they won't take the vaccine."[20]

Mike Wallace with the television news program "60 Minutes" interviewed CDC scientist Dr. Michael Hattwick, the man who "directed the surveillance team for the swine flu program at the CDC. His job was to find out what possible complications could arise from taking the shot and to report his findings to those in charge."[21] Hattwick told Wallace that he knew ahead of time and he had informed his superiors "that there had been case reports of neurological disorders, neurological illness, apparently associated with the injection of influenza vaccine."

Wallace asked, "What would you say if I told you that your superiors say that you never told them about the possibility of neurological complications?" Hattwick responded, "That's nonsense. I can't believe that they would say that they did not know that there were neurological illnesses associated with influenza vaccination. That simply is not true. We did know that."

Wallace also pointed out the CDC's claim that "important persons" such as President Ford, Henry Kissinger, Elton John, Muhammad [Ali], Mary Tyler Moore, Rudolf Nureyev, Walter Cronkite, Ralph Nader, and Edward Kennedy had taken the shot. Moore told Wallace on camera that she had refused the shot and that her doctor was "delighted" that she had done so.[22]

The *Washington Post* reported, "In the end, more than 40 million people had been inoculated against an epidemic that never occurred."[23]

Big debacles require big scapegoats. Joseph A. Califano, secretary of the then-Department of Health, Education and Welfare, asked for Dr. Sencer's resignation in February 1977.[24]

On a related note, Dr. Archie Kalokerinos stated in a 1995 interview that President Ford's publicized receipt of the Swine Flu vaccine was staged. "Now there is no doubt he did not have swine flu vaccine. They would not have given it to him, no way!"[25] Thomas Stone, MD, seconded the opinion of Kalokerinos, suggesting that President Ford's flu vaccine was nothing more than saline.[26]

The doctors' claim is not, as of yet, verified, but it makes sense. Killing a sitting president with a flu vaccine would destroy a multibillion-dollar industry. Not a risk the industry would be willing to take. Injuring and killing American citizens, however, that's just the cost of doing business.

Twenty years later, the FDA let other nations do the killing when it did not approve the Urabe strain of the mumps vaccine. Dr. Andrew Wakefield detailed the disaster in a 2015 presentation:

> [Urabe AM9] came from Japan and it caused meningitis. Interestingly, when used alone as the single monovalent mumps vaccine, it didn't cause injuries. When it was put in MMR it caused meningitis at a rate of more than 1 in 2000. This is a fascinating observation right off the bat. 1 and 1 and 1 doesn't equal 3. It's something very different. And this meningitis from the mumps vaccine was recognized in Ontario where they introduced it and they withdrew it rapidly. But the British government wanted that vaccine used in the UK because it was made by the home team, GlaxoSmithKline. [A Canadian whistleblower warned:] "Don't touch it. It's causing meningitis at an unacceptable rate." They ignored him completely; the only thing that changed was the name. It was called TriVirix in Canada and they changed the name to Pluserix in the UK. And they introduced it. GlaxoSmithKline—SmithKline Beechem at the time—got 85% of the market. Four years later, after meningitis had occurred in exactly the same way, it had to be rapidly withdrawn. . . . At that point, the vaccine should have been destroyed. . . . Was it? No. It was shipped to developing countries like Brazil, where it was used in a mass vaccination campaign. And not surprisingly, there was an epidemic of meningitis.[27]

Wakefield has a personal interest in the Urabe-containing jab because

> [s]ome of the 12 children whose medical history featured in the controversial 1998 Lancet paper, drawn up by Dr. Wakefield and his colleagues

and which suggested a possible link between the jab and bowel disease and regressive autism, had received the Urabe-strain vaccine. . . .[28]

In addition, Professor Denis McDevitt, the man who chaired the General Medical Council's disciplinary panel,

> . . . once sat on the government advisory committee that looked at adverse reactions to vaccinations and immunisations and considered issues of MMR safety. He attended meetings that discussed warnings from other countries about an early form of the triple jab, using the Urabe strain of mumps virus, which caused encephalitis and meningitis.[29]

The British website Child Health Safety stated that as of 2009, ". . . organisations like UNICEF continue supplying urabe strain containing MMR vaccine to the more adverse reaction vulnerable and less well nourished third world children . . . because it is cheaper than safer alternatives . . ."[30]

In 2003, Congressman Dan Burton submitted a 30,000-word congressional record titled Mercury in Medicine Report, the result of a three-year investigation initiated by the Committee on Government Reform. The primary focus of the report was the known risks associated with mercury in vaccines. The report briefly mentioned recent changes in the vaccine policy to illustrate the fact that vaccines are not nearly as safe or effective as industry and government claim:

> On three occasions in the last 15 years, changes have been made to vaccine policies to reduce the risk of serious adverse effects. First, a transition from oral polio vaccine to injected polio was accomplished in the United States to reduce the transmission of vaccine-induced polio. Second, an acellular pertussis vaccine was developed and a transition from DTP to DTaP was accomplished to reduce the risk of pertussis-induced seizures in children. And third, when the Rotashield vaccine for rotavirus was linked to a serious bowel condition (intersucception), it was removed from the US market.[31]

Vaccine manufacturers and government officials are well aware that there is no such thing as an entirely safe vaccine. The 1986 National Childhood Vaccine Injury Act was enacted because vaccine injury or death may be "unavoidable even though the vaccine was properly prepared and accompanied by proper directions and warnings."[32]

In 2000, the Institute of Medicine (IOM) signed a CDC contract to study some of the numerous health conditions that scientists had suggested were linked to vaccines, including: arthritis, asthma, chronic allergy conditions, cancer, chronic fatigue syndrome, inflammatory bowel disease, multiple sclerosis, diabetes, influenza, autism, attention deficit disorder and other learning disorders, encephalitis, seizure disorder, generalized muscle weakness and fatigue, SIDS, and "unexplained death."

The contract also included potential study of the following mechanisms, components, tissues, and contaminants:

Hypothesized Mechanisms

1. Autoimmune overload hypothesized in persons who receive multiple vaccines (e.g., infant and military vaccine schedule).
2. Genetic susceptibility hypothesized as reason why some people get chronic effects.
3. Children's immune system immature and not as well understood compared to adults and so childhood immunization recommendations are hypothesized to be unsafe.

Vaccine Additives/components

1. Chemical additives are not natural and are hypothesized to be unsafe.
   a. Any chemical additive is potentially unsafe—all vaccines.
   b. Thimerosal—all vaccines with thimerosal (e.g., hep B) hypothesized that cumulative levels of mercury found in vaccines can cause brain damage and mental retardation.
   c. Alum—all vaccines with Alum adjuvant, theorized that it can cause Macrophagic Myofascitis [sic] (MMF), a potential syndrome with weakness, myalgia, and arthralgia.
2. Tissue
   a. Animal tissues used in vaccine preparation hypothesized that they may cause chronic effects (e.g., reverse transcriptase in chick cells for MMR and influenza vaccine; SV40 in monkey kidney cells in OPV).
   b. Gelatin—may be bovine-derived and therefore hypothesized vaccine risk for transmitting new variant Creutzfeldt Jakob Disease/Bovine Spongiform Encephalitis (mad cow disease).

Vaccine Contaminants

1. SV40 and polio vaccine were known to be present in early stocks of IPV in the late 1950s early 1960s; some theorize that it may be the cause of rare malignancy's [sic] in persons that received IPV during this time.
2. HIV early OPV trials in Africa hypothesized to have been prepared with African Green Monkey kidney cells contaminated with SIV causing the spread of HIV in Africa.

3. Reverse Transcriptase—concern that it may be present in some vaccines and some imply that it could change DNA structure.[33]

The FDA website informs the public that

The first review by [IOM Immunization Safety Review Committee] focused on a potential link between autism and the combined mumps, measles, and rubella vaccine. The second review focused on a potential relationship between thimerosal use in vaccines and neurodevelopmental disorders (IOM 2001).[34]

The FDA fails to inform the public that the committee disbanded in 2004 after it issued its eighth and final report in which it reversed its previous position by claiming there was no association between vaccines and autism. Only later did the public learn that the IOM's report was directed by CDC mandate, not science (more in later chapters).

In 2010, Karen Midthun, MD, director of the FDA's Center for Biologics Evaluation and Research, addressed the International Conference of Drug Regulatory Authorities (ICDRA). Her presentation documented several of the problems the CDC referred to as "hypothetical" in its contract with the IOM in 2000.[35] Louise Kuo Habakus posted a 2016 article on the *Fearless Parent* website titled "Do Vaccines Cause Cancer?" in which she summarized the text from several slides Dr. Midthun used in her presentation:

Stringent regulatory requirements in place to ensure, **to the extent possible**, that products are **"free"** of adventitious agents. (slide #4)

New technologies have the potential to detect adventitious agents **not previously known or detected** . . . (slide #10)

Formalin inactivation did not completely inactivate SV40 (slide #11)

More sensitive PCR assay showed that **previously undetectable** quantities of reverse transcriptase [from endogenous avian retrovirus] **were present in some vaccines** (e.g., measles) produced in avian cells. (slide #11)

[B]enefits of vaccination **far outweigh any remote risk** of vCJD [human form of mad cow disease; emphasis added by Habakus].[36] (slide #13)

Habakus asks readers to note the

repeated use of quotations around "free" of adventitious agents . . . their admission that they missed adventitious agents in the past and that new agents are being discovered . . . and the risk/reward tradeoff they're making for us.[37]

Perhaps Midthun would do well to inform her FDA colleague, Dr. Norman Baylor, that his presentation to parents on vaccine safety, as discussed in Chapter 5, falls short on facts and long on fantasy—fantasy that medical professionals like Dr. Kalokerinos believed early in their careers. Such belief is hard to maintain while watching up to half of vaccinated children fall ill and die. Late in his life, Kalokerinos summarized his experience:

> My final conclusion after forty years or more in this business is that the unofficial policy of the World Health Organisation and the unofficial policy of Save the Children's Fund and almost all those organisations is one of murder and genocide. They want to make it appear as if they are saving these kids, but in actual fact they don't. I am talking of those at the very top. Beneath that level is another level of doctors and health workers, like myself, who don't really understand what they are doing. But I cannot see any other possible explanation: It is murder and it is genocide. And I tell you what: when the black races really wake up to what we have done to them they are not going to thank us very much.[38]

Kalokerinos charges top public health officials with premeditated murder and genocide, a charge that many if not most people will find laughable. But the parents of countless vaccine-injured or killed children in developed countries aren't laughing. And while the number of vaccine-injured or killed children in developed countries is disturbing, it is but a small fraction of the injured or killed in developing countries where the effects of poverty result in children living in a chronically immunocompromised state. Whether those injuries or deaths are due to noble or nefarious intentions is a question of utmost importance, but in the end, the injured were injured and the dead are dead.

Chapter Nine

HERD IMMUNITY: ARTIFACT, CONTRIVANCE, AND CONTROL

"The tendency of a mass vaccination program is to herd people. People are not cattle or sheep. They should not be herded. A mass vaccination program carries a built-in temptation to oversimplify the problem; . . . to discourage or silence scholarly, thoughtful and cautious opposition; . . . to whip up an enthusiasm among citizens that can carry with it the seeds of impatience, if not intolerance; to extend the concept of the police power of the state in quarantine far beyond its proper limitation . . . .[1]
—Suzanne Humphries, MD

Prepare to enter yet again the inner sanctum of The Church of Vaccinology. Prepare for another sip from the Holy Grail. Prepare to worship yet another golden calf—a golden calf responsible for filling the church's coffers with billions of dollars in profits, a golden calf that combines unique human beings with unique genetics, medical conditions, and minds and then transforms each and every soul into an eight-billion-member herd.

Church administrators have branded the name of the calf deeply within the minds of virtually every member of The Herd. Let us praise the holy name of the golden calf: Herd Immunity. The doctrine of herd immunity is both a relic from a scientifically primitive time as well as a talisman held up for veneration and worship in the modern era—an era that one day will also be viewed as primitive.

The Church of Vaccinology was founded in a former era—an era that had barely grasped the concept of germs. It was observed that humans and animals gained a state of immunity following disease outbreaks. The great thinkers of the era surmised that if one germ is responsible for one disease, then one pharmaceutical compound could protect one person from that disease. From that line of simplistic thinking, it was not a huge leap to conclude that one vaccine administered to all people may artificially replicate immunity conferred by natural means. Such was the state of the science during the smallpox epidemics of the 1800s.

In 1923, scientists from the University of Manchester studied "The Problem of Herd-Immunity" in their immunization research on mice. They referred to "recent reports on experimental epidemiology from the Rockefeller Institute," which led them "to believe that the question of immunity as an attribute of a herd should be studied as a separate problem, closely related to, but in many ways distinct from, the problem of the immunity of an individual host."[2]

In 2011, Paul Fine, Ken Eames, and David L. Heyman, scientists from the London School of Hygiene and Tropical Medicine, published an article in the Oxford journal *Clinical Infectious Diseases* in which they provided "a rough guide" of the history and concept of herd immunity. Though coined almost a century ago, the term *herd immunity* "was not widely used until recent decades, its use stimulated by the increasing use of vaccines, discussions of disease eradication, and analyses of the costs and benefits of vaccination programs."[3] The theory of vaccine-induced herd immunity gained traction in the 1970s, when scientists calculated and diagrammed decreased disease incidence based on increased vaccination rates.[4, 5]

Whereas the vaccines-are-safe-and-effective dogma assures parents and patients that vaccines safely prevent disease, the doctrine of herd immunity persuades parents and patients that they have a social obligation to vaccinate, that those who fail to vaccinate are "freeloaders"—people who freely reap the benefits of vaccines while failing to assume their share of vaccine risks. The two doctrines have now combined in an irrational yet powerful third doctrine: vaccines protect vaccine recipients but only if everyone else vaccinates. Thus, the unvaccinated have morphed from freeloaders into diseased and filthy child abusers, child killers, and murderers. It is this third doctrine that vaccine believers and sociopaths wield to justify discrimination, mandatory vaccination, and just plain nasty behavior.

By comparison, ancient believers once threatened to kill nonbelievers to help them see the value of converting to the religion of their more righteous oppressors. Modern vaccine believers believe their salvation lies in the conversion and baptism by vaccination of all of humanity. Thus, believers view the unvaccinated not only as vectors of disease but also as the indispensible key to their own salvation from the ever-threatening hell of infectious disease.

In truth, the third doctrine is a blatant disavowal of the doctrine of vaccine safety and efficacy, but vaccine sociopaths have long since banished Truth from fellowship in The Church of Vaccinology.

Paul Fine and his fellow British scientists documented several recent disease outbreaks, not due to "freeloaders," but due to the failure of vaccines to achieve herd immunity. Of these failures, the researchers concluded:

> . . . there is a need for immunization programs to maintain high vaccine coverage, together with surveillance and outbreak response capabilities, as

numbers of susceptible individuals accumulate in older age groups. Herd immunity implies a lasting programmatic responsibility to the public.[6]

Their conclusion is one of believers still locked in a vaccine paradigm conceived and commercialized in the 1800s. The only possible solution such individuals can see to the problem of vaccine failure is the injection of more vaccines.

The problem of the failure of vaccines to measure up to the reality of natural herd immunity is only one of many problems associated with the practice of contrived herd immunity. An equal if not greater problem lies in the armies of pharma-funded scientists who are unable to even consider that the practice of vaccination often results in more harm than good. Such a concept blasphemes yet another sacred cow of the vaccine paradigm: the sacrificial offering of untold numbers of vaccine damaged or dead in the service of "the greater good."

Many laboratory scientists and practicing medical professionals have concluded that the greater good doctrine is a smokescreen for what Eric Gladen, the producer of the documentary film *Trace Amounts*, refers to as "the greater greed." Members of the American Association of Physicians and Surgeons are included in this group. Executive Director Jane Orient, MD, argues against the greater good dogma in a 1999 letter to Congress:

> Measles, mumps, rubella, hepatitis B, and the whole panoply of childhood diseases are a far less serious threat than having a large fraction (say 10%) of a generation afflicted with learning disability and/or uncontrollable aggressive behavior because of an impassioned crusade for universal vaccination.[7]

More recently, Physicians for Informed Consent (PIC) issued a press release in which the organization highlighted "the greater greed" ethos as perpetrated upon the American public with the MMR vaccine, stating:

> There is a five-fold higher risk of seizures from the MMR vaccine than seizures from measles, and a significant portion of MMR-vaccine seizures cause permanent harm. For example, 5% of febrile seizures result in epilepsy, a chronic brain disorder that leads to recurring seizures. Annually, about 300 MMR-vaccine seizures (5% of 5,700) will lead to epilepsy.

Dr. Shira Miller, PIC president and founder, concluded:

> In the United States, measles is generally a benign, short-term viral infection; 99.99% of measles cases fully recover. As it has not been proven

that the MMR vaccine is safer than measles, there is insufficient evidence to demonstrate that mandatory measles mass vaccination results in a net public health benefit in the United States.[8]

In spite of facts such as these, few vaccine-informed medical professionals are willing to risk the sanctions meted out to those who expose the vaccine paradigm for what it is: a fraud and an illusion. Yet, their numbers are increasing and their message shines ever more light on the darkness of the paradigm. Former believers are stepping forth and speaking their truth.

Kelly Brogan, MD, was once a believer in pharmaceutical-based medicine. Her research and her clinical practice as a psychiatrist led her to the realization that chemicals in vaccines and other drugs are often brought to market by fraud and corruption and often do more harm than good. She, like many others, realized that human cells, tissues, and systems function by means of complex webs of interrelationships. Yes, injecting antigens and accompanying toxicants directly into an infant's body may increase serum antibody levels, but doing so also results in a cascade of cellular and systemic reactions with immediate and lifelong consequences. Brogan wrote in her best-selling 2016 book, *A Mind of Your Own*,

> Is it possible that vaccinology has applied a reductionist—one disease, one drug/vaccine—model to an evolutionarily adapted system with built-in complexities we have barely begun to appreciate? Is it possible that we have misunderstood immunity, or are still fundamentally learning about its most basic principles? If we are to accept that billions of years have gone into priming our physiology for interface with microbes, then we must acknowledge that there is more to immunity than simply jacking up antibody levels.[9]

Brogan further explained:

> Vaccines were designed before we knew about DNA, viruses that contaminate cells used to produce them (SV40, retroviruses), the microbiome, or how toxic one chemical can be to one person while leaving another unscathed. One-size-fits-all medicine is no longer appropriate, and we just don't know how to determine who might be at risk for adverse effects ranging from psychiatric conditions to death.[10]

Suzanne Humphries, MD, was once enjoying her career as a nephrologist when she objected to the routine vaccination of her patients who were suffering from severe kidney disease. From that experience, she launched into extensive research that led to discover that as much as scientists know about human functioning, they still have much to learn. In 2015, Humphries coauthored the book *Dissolving Illusions*, in which she wrote,

> Nobody—not even the most educated immunologists—understands or can describe the complete cascade of events that occurs after injecting a vaccine. If physicians realized how little is known today about the immune system and vaccines, they would be duty bound to tell patients that there are no accurate scientific answers.[11]

Christopher J. Gill, MD, Boston University associate professor of global health, confirmed Humphries's statement when he admitted that vaccine scientists don't know what they are doing. Addressing the "startling global resurgence of pertussis, or whooping cough, in recent years . . .," Gill said:

> This disease is back because we didn't really understand how our immune defenses against whooping cough worked, and did not understand how the vaccines needed to work to prevent it. Instead we layered assumptions upon assumptions, and now find ourselves in the uncomfortable position of admitting that we may [have] made some crucial errors. This is definitely not where we thought we'd be in 2017.[12]

Yes, human understanding of complex biological processes is yet in its infancy, and it's nothing but hubris that allows scientists to ignorantly think that they can imitate natural immunity by injecting scores of foreign substances into human beings to raise targeted antibody levels without disrupting or destroying cells, tissues, systems, and processes. Immunologist and author Tetyana Obukhanych states as much in a 2012 interview:

> We would expect that vaccinated individuals would not be involved (or very minimally involved) in any outbreak of an infectious disease for which they have been vaccinated. Yet, when outbreaks are analyzed, it becomes apparent that most often this is not the case. Vaccinated individuals are indeed very frequently involved and constitute a high proportion of disease cases.
>
> I think this is happening because vaccination does not engage the genuine mechanism of immunity. Vaccination typically engages the immune response—that is, everything that immunologists would theoretically "want" to see being engaged in the immune system. But apparently this is not enough to confer robust protection that matches natural immunity. Our knowledge of the immune system is far from being complete.[13]

Like biological systems and processes, the doctrines of herd immunity, safety, efficacy, and the greater good are also interrelated. A problem in one is a problem in all. Following is what is certainly a partial list of the multiple problems that many modern vaccine enthusiasts ignore at their peril as well as the peril of their families and the human race:

1. Vaccination is not the same as immunization, and vaccine-induced immunity is not the same as natural immunity. Natural immunity results in lifelong immunity to a disease. Vaccine-induced immunity results in an elevated serum antibody level, which at best provides an incomplete and temporary form of immunity.

2. Vaccines are the same, while people are different. Treating all people as if they were the same, regardless of genetic vulnerabilities, past vaccine reactions, or a host of other factors is morally and scientifically indefensible.

3. Subsets of the population are "nonresponders" or "poor responders," which means vaccine-induced herd immunity is unachievable.

4. Artificially induced elevated antibody levels are just that: artificial. The human organism works to return antibody titers to their natural levels, which means that whatever immunity was achieved with the elevated antibodies is lost with the body's return to a natural state. This means that the majority of The Herd may well be fully vaccinated, but only a fraction is immunized in any given moment. Hence the need for multiple "boosters." The industry is well aware of this fact and is working in collaboration with the US government to implement a profit-driven womb-to-tomb vaccination program (more in Chapter 24).

5. The efficacy of vaccines is known to decrease with every booster, while the risk of harm increases with every booster.

6. Natural immunity exposes a person to the risk of disease once in a lifetime. Temporary vaccine-induced immunity exposes a person to the risk of disease every time the pathogen is reintroduced into the body and every time the antibody titers return to their natural levels. Thus, over a lifetime, vaccinated individuals pose a much greater risk to herd immunity than do individuals who possess natural herd immunity.

7. Immunologists tend to view disease outbreaks in vaccinated individuals as the only negative measure of vaccine efficacy. But when measured holistically, efficacious vaccines may be more harmful than vaccine failures due to the fact that vaccination-induced reduction in disease outbreaks often results in increased rates of related and apparently unrelated diseases. One of many examples is found in the relationship between the chickenpox vaccine and shingles. The increased incidence of shingles is directly related to the "success" of

the chickenpox vaccine and was, in fact, predicted prior to the vaccine's commercialization.[14]

8. Natural immunity not only confers up to lifelong immunity against disease, it also confers numerous additional health benefits, including a more robust immune system and increased protection against cancer, heart disease, etc. This means that vaccination increases one's risk of contracting several serious and life-threatening diseases.

9. Temporary vaccine-induced immunity has the potential to turn relatively harmless childhood diseases into more dangerous diseases when contracted by adolescents or adults. This is true for mumps, measles, and chickenpox.

10. A percentage of vaccinees contract the disease the vaccines are meant to protect against, and some contract more serious forms of the disease because they were vaccinated.

11. Breast milk is Mother Nature's natural form of immunization. Breast milk provides natural immunity to a baby by working in concert with the infant's natural anti-inflammatory state. Aluminum, toxic to both brain and kidneys, is added to vaccines to create an unnatural and unhealthy inflammatory state to increase antibody titers.[15]

    The natural immunity of pregnant and breast-feeding mothers protects unborn and breast-feeding children. Vaccine-induced immunity in mothers provides no such protection to their babies through their breast milk. This means that vaccination increases the risk of illness or death to children of vaccinated mothers. Suzanne Humphries, MD, explains this point in further detail in her article titled "Herd Immunity: Flawed Science and Mass Vaccination Failures":

    > Since most vaccines are delivered by injection, the mucous membranes are bypassed and thus blood antibodies are produced but not mucosal antibodies. Mucosal exposure is what contributes to the production of antibodies in the mammary gland. A child's exposure to the virus while being breastfed by a naturally immune mother would lead to an asymptomatic infection that results in long-term immunity to that virus. Vaccinated mothers have lower levels of virus-specific antibodies in the serum and milk compared to naturally immune mothers and thus their infants are unprotected.[16]

12. Countless mothers have helplessly watched their babies lose the ability to breast-feed following infant vaccinations, resulting in reduced breast milk intake and increased formula intake. Breast milk contributes to

natural immunity. Formula contributes to sickness and death (more in Chapter 10).

13. Live virus vaccines shed, which means that recently vaccinated individuals are disease vectors. Live virus vaccines include influenza, measles, rubella, rotavirus, chickenpox, and the polioviruses in the oral polio vaccine. Individuals who contract these diseases by natural means are also disease vectors exactly one time in their lives. Vaccinated individuals are disease vectors every time they are revaccinated. In 2014, the National Vaccine Information Center treated the subject of "Vaccine Strain Virus Infection, Shedding & Transmission" in a 42-page referenced report titled "The Emerging Risks of Live Virus & Virus Vectored Vaccines."[17]

    Inasmuch as "[t]here is no active surveillance and testing for evidence of vaccine strain live virus shedding, transmission and infection among populations routinely being given multiple doses of live virus vaccines, including measles vaccine,"[18] public health officials have no idea whether disease outbreaks originate with vaccinated or vaccine-free individuals. And inasmuch as vaccinated individuals are exposed to live viruses every time they are revaccinated, they are a much more likely source of disease outbreaks than are unvaccinated individuals. Hospital policy supports this statement by prohibiting recently vaccinated individuals from visiting immunocompromised patients.

14. Just as the introduction of GMOs into the environment and the food supply includes countless known and unknown risks, the introduction of GMO-containing vaccines also includes countless known and unknown risks.

15. Vaccine strains of live viruses are laboratory-created novel life forms. Introducing vaccine strains directly into the bodies of vaccine recipients and indirectly through viral shedding spreads novel diseases, which presents myriad potential consequences.

16. Attenuated live virus vaccines have regained virulence, resulting in disease outbreaks.

17. Just as bacteria evolve and develop resistance to the pressure placed upon them by antibiotics, germs targeted by vaccines evolve, shift, and develop resistance to vaccines as well as resistance to antibiotics, potentially resulting in diseases of greater pathogenicity or lethality—diseases that never would have come into existence without the pressure placed upon them by vaccines. Jacob M. Puliyel, MD, head of pediatrics at St. Stephen's Hospital in Delhi, India, addressed strain shift and antibiotic resistance in a rebuttal to an article published in *The Guardian* in 2010. "The pneumococcus strains prevalent in India are nearly all sensitive to inexpensive antibiotics like penicillin," wrote the pediatrician.He added:

In the US which has been using the pneumococcal vaccine for some years now, there has been a strain shift—strains covered in the vaccine are being replaced by other strains. Ominously the new strains are more antibiotic resistant. . . . Vaccine has simply made the problem of pneumococcal disease worse.[19]

18. Irrespective of vaccine-induced immunity or efficacy, all vaccines result in various levels of vaccine injury. The question is not if vaccines injure recipients; the question is to what degree vaccines injure recipients. To believe otherwise is magical thinking.

19. The greater the number of vaccines administered, the greater the injury to vaccine recipients. To believe otherwise is more mystical thinking.

20. Long-term disease prevention or eradication results in population-wide loss of immunity, placing The Herd at risk of accidental or intentional reintroduction of pathogens. In other words, eradication destroys natural herd immunity. The only solution in such a scenario is to continue vaccinating everyone against such diseases or participate in an endless cycle of stockpiling, trashing, and stockpiling vaccines (more in Chapter 24).

21. Many vaccines simply don't do what the public has been taught they do—they don't protect against the spread of disease. On occasion, even the CDC and the American Academy of Pediatrics acknowledge this fact, as they did in June 2016, when they advised pediatricians to stop using the worthless ". . . live attenuated influenza vaccine (LAIV). . . ."[20]

22. Vaccine-based disease prevention blinds humanity to the powerful role that hygiene, sanitation, nutrition, and healthy lifestyles play in disease prevention. It also blinds public health officials to the fact that people who are suffering and dying from poor nutrition, etc., are by definition immunocompromised, and such people are far more likely to sustain vaccine injuries or death than are healthy individuals.

23. Vaccine-based disease prevention misappropriates billions of dollars in research funding and public health policy—money that would be more wisely spent on an increased understanding of the role of natural protective factors. An example of this is found in the development of the meningococcal vaccine to prevent meningitis. According to the CDC's *Pink Book*, the incidence of this disease in the USA is less than 1 in 300,000 people, while it is epidemic in sub-Saharan Africa.[21]

Obviously, vaccinating to prevent this disease in the USA is insanity. Wouldn't it make more sense to export what is already working in the USA: good hygiene, nutrition, and sanitation practices to disease ridden areas—factors that reduce the incidence of virtually all diseases—rather than export yet another problem-laden vaccine?

24. Vaccine-based disease prevention also casts aside effective and inexpensive treatments in favor of dangerous and expensive vaccines. Quoting again the Indian pediatrician Dr. Puliyel:

> An analysis in the *Lancet* showed how the Pneumococcal vaccine reduces only 4 cases of pneumonia per 1000 children. . . . The cost for vaccinating 1000 children comes to $12,750. . . . Treating the 4 cases of pneumonia in India using WHO protocol, would cost $1. . . .[22]

25. The doctrines of herd immunity and vaccine safety and efficacy prevent the CDC and others from conducting much-needed research into vaccine safety. Those doctrines led to the IOM's 2004 statement to stop conducting research into the relationship vaccines share with autism and several other disorders. Those doctrines disseminate from the government to medical education, medical journals, and into the minds of practitioners leaving them unable to provide informed consent, unable to exercise sound clinical judgment before vaccinating their patients largely blind to the reality of vaccine injury, and also unable to provide effective treatment for those who suffer vaccine injury at their hands.

26. Vaccine-based disease prevention places the health and welfare of every human being including fetuses, newborns, women of reproductive age, and the elderly in the hands of criminally run, profit-driven corporations and their counterparts in government regulatory agencies.

Few people in history have more experience related to vaccines and corruption in government than the recently deceased Dr. Shiv Chopra, whose résumé includes: Microbiologist, Vaccination Researcher & Specialist, Former Senior Scientific Advisor on Vaccinations for Health Canada, and author of *Corrupt to the Core: Memoirs of a Health Canada Whistleblower*. Orthopedic surgeon Dave Janda, MD, interviewed Chopra in July 2016 starting with what might be the granddaddy of all vaccine questions: "Are there any vaccine programs that have been beneficial to society?" Chopra responded, "None."[23]

Russell Blaylock, MD, an outspoken critic of concrete-thinking vaccinologists, states, "Herd immunity is mostly a myth and applies only to natural immunity—that is, contracting the infection itself." The neurosurgeon holds a dim view of vaccine architects who believe that common people are too dim-witted to understand the miracle and the necessity of vaccines:

> A growing number are made of those with a collectivist worldview and see themselves as a core of elite wise men and women who should tell the rest of us what we should do in all aspects of our lives. They see us as ignorant

cattle, who are unable to understand the virtues of their plan for America and the World. Like children, we must be made to take our medicine— since, in their view, we have no concept of the true benefit of the bad-tasting medicine we are to be fed.[24]

Michael Gaeta, a doctor of acupuncture, has facilitated hundreds of presentations on what he calls the "vaccine scam." He asks the question, "Is it truly so that vaccinating protects others, and that failing to vaccinate endangers others?" to which he responds:

For the precious few with the courage to question the forced vaccination propaganda, and accept the truth, based on credible, non-CDC science, [the answer] is no, or, more accurately, absolutely not.

Vaccine-induced herd or community immunity is scientifically impossible. It is a brilliant piece of marketing, using guilt to coerce behavior and drive drug sales. It is twisted genius in action, making intelligent, independent-thinking people ignore their honest, well-founded vaccine skepticism, and causing the rest to accept unlimited vaccinations without question.[25]

Marcella Piper-Terry is a vaccine researcher, founder of VaxTruth.org, and mother of a daughter who recovered from autism with biomedical treatments. According to Piper-Terry,

There is no such thing as vaccine-induced herd immunity. It doesn't exist. It never has. The vast majority of adults have ZERO immunity from vaccines and we have not been having huge outbreaks of disease. Let's please just stop talking about how we're going to lose herd immunity if we stop vaccinating. We can't lose what we've never had.[26]

Janet Levatin, MD, Board Certified Pediatrician and Clinical Instructor in Pediatrics at Harvard Medical School, assumes a more moderate position than Chopra, Blaylock, Gaeta, and Piper-Terry, but even she has come to the conclusion that the modern vaccine schedule has jabbed the beloved doctrine of the greater good beyond "the crossover point":

We have arrived at—indeed we have passed—the crossover point, that point at which we realize that the preventive measures we were prescribed cause more damage than the problems they were intended to prevent. When we realize we have crossed that point, it is time for us to inform ourselves as fully as possible and assume responsibility for our own healthcare and the healthcare of our children.[27]

It's long past time for scientists to move beyond the reductionist science of the 1800s and their religious faith in the doctrines of herd immunity, the greater good, and vaccine safety and efficacy to justify the scientifically insupportable vaccine epidemic in the 21st century.

Previous chapters provided an introduction into the role the medical establishment plays in the government-pharma industrial complex. The following chapter takes a closer look at some of the numerous business relationships industry shares with an organization that claims to be "Dedicated to the health of all children."

Chapter Ten

AMERICAN ACADEMY OF PEDIATRICS: PARENTAL DISCRETION ADVISED

Now we have a generation of pediatricians, who face perhaps the greatest iatrogenic accident in the history of pediatrics, who actually need to be deprogrammed to understand what the true nature of all neuro-behavioral problems are that they confront without any understanding of etiology or potential interventions.[1]
—Ken Stoller, MD

The American Academy of Pediatrics portrays itself as a medical trade organization dedicated to providing the highest standards of childhood medical care. Its mission statement reads: "The mission of the American Academy of Pediatrics (AAP) is to attain optimal physical, mental, and social health and well being for all infants, children, adolescents, and young adults."[2]

This noble statement would be difficult to realize under the best of circumstances, but considering the fact that AAP members share a business relationship with numerous corporations that market unhealthy and dangerous products, its mission crosses the line into fantasy. The boundaries between the medical establishment—of which the AAP is part—and the industry targeting America's youngest citizens are permeable with members, money, and influence flowing freely between them.

The AAP's primary conflicts of interest lie with vaccine manufacturers. But the 64,000-member guild also profits from its enmeshed relationship with other industries as evidenced in a bizarre 2016 article published in the AAP's journal *Pediatrics* in which Jessica Martucci and Anne Barnhill warn pediatricians of the "Unintended Consequences of Invoking the 'Natural' in Breastfeeding Promotion." The authors wrote,

We are concerned about breastfeeding promotion that praises breastfeeding as the "natural" way to feed infants. This messaging plays into a powerful perspective that "natural" approaches to health are better, a view examined in a recent report by the Nuffield Council on Bioethics. Promoting breastfeeding as "natural" may be ethically problematic, and, even more troublingly, it may bolster this belief that "natural" approaches are presumptively healthier. This may ultimately challenge public health's aims in other contexts, particularly childhood vaccination.[3]

If the AAP is "concerned about breastfeeding promotion that praises breastfeeding as the 'natural' way to feed infants," then it's high time for parents and patients to be concerned about the AAP. And when the AAP uses quotation marks around the word natural—as if to suggest that breast-feeding isn't natural—then it's time for parents to mistrust the AAP. And when the promotion of breast-feeding is seen as "ethically problematic," then it's time for the public to be outraged at the AAP. And finally when the AAP connects this ridiculous message with the fear of parents who "challenge public health's aims in other contexts, particularly childhood vaccination," then it's time for pediatricians, parents, and the general public to wake up to the realization that the AAP has sold out to Big Pharma and Big Business in a big way.

Publishing such an outrageous article may feel like betrayal to those who associate the name American Academy of Pediatrics with the health and well-being of infants and toddlers. But the betrayal didn't start in 2016. The AAP has been sucking up to companies that manufacture infant formula and numerous other products for quite some time; so long in fact, it probably feels "natural" to those sucking on the corporate teat.

In 1995, Naomi Baumslag, MD, MPH, and Dia Michels published a book titled *Milk, Money, and Madness: The Culture and Politics of Breastfeeding*. They authors stated that formula manufacturers

> . . . donate $1 million annually to the American Academy of Pediatrics in the form of a renewable grant that has already netted the AAP $8 million. The formula industry also contributed at least $3 million toward the building costs of the AAP headquarters.[4]

In 2001, three formula manufacturers—Ross, McNeil, and Johnson & Johnson— ". . . were the top three corporate supporters of the academy's $65 million operating budget, . . . each giving $500,000 or more."[5]

In 2002, the AAP released a book written by some of its members. The *New Mother's Guide to Breastfeeding* briefly mentioned infant formula, but the numerous benefits of breast-feeding was the primary message. Soon after, AAP management sold 300,000 special edition copies of the book to the Ross Products unit of Abbott Laboratories, the makers of Similac. The book cover included both the Similac name and the Similac teddy bear logo. According to the *New York Times*, the authors of the book "were stunned" and expressed "outrage" to learn that AAP had slapped a formula maker's name and logo on their book:

> "For those of us who wrote the book, this is thievery," said Dr. Lawrence M. Gartner, the former chairman of the University of Chicago's pediatrics department and chairman of the academy's executive committee on breast-feeding. "The impression that people have when they see the book is that Ross is a supporter. This corrupts efforts to promote breast-feeding."[6]

Dr. Joe M. Sanders, the academy's executive director, agreed with Gartner's assessment, sort of, that is. "Ten years ago, this probably would not have been acceptable, but things change," said Sanders.[7]

Apparently, the things Sanders was referring to are morals and ethics, and apparently Gartner and his colleagues had missed the memo, and apparently Sanders had missed the 1981 memo from the World Health Organization when it "adopted a code banning formula advertising and free distribution by doctors and in hospitals."[8]

Why would the WHO ban a practice that's still going on in many American hospitals more than 30 years later? Because in many developing countries, breast-feeding is far more than a mother's choice; it is literally a matter of life and death. The British nonprofit organization Save the Children crunched the numbers, and they are nothing less than astonishing. Their research ". . . estimates that 830,000 newborn deaths could be prevented every year if all infants were given breast milk in the first hour of life." And babies who are fed breast milk exclusively ". . . for the first six months . . . are protected against major childhood diseases." By contrast, "[a] child who is not breastfed is 15 times more likely to die from pneumonia and 11 times more likely to die from diarrhoea." The organization states that breast-feeding is "the most effective of all ways to prevent the diseases and malnutrition that can cause child deaths."[9] The frightening but unstated implication of the Save the Children report is that baby formula kills babies.

In the same year the report was published—2013—the American Academy of Pediatrics entered into a business relationship with Mead Johnson, the maker of Enfamil. Since then, thousands of American mothers of newborns leave the hospital with their babies in one arm and gift bags of formula stamped with both Enfamil's and AAP's names and logos in the other. The *New York Times* writer Kimberly Seals Allers is not impressed with the arrangement. "By placing its logo on tags attached to Enfamil's hospital discharge bags," Allers wrote, the A.A.P. is effectively endorsing both the formula those bags contain and the decision to distribute them (as direct-to-consumer a marketing strategy as it is possible to get). It is a decision that is inconsistent with its own policies, and with its stated "dedication to the health of all children."[10]

The AAP is not particular when it comes to sucking on synthetic breasts. Again from the same *New York Times* article:

The A.A.P. has a financial relationship with several companies that manufacture formula (among other products). Enfamil's maker, Mead Johnson, currently supports a grant for the academy's educational perinatal pediatrics conferences, conducted for training physicians specializing in newborn care. Mead Johnson also supports the organization's annual Neonatal Education Awards. Abbott Nutrition, the maker of Similac, is another big supporter of the A.A.P., donating toward the academy's journal, *Pediatrics in Review*, through an educational grant. The Nestlé Nutrition Institute, the parent company of the infant formula maker Gerber, funds the American Academy of Pediatrics' Healthy Active Living for Families program.[11]

On a side note, the AAP is not the only medical trade organization that profits from selling its logo and reputation to industry. According to Sheldon Rampton and John Stauber, authors of *Trust Us We're Experts: How Industry Manipulates Science and Gambles with Your Future,*

Bristol-Myers Squibb paid $600,000 to the American Heart Association for the right to display AHA's name and logo in ads for its cholesterol-lowering drug Pravachol. Smith Kline Beecham paid the American Cancer Society $1 million for the right to use its logo in ads for Beecham's Nicoderm CQ and Nicorette anti-smoking ads.[12]

To be fair, the AAP is not alone in its proficiency at giving breast-feeding advice that, in a word, sucks. Ten CDC researchers with the National Centers for Immunization and Respiratory Disease were stymied at the power of natural breast milk to reduce babies' unnatural antibody response to rotavirus vaccines. The only solution they could identify was "delaying breast-feeding at the time of immunization."[13] Such irony! Ten scientists so intent on immunizing babies with an unnatural, temporary, incomplete, and dangerous form of immunity that they would ask mothers to temporarily stop immunizing their babies with natural, safe, and effective breast milk.

Dissuading mothers from thinking of breast-feeding as natural and advising mothers to delay breast-feeding is anti-mother, anti-baby and pro-industry. But the industry relationship that results in bad breast-feeding advice is just the beginning of bad relationships and bad advice.

Nearly twenty years ago, the AAP made available to the public a list of corporations that had donated to its "Friends of Children Fund." The total figure for the 1996–1997 fiscal year came over $2 million, and donors included:

> . . . Procter & Gamble, Gerber, Infant Formula Council, McNeil Consumer Products Company, National Cattlemen's Beef Association, Johnson & Johnson Consumer Products, Abbott Laboratories, Wyeth-Lederle Vaccine & Pediatrics, Mead Johnson Nutritionals, SmithKline Beecham Pharmaceuticals, Schering Corp., Rhone-Poulenc Rorer, Food Marketing Institute, Sugar Association, International Food Information Council, Merck Vaccine Division, and others.[14]

Suffice it to say that at least some of the AAP's friends are not friends to children. But this list is just the tip of the iceberg. As will be discussed later, industry co-opted medicine a century ago, and since that time, the two have become ever more enmeshed. Even referring to the AAP strengthens the illusion that it is separate from industry. It's not. The AAP acknowledges as much in the "AAP Policy on Conflict of Interest and Relationships with Industry and Other Organizations." The opening paragraph recites the standard AAP mission baloney before addressing what Paul Harvey would have called "the rest of the story." Rather than restrict members from conflicts of interest, it merely requires that members disclose such relationships.[15]

It couldn't possibly ask more of its members because conflicts of interests are the lifeblood of the AAP. In 2002, the *New York Times* asked Dr. Joe M. Sanders, former AAP executive director, how much Ross—the maker of Similac—had paid for its 300,000 special edition AAP-endorsed books. Sanders declined to answer. Similarly, when the *Times* asked Sanders for specific donation amounts it had accepted from Ross, McNeil, and Johnson & Johnson, Sanders refused to answer.[16] Apparently, the AAP's conflict of interest policy applies only to its members, not to the organization. This may explain why there appears to be a virtual media blackout on the AAP's financial dealings in more recent years.

Richard Gale exposed additional AAP conflicts of interest beyond the fake breast milk industry in a 2012 article posted on the CounterPunch website titled "Why Does the American Academy of Pediatrics Put Corporate Profits Ahead of Children's Health?"[17] The answer is found in the question: "Corporate Profits," but the depravity of the AAP in pursuing profits is beyond disturbing.

In 2011, the AAP dropped the minimum age at which children can be diagnosed with ADHD, a set of symptoms the incidence of which exploded in the 1990s, concurrent with the greatly expanded AAP-endorsed vaccine schedule.[18] That means of course that millions of children—many already vaccine injured—will swallow even more chemicals at an earlier age leading to what will be for many a lifetime on the pharmaceutical industry's chemical treadmill. Is the AAP's change in ADHD-related recommendations due to science or to conflicts of interest? According to Gale, "the AAP's chairman for ADHD guidelines, Dr. Mark Wolraich, is a consultant for psychotropic drug companies including Shire Pharmaceutical, Eli Lilly, Shinogi and Next Wave Pharmaceuticals."[19]

The AAP also reduced its minimum recommended age at which children can receive statin drugs from 10 to 8, effectively strengthening the dangerous message to American providers, parents, and children that dangerous chemicals are the solution to dangerous diets and lifestyles. Is it possible that the AAP's more than $1.4 million relationship with the statin makers Merck, Abbott, and Bristol Myers might have played an eensy-weensy role in the AAP's profit-generating recommendation?[20]

In the fall of 2012, California was gearing up for its vote on the labeling of GMO foods. On October 22nd, two weeks before the vote, *Pediatrics* published a "Clinical Report" titled "Organic Foods: Health and Environmental Advantages and Disadvantages." The report would have been more accurately titled "Advantages and Disadvantages of Organic vs. GMO Foods." Essentially a policy statement, the authors provided the basis upon which guild members should respond to patient questions regarding food choices—questions that were no doubt increasing with the pending vote. The report had the potential to faithfully address the conflicting evidence, and, at the very least, it could have advised doctors to adhere to the precautionary principle regarding GMOs and attendant poisons, but it did neither. Instead, it left pediatricians with a mealy-mouthed and spineless message for patients, offering them no protection from the $46 million agrochemical and junk food industries' media blitz. The following quotation is characteristic of the entire article:

> Current evidence does not support any meaningful nutritional benefits or deficits from eating organic compared to conventionally grown foods, and there are no well-powered human studies that directly demonstrate health benefits or disease protection as a result of consuming an organic diet.[21]

The report provided tacit support for the GMO industry with its claim that organic milk has no particular health benefits over milk derived from cows injected with the genetically modified bovine growth hormone (rBGH), in spite of the fact that the industry went to great and fraudulent lengths to cover up the health risks associated with rBGH.[22] The AAP also missed the opportunity to take a stance that could have protected children from the primary reason GMOs exist: to increase the sale and profits from pesticides. By failing to oppose an industry based on fraud and corruption, an industry that is responsible for the destruction of genetically diverse ecosystems, environmental poisoning, displacement of millions of farmers, and the health crisis facing the USA and much of the rest of the world is unconscionable, and if AAP membership had any integrity, it would have walked away from the AAP in 2012. But when it comes to conflicts of interest involving bread and butter, the AAP is more focused on its primary bread-and-butter product: vaccines.

At first glance, it would appear that pediatricians and vaccines are a match made in heaven—a mandated, liability-free product, an expanding product line delivered to an expanding demographic market, financial perks for high rates of compliance, and the certain public belief that vaccines safely and effectively protect children from infectious disease. What could possibly go wrong with such an arrangement?

CBS News journalist Sharyl Attkisson answered that question in 2008 when she exposed numerous conflicts of interest in the AAP, the vaccine-pushing organization Every Child By Two, and the king of conflicts of interest, Dr. Paul Offit. According to Attkisson, the vaccine manufacturer Wyeth gave the AAP $342,000. Merck's "contribution" was $433,000, and "Sanofi Aventis, maker of 17 vaccines . . ." was "[a]nother top donor." Offit held "a $1.5 million dollar research chair at Children's Hospital, funded by Merck," and he made untold millions on the sale of his patented Rotateq vaccine. Every Child By Two refused to tell CBS News how much Pharma money it accepts. Of course, the AAP, Every Child By Two, and Offit told Attkisson that the money they receive "doesn't sway their opinions." All refused to be interviewed on camera.[23]

Attkisson's conclusion that the medical-industrial complex poses "a serious risk for conflict of interest" demonstrates journalistic restraint, but it minimizes the truth: the shared relationship between industry and medicine *is* a serious conflict of interest. Period.

On June 15th, 2000, the US House of Representatives' Committee on Government Reform highlighted a few of those conflicts in a report titled "Conflicts of Interest in Vaccine Policy Making." As the report reveals, the AAP is far from alone and is also far from the worst offender. The American Academy of Family Pediatrics takes money from:

> Abbott Laboratories, American Home Products Corporation, Aventis, Bayer Corporation, bioMerieux, Boehringer Ingelheim Chemicals Co., Bristol-Myers Squibb Company, Eli Lilly and Company, Forest

Laboratories, G.D. Searle & Co., Glaxo Wellcome plc, Janssen Pharmaceutica, Lederle Laboratories, Merck & Co., Muro Pharmaceuticals, Novartis, Novo Nordisk A/S, Ortho-McNeil Pharmaceuticals, Otsuka America Pharmaceutical, Inc., Pasteur Merieux Connaught, Pfizer, Inc., Pharmacia, Schering AG, Schwarz Pharma, Inc., SmithKline Beecham, Solvay S.A., Warner-Lambert Company, and Wyeth-Ayerst Laboratories.[24]

The American College of Obstetricians and Gynecologists, American Medical Association, Infectious Disease Society of America, and Biotechnology Industry Organization stuff their pockets from numerous contributors, as well.[25]

Corporate contributions to medical guilds such as the AAP are anything but gifts. They're investments. Which means they expect to receive more in return than they donate through the implementation of business-friendly policies. When it comes to vaccines, the AAP is so friendly, it's sickening . . . literally.

In 2005, AAP's flagship journal, *Pediatrics*, published an article so industry-friendly it could have been written by vaccine manufacturers. The opening statement reads: "The American Academy of Pediatrics strongly endorses universal immunization."[26] "Universal immunization" is a phrase taken straight from The Church of Vaccinology's most holy scriptures. All vaccines, all the time, all ages. "Universal immunization" is a crusade that makes the medieval ones look like modern-day backsliding, bar hopping, go-to-church-twice-a-year Christians. By endorsing the "universal immunization" of children, the AAP simultaneously endorses a sociopathic vaccine industry while making a mockery of its trademarked slogan: "Dedicated to the health of all children."

To its credit, however, the article included the fact that "[f]our percent of pediatricians had refused permission for an immunization for their own children younger than 11 years."[27] Yet, having made that statement, it ignored the question of why those pediatricians would oppose the vaccine paradigm, program, and schedule. Instead, it focused solely on the problem of parents who resist or refuse to vaccinate their children. Is it possible that vaccine-informed pediatricians realize that the policy of universal immunizations is at best irresponsible and at worst sociopathic? Do AAP executive management members realize that vaccine manufacturers exclude sick and otherwise vulnerable children from vaccine trials?[28] Certainly, the manufacturers are aware that the AAP's universal immunization policy will likely injure the same children scientists exclude from their vaccine trials. In 2015, researchers Soriano, Nesher, and Shoenfeld addressed this problem in a paper published in the journal *Pharmacological Research*. They concluded, "Because of such selection bias, the occurrence of serious adverse reactions resulting from vaccinations in real life where vaccines are mandated to all individuals regardless of their susceptibility factors may be considerably underestimated."[29]

One egregious example of this scenario plays out in neonatal intensive care units across the nation. Low birth weight premature infants—babies who are fighting for their lives—are injected with vaccines according to the standard schedule. Due to the AAP's callous universal immunization policy, this medical guild bears at least part of the responsibility for the injuries and deaths that follow.

Certainly, the trauma to medical professionals who are mandated to vaccinate fragile infants is also considerable. A pediatric care unit nurse voiced her trauma to Dr. Andrew Wakefield, a man who recognized twenty years ago the catastrophic results of "universal vaccination." She said, "I can no longer work in there because we are mandated to give these premature, underweight babies the full vaccine schedule and they go into respiratory arrest."[30]

In addition to sharing dogma and money with the vaccine industry, the AAP also shares its influence in legislative processes. The wave of coercive vaccination legislation currently sweeping the country rides, in part, upon the influence and blessing of the corporate-sponsored AAP. As will be discussed later, AAP representatives are also deeply involved in governmental vaccine policy.

Pediatrician Kenneth Stoller was so disgusted with the AAP's approach to the autism epidemic and its refusal to protect babies from thimerosal in vaccines, he informed the AAP by letter that he could no longer continue his fellowship. "It is a token protest," Stoller wrote, "but it has to begin with someone."[31] If all pediatricians were true to their oath, they would follow Stoller's lead and throw the AAP, its products, and promotions into the world's largest biohazard garbage dump.

If conflicts of interest were a disease and if life were fair, most American medical guilds would be on their deathbeds and American children would be healthier. Unfortunately, the guilds prosper while disorders and diseases strike ever-greater numbers of children. The USA has one of the highest infant mortality rates in the developed world, and one in six of those who survive will be diagnosed with disabling medical conditions and learning disorders. According to the National Institute of Mental Health, 49.5% of American adolescents have been diagnosed with a mental disorder and an estimated 22% of those had severe impairment.[32] There is no doubt that the AAP's complicity with a corrupt industry and corrupt government is a contributing factor in the health crisis striking so many of the young people it professes to serve.

Chapter Eleven

CONFLICTS OF
INTEREST IN EVERY JAB

*Can physicians be so stupid as to trust these rubber stamp
committees whose members have such questionable
vested interests and conflicts of interest?*[1]
—Thomas Stone, MD

The business of vaccines is the business of government.[2]
—John Rappoport

The story of vaccines is the story of corruption, deception, and conflicts of
interest, CDC for short, and the multibillion-dollar pharmaceutical industry lies at the heart of the evil. The government, medical establishment, and
corporate-owned media all act out the roles assigned to them by Big Pharma. In
exchange, they receive money, influence, power, and control from the industry.
Elite members with multiple ties to industry meet behind closed doors to create
and implement strategies to increase their profit and power. These people form
what will be referred to as "the insiders." When the doors are opened to the
public, they present profit-producing plans and policies under the guise of public health to everyone else—"the outsiders"—including public health officials,
medical professionals, and media. Vaccine believers and sociopaths exist in both
the insiders and the outsiders groups. As stated in the introduction, both believers and sociopaths can and do commit sociopathic acts. Believers commit such
acts with the belief that they are serving the public. Examples include advancing
mandatory vaccination legislation, removing children from vaccine informed
parents, vaccinating sick or otherwise immunocompromised individuals, or
giving multiple vaccinations at once. Sociopaths commit the same or other acts
with no illusion of noble intent.

The pharmaceutical industry—which includes the vaccine industry—heads
up the government's role in increasing profit margin and power. Election results
and appointments are often determined by proven loyalty to the industry. This

holds true for US presidents, cabinet members and officials in all three branches of government, and their departments, agencies, and committees.

The Bush family's loyalty to the vaccine industry is second to none. George H. W. Bush sat on the Eli Lilly board in the 1970s. And during George W. Bush's stint as US President, Mitch Daniels, a former Eli Lilly executive, served as White House budget director. Eli Lilly CEO Sidney Taurel served on the president's homeland security advisory council.[3]

In December 2002, the influence of Eli Lilly over government policy made the news. US citizens were more than willing to give up their constitutional rights with the passage of the Homeland Security Act that created the Homeland Security Department, but when an unidentified person slipped in a rider that would immunize Eli Lilly from hundreds of pending lawsuits filed by parents of children injured by Eli Lilly's thimerosal in vaccines, the public was outraged. House Majority Leader Dick Armey finally fessed up to adding the rider. Representative Dan Burton, grandfather of an autistic grandson, asked Armey, "Who told you to put it in?" Armey replied, " . . . they asked me to do it at the White House . . ." Some surmised that "the outgoing majority leader [was] the perfect fall guy to take the heat and shield the White House from embarrassment." According to the *New York Times*, "It's a claim both the White House and Armey deny."[4]

The claim, however, is likely true. In 2005, activist Robert F. Kennedy, Jr., published an article in *Salon* titled "Deadly Immunity." Among other things, Kennedy pins the deed and the motive on

> Senate Majority Leader Bill Frist, who has received $873,000 in contributions from the pharmaceutical industry, [and] has been working to immunize vaccine makers from liability in 4,200 lawsuits that have been filed by the parents of injured children. On five separate occasions, Frist has tried to seal all of the government's vaccine-related documents—including the Simpsonwood transcripts—and shield Eli Lilly, the developer of thimerosal, from subpoenas. In 2002, the day after Frist quietly slipped a rider known as the "Eli Lilly Protection Act" into a homeland security bill, the company contributed $10,000 to his campaign and bought 5,000 copies of his book on bioterrorism.[5]

Numerous news outlets carried the mysterious and dramatic Lilly rider story. A *New York Times* Opinion piece expressed indignation against the government officials who would exploit the public for private gain: "The politicians with their hands out and the fat cats with plenty of green to spread around have carried the day. Nothing is too serious to exploit, not even the defense of the homeland during a time of terror."[6]

At the same time the rider fiasco blew up the press, George W. Bush set off another bomb when he announced his "'ambitious plan to inoculate as many as 11 million military personnel and emergency responders with the smallpox vaccine." According to the *Washington Post*, Bush "characterized the unprecedented program as a precaution aimed at protecting front-line personnel and improving response capabilities to a biological attack."[7]

In a rare admission of vaccine risk, federal officials said they were "not recommending everyone get the shot, made from live vaccinia that causes side effects ranging from a fever and rash to brain swelling and, rarely, death."[8] In addition, "Several of Bush's health advisers said they did not know how the president arrived at the notion of providing unlicensed vaccine to those Americans who 'insist' upon being inoculated."[9] Considering the Bush family's two-generation love affair with vaccine industry movers and shakers, it appears entirely plausible that both the Eli Lilly rider and the smallpox vaccine farce had far more to do with protecting industry profits than protecting American troops and citizens.

Parent activists, already angry at the role the government played in injuring their children, "mounted a letter writing campaign, and chastised Senator Frist and the Republican leadership in an advertisement in the Congressional newspaper *Roll Call*, Congress, in a bi-partisan vote, repealed the provision in 2003."[10]

During her two decades at *The New England Journal of Medicine*, Dr. Marcia Angell had a front-row seat on the growing corruption of the pharmaceutical industry. Angell summed up the relationship between Pharma and government and the impact of that relationship on American consumers in the introduction to her book *The Truth About Drug Companies*:

> Drug companies have the largest lobby in Washington, and they give copiously to political campaigns. Legislators are now so beholden to the pharmaceutical industry that it will be . . . difficult to break its lock on them. . . .
>
> The fact is that this industry is taking us for a ride, and there will be no real reform without an aroused and determined public to make it happen.[11]

Laurie Powell once served the pharmaceutical industry as a marketing communications specialist. The former insider now speaks out against the abuses in the pharmaceutical-based health care system including "Big Pharma's silent hold over the US government." In a 2016 article, Powell wrote, "Lobbying expenditures by the pharmaceutical industry have been increasing every year and hit an all-time high of $273 million in 2009." Political leaders have stated that Pharma money does not influence their work. Powell disagrees, saying it's nothing but "[p]olitical payback" that results in "cancer treatments [that] can cost

600 times more in the US than in other countries. . . ." Payback also ensures that the government continue to spend exorbitant amounts on patented drugs that could be purchased for a fraction of the price with generics. Powell also states that Pharma money played a role in the creation of the National Vaccine Injury Compensation Act, which shielded manufacturers from liability.[12]

According to *CalWatchdog*, an investigative news service focused on government transparency, California Assemblyman Henry Perea provides a good example of a system based on political payback. In exchange for favorable legislation, Perea received "tens of thousands of dollars in luxury goods, entertainment and travel . . ." to several locations including Italy, Chile, Israel, Central America, and Maui.[13]

As far as the pharmaceutical industry is concerned, Perea's a cheap trick. The golden boy of the Golden State is Senator Richard Pan, the pediatrician who lined his campaign pockets with more than $95,000 from Big Pharma.[14] Credited with the deceitful passage of SB 277, Pan has proven to be a valuable asset to the industry and a dangerous enemy to truth and freedom. He also proved to be a coward when Dr. Andrew Wakefield and associates attempted to meet with Pan in the California State Capitol on May 9, 2016. Pan ran from them "like the Pink Panther."[15] He might have be able run a lot faster if his pockets had not been stuffed full of industry money.

In 2015, the Australian parliament passed a law that makes "benefits, rebates and the Family Tax Benefit A" conditional on vaccination status. The law is dubbed "No Jab, No Pay."[16] New York State Senator Kemp Hannon, chair of the State Health Committee, provides an example of what might be called "No Pay, No Jab." The *New York Daily News* reported in 2015 that Hannon "has up to $130,000 in investments in pharmaceutical and other health-related companies. . . . In addition to his investments, Hannon over the past four years also received more than $420,000 from pharmaceutical and other medical interests. . . ."[17] Hannon is also the "author of the recently passed law that will require all seventh and twelfth graders in the state to get meningitis shots."[18]

Hannon's business relationship with Pharma is but a microcosm of the entire government-industrial relationship that functions on the same "No Pay, No Jab" principle. The Department of Health and Human Services (HHS) exploits that principle on a colossal level.

The US White House website states that the HHS, an $80.1 billion department, "is the principal Federal agency charged with protecting the health of all Americans and providing essential human services."[19]

The FDA and the CDC are the two HHS agencies most commonly associated with vaccine licensing, safety analysis, and promotion. A brief review of the organizational makeup of HHS demonstrates that, in addition to the FDA and

CDC, vaccine policy and implementation involve numerous agencies, organizations, trade groups, and corporations. The National Vaccine Program Office (NVPO),

> located in the Office of the Assistant Secretary for Health (ASH), Office of the Secretary (OS), US Department of Health and Human Services (HHS) . . . is responsible for coordinating and ensuring collaboration among the many federal agencies involved in vaccine and immunization activities.[20]

The "many federal agencies" NVPO refers to include the CDC, FDA, Agency for Healthcare Research and Quality (AHRQ), Centers for Medicare and Medicaid Services (CMS), Health Resources and Services Administration (HRSA), and National Institutes of Health (NIH).[21] NVPO lists numerous other partners stating, "Each of our partners contributes by informing NVPO's work and helping to meet the goals set forth in the National Vaccine Plan."[22]

Partners within HHS include the National Vaccine Injury Compensation Program (NVICP), Biomedical Advanced Research and Development Authority (BARDA), Assistant Secretary for Preparedness and Response (ASPR), and Office of the General Counsel (OGC). Other Federal agencies include the Department of Defense (DoD), US Agency for International Development (USAID), and Veterans Health Administration (VHA), Department of Veterans Affairs (VA). "State and Local Partners" include the National Association of County and City Health (NACCHO), Association of State and Territorial Health (ASTHO), and Association of Immunization Managers (AIM). "Global Partners and Non-governmental Organizations (NGOs)" include the World Health Organization (WHO), Public Health Agency of Canada, GAVI Alliance (GAVI), and the Gates Foundation. And finally, industry partners include Pharmaceutical Research and Manufacturers of America (PhRMA), Biotechnology Innovation Organization (BIO), and America's Health Insurance Plans (AHIP).[23]

As to the deceptive heading "State and Local Partners," the word *state* implies state governmental. The names "National Association of County and City Health Officials" as well as the "Association of State and Territorial Health Officials" give the impression that these organizations are government organizations. By including the Association of Immunization Managers under the "State and Local Partners" heading and under the other two organizations, one is left with the incorrect impression that it too is a government organization. These organizations are registered as independent nonprofit organizations, not government bodies.[24, 25, 26] But their independence is a sham. All three are heavily funded by the federal government and/or corporate funders. All three are designed to keep local vaccinators marching lockstep with federal policy. All three promote legislation designed to decrease the right of citizens to exercise personal belief exemptions to vaccinations. All three lobby legislators or support "State Legislative Liaisons" to this end.[27, 28, 29, 30]

Nearly 40 organizations fund the National Association of County & City Health Officials including the CDC and The Association of State and Territorial Health Officials.[31] The Association of State and Territorial Health Officials corporate alliance partners include, among others: Merck, GlaxoSmithKline, PhRMA, and Sanofi Pasteur.[32] The AIM Corporate Alliance Program gives corporate allies graded levels of access to AIM members based on donation amounts; $25,000 or more is the "Suggested Support" amount to be granted maximum Platinum level access.[33] A few of AIM's partners include: Pfizer, Sanofi Pasteur, AstraZeneca, GlaxoSmithKline, and Seqirus, "the second largest influenza vaccine company in the world."[34] [35]

The World Health Organization, GAVI Alliance, and the Gates Foundation have strong financial interests in aggressive vaccine policy. Miloud Kaddar, Senior Advisor and Health Economist to the WHO, presented a slide slow titled "Global Vaccine Market Features and Trends." Bullet points include:

- Global [vaccine] market projected to rise to USD 100 B by 2025
- More than 120 new products in the development pipeline
- 60 are of importance for developing countries
- Newer and more expensive vaccines are coming into the market faster than ever before.

A pie chart shows the "[g]lobal vaccine leaders" and their "[m]ajor focus on new vaccine development for industrialised country markets." The self-identified Health Economist lists the "[t]op product sales in 2010": Prevnar-13, Proquad, Gardasil, Prevnar ("7-valent pnenumococcal conjugate vaccine"), Fluzone, Infanrix and Pediarix, bringing in a total of $7.75 billion in sales. Kaddar reviews the importance of "Vaccine Market Growth Factors" including:

- Importance of communicable diseases and new threats
- Cost effectiveness of immunizations
- New funding opportunities (Gov, PPP, donors, Foundations)
- New research techniques and manufacturing technologies
- Increasing demand, new target population, larger emerging markets
- Higher prices, improved profitability for the industry ("blockbuster vaccines").

He identifies the "new trend" for multinational corporations to target "[e]merging markets such as Mexico, Brazil, Turkey, Indonesia, Russia, China and India" with "innovative vaccines" marketed by "MNC [multinational corporations] representatives" using a "Pharma like model." Finally, Kaddar mentions "[r]isk sharing with countries and funders,"[36] a concept that the Indian pediatrician Jacob Puliyel, MD, discusses in greater detail.

Puliyel is pro-vaccine but anti ". . . ill-conceived national vaccine policies." According to the doctor:

> Such policies are promoted by the powerful VACCINE INDUSTRY; its profit-sharing stakeholders in government, academia and so-called nonprofits—such as the Bill and Melinda Gates Foundation and The Global Alliance for Vaccines and Immunization (GAVI) whose board of directors includes vaccine manufacturers [emphasis in original].

Puliyel cites GAVI's use of "subsidies" to:

> entice governments in underdeveloped countries to include vaccines of questionable health benefit. Once these vaccines are added to the country's national immunization program, GAVI withdraws the "subsidies" putting the entire cost burden on poor countries. This "bait and switch" marketing strategy has been developed by vaccine stakeholders masquerading as "Advocates."[37]

In addition, the Bill & Melinda Gates Foundation (BMGF) vaccine funds are tied to "a binding confidentiality clause aimed at stifling and controlling" national level vaccine organizations.[38]

In 2016, Global Justice Now, a UK-based organization that ". . . campaigns for a world where resources are controlled by the many, not the few," published a heavily referenced, 54-page report titled "Gated Development: Is the Gates Foundation always a force for good?" The short answer is no. The BMGF is an enormous entity with a hold over the policies and politics of both governments and organizations such as the WHO. According to the report, "The BMGF provided 11 per cent of the WHO's entire budget in 2015 . . . ." The report fleshes out Dr. Puliyel's assertion that both the BMGF and its Global Alliance for Vaccines and Immunization is filled with industry executives from "the International Federation of Pharmaceutical Manufacturers, which involves **GlaxoSmithKline**, **Merck**, **Novartis**, and **Pfizer**, among others . . ." [emphasis in original].

As many other critics have noted, the report declares that global health initiatives sponsored by BMGF must focus more on the causes of infectious disease such as poverty, poor sanitation, malnutrition, etc., and less on vaccines. Global Justice Now argues that

. . . the BMGF's programmes are—overall—detrimental to promoting economic development and global justice. The world is being sold a myth that private philanthropy holds many of the solutions to the world's problems, when in fact it is pushing the world in many wrong directions.[39]

Finally, a word about the National Vaccine Program Office "Industry Partners" is in order. According to the Pharmaceutical Research and Manufacturers of America website, PhRMA consists of more than 50 member companies including major vaccine manufacturers.[40] The Biotechnology Innovation Organization bills itself "As the world's largest biotechnology trade association" with a membership of nearly 3,000 biotech companies.[41, 42] Several vaccines contain genetically modified ingredients, and many more are in development.[43] The American Association of Health Plans (AAHP) accepted $190 million to conceal the information in the CDC's Vaccine Safety Datalink[44] (more on the Vaccine Safety Datalink in coming chapters).

The collaboration of several governmental organizations responsible for the implementation of vaccination policy is most impressive. That collaboration is evident in the National Vaccine Advisory Committee's National Adult Immunization Plan. In addition to the CDC and the FDA, the plan to increase vaccination compliance in adults involves the participation of the Health Care Financing Administration (HCFA), Health Resources and Services Administration (HRSA), Office of Public Health Science (OPHS)/ National Vaccine Program Office (NVPO), Agency for Health Care Policy and Research (AHCPR), Open Access Scholarly Publishers Association (OASPA), Administration for Children and Families (ACF), Administration on Aging (AoA), Indian Health Service (IHS), Office for Civil Rights (OCR), Office of Mental Health (OMH), Substance Abuse and Mental Health Services Administration (SAMHSA), Office of the Surgeon General (OSG), Office of the Secretary (OS), and the National Institutes of Health (NIH)[45] (more on the National Adult Immunization Plan in Chapter 25).

The NVPO published a 58-page document detailing the goals, objectives, and strategies of the National Vaccine Plan.[46] The plan is clear: the future for both the American and the global Herds includes more vaccines and more propaganda than ever before. Considering the fact that government has partnered with the multibillion-dollar vaccine industry and the fact that vaccine industry growth is predicted to explode in future years, no other outcome can be anticipated.

The public-private partnership is plainly visible in the makeup of the National Vaccine Advisory Committee, which is nested in the National Vaccine

Program Office under the jurisdiction of Health and Human Services. The committee is made up of 15 members, 11 "Liaison Representatives," and "13 Ex Officio Members." The liaison representatives hail from

> Advisory Committee on Immunization Practice (ACIP) (CDC), Advisory Commission on Childhood Vaccines (HRSA), America's Health Insurance Plans (AHIP), American Immunization Registry Association (AIRA), Association of Immunization Managers (AIM), Association of State and Territorial Officials (ASTHO), National Association of County and City Health Officials, Pan American Health Organization/World Health Organization (PAHO/WHO), Public Health Agency of Canada, Vaccines and Related Biological Products Advisory Committee. [47]

The 13 ex officio members represent

> Agency for Healthcare Research and Quality, Assistant Secretary for Preparedness and Response (ASPR), Centers for Disease Control and Prevention, Centers for Medicaid and Medicare Services (CMS), Department of Defense (DoD), Food and Drug Administration (FDA), Health Resources and Services Administration (HRSA), Indian Health Service (IHS), National Institutes of Health (NIH), US Department of Veterans Affairs (VA), US Department of Agriculture. [48]

Walter A. Orenstein, MD, served as NVAC Chair from 2011 to 2016. In 2000, Orenstein participated in the secret and illegal Simpsonwood meeting (more in Chapter 15). Bruce G. Gellin, MD, MPH, serves as the NVAC executive secretary. Gellin also serves as the deputy assistant secretary for health and director of the National Vaccine Program Office (NVPO) at HHS and "is the principle technical, strategic and policy advisor to the Assistant Secretary for Health on all aspects of the National Vaccine Program." Gellin's vitae reads like a veritable who's who of global vaccination policy leadership, false flag epidemics, and catastrophes involving among other things the 2005 Bird Flu nonevent and the contrived 2009 H1N1 influenza "pandemic." He addresses the issue of "vaccine hesitancy," a term vaccine believers and sociopaths use to describe the resistance of the vaccine informed to worship in The Church of Vaccinology. He is a coordinator of the research and development focus of the Decade of Vaccines Collaboration, which treats the effects of poverty with vaccines rather than address poverty and malnutrition. As a Warren Weaver Fellow at the Rockefeller Foundation, Gellin apparently became indoctrinated in the misguided concept that vaccines are the cornerstone of public health initiatives and a panacea for immunocompromised children in developing countries. He spreads his vaccine indoctrination to both domestic and international audiences. His apparent belief in the vaccine paradigm plays a part in the content of over a dozen medical journals as well as the Encyclopedia Britannica.[49]

NVAC membership is decidedly biased in favor of vaccinating Americans and the rest of the world with or without the consent of vaccine-informed individuals. Such bias destroys scientific objectivity. Like any other quota-driven salesperson, the sales strategy of the NVAC is to sell citizens on the benefits of vaccines while downplaying or denying the risks.

In 2010, Health & Human Services Secretary Kathleen Sebelius demonstrated the extent to which HHS would go to sell consumers on vaccines. The monthly magazine *Reader's Digest* wrote up its interview with Sebelius in an article titled "H1N1: The Report Card." RD asked Sebelius, "What can be done about public mistrust of vaccines?" She replied,

> There are groups out there that insist that vaccines are responsible for a variety of problems despite all scientific evidence to the contrary. We have reached out to media outlets to try to get them to not give the views of these people equal weight in their reporting to what science has shown and continues to show about the safety of vaccines.[50]

The government not only censors the media's reporting of information from "groups out there," it also censored its own H1N1 statistics, as former CBS investigative journalist Sharyl Attkisson revealed in an interview with independent journalist Jon Rappoport. Attkisson had discovered that the CDC had stopped counting the number of H1N1 cases in the USA. She shared the details with Rappoport:

> We discovered through our FOI efforts that before the CDC mysteriously stopped counting Swine Flu cases, they had learned that almost none of the cases they had counted as Swine Flu was, in fact, Swine Flu or any sort of flu at all! The interest in the story from one [CBS] executive was very enthusiastic. He said it was "the most original story" he'd seen on the whole Swine Flu epidemic. But others pushed to stop it and, in the end, no broadcast wanted to touch it. We aired numerous stories pumping up the idea of an epidemic, but not the one that would shed original, new light on all the hype. It was fair, accurate, legally approved and a heck of a story.[51]

Attkisson provided further examples of media censorship in her book *Stonewalled: My Fight for Truth Against the Forces of Obstruction, Intimidation, and Harassment in Obama's Washington:*

Some of the hardest pushback I ever receive comes after [executive director Jim Murphy] assigns me to look into the reported cover-up of adverse effects of various prescription drugs and military vaccinations. That series of reports leads me to investigate related stories about childhood vaccinations and their links to harmful side effects, including brain damage and autism. At the time, the Bush administration is marching in lockstep with the pharmaceutical industry in denying problems with the prescription drugs at issue as well as both military and childhood vaccines.[52]

Attkisson is not opposed to the government's desire "to want their side of the story told. . . ." Her beef is with government censorship. The stonewalled journalist wrote, "They don't want Americans to know about the many controversies or hear from the scientists doing peer-reviewed, published research that contradicts the official party line."[53]

Attkisson's experience with government censorship was largely invisible to the public. In 2016, the entire world witnessed censorship surrounding the release of the documentary film *Vaxxed: From Cover-up to Catastrophe*, a film that details the story of Dr. William Thompson, the CDC whistleblower. Robert De Niro had pulled *Vaxxed* from the lineup at his Tribeca Film Festival due to pressure from unnamed sources. The media celebrated De Niro's move and then recycled its tirades against Andrew Wakefield, the film's director. Omitted from their tirades was the fact that the film told the real story of the real William Thompson who had provided US Representative Bill Posey with thousands of documents, which exposed years of CDC fraud and cover-up. Less than two weeks later, Hunter Todd, Chairman and Founding Director of Houston's annual WorldFest film festival, pulled *Vaxxed* from its lineup, as well. On April 5, Todd sent a message to Philippe Diaz, Chairman of Cinema Libre, distributor of *Vaxxed*. Todd described "very threatening calls" from "high Houston government officials" and threats of "severe action against the festival if we showed it. . . ." Todd wrote matter-of-factly, "It is done, it is out and we have been censored. . . . There are some very powerful forces against this project."[54] Two days later, the *Houston Chronicle* named the source of the threats as Houston Mayor Sylvester Turner.[55]

Returning to the question *Reader's Digest* asked HHS Secretary Kathleen Sebelius, "What can be done about public mistrust of vaccines?" The US government's answer is clear: Thou shalt speak no evil of the vaccine paradigm, the vaccine clergy, the vaccine schedule, or vaccine ingredients. Heretics will be punished and silenced. Their reputations and careers will be destroyed by vaccine crusaders who will employ lies, threats, and smear campaigns.

Just as HHS has a vaccine advisory committee, the CDC and FDA also have committees that make recommendations on vaccine-related matters. The CDC claims, "Stringent measures and rigorous screening are used to avoid both real and apparent conflicts of interest" in its vaccine advisory committee.[56]

On June 14, 2000, Linda A. Suydam, FDA senior associate commissioner, testified before the House Committee on Government Reform. She described the FDA advisory committees and assured government officials "that advisory committee recommendations are based on the best possible science and are free from bias."[57] The following day, the same committee before which Suydam had testified submitted a Majority Staff Report titled "Conflicts of Interest in Vaccine Policy Making." The report focused

> . . . on two influential advisory committees utilized by Federal regulators to provide expert advice on vaccine policy:
>
> 1. The FDA's Vaccines and Related Biological Products Advisory Committee (VRBPAC); and
> 2. The CDC's Advisory Committee on Immunizations Practices (ACIP).
>
> The VRBPAC advises the FDA on the licensing of new vaccines, while the ACIP advises the CDC on guidelines to be issued to doctors and the states for the appropriate use of vaccines. [58]

The damning report summarized its findings as follows:

> Members of the advisory committees are required to disclose any financial conflicts of interest and recuse themselves from participating in decisions in which they have an interest. The Committee's investigation has determined that conflict of interest rules employed by the FDA and the CDC have been weak, enforcement has been lax, and committee members with substantial ties to pharmaceutical companies have been given waivers to participate in committee proceedings.[59]

The conflicts of interest in the FDA's advisory panel are a reflection of the conflicts of interest held by the FDA commissioner, Robert M. Califf, MD, whose

> . . . salary is contractually underwritten in part by several large pharmaceutical companies, including Merck, Bristol-Myers Squibb, Eli Lilly and Novartis. He also receives as much as $100,000 a year in consulting fees from some of those companies, and from others, according to his 2014 conflict of interest disclosure. . . .[60]

Califf refers to his cozy business relationship with industry as "collaboration" and views such relationships as assets. He states how "useful" it is ". . . to have someone [leading the FDA] who understands how companies operate because you're interacting with them all the time."[61]

It's also useful for the public to understand that the FDA not only understands how pharmaceutical companies operate, it also operates with a similar criminal culture. In 2012, members of Congress and the Office of Special Counsel (OSC) became aware that FDA managers bully and intimidate employees who attempt to protect the public from unsafe products. One of their tactics includes an email surveillance program. In 2009, scientists working in the FDA's Center for Devices and Radiological Health wrote to President Obama claiming that top FDA managers "committed the most outrageous misconduct by ordering, coercing and intimidating FDA physicians and scientists to recommend approval, and then retaliating when the physicians and scientists refused to go along."[62] Some of the scientists were fired from their jobs, prompting another letter to the president. The scientists wrote,

> It has been brought to our attention that FDA management may have just recently ordered the FDA Office of Criminal Investigations (OCI) to investigate us, rather than the managers who have engaged in wrongdoing! It is an outrage that our own Agency would step up the retaliation to such a level because we have reported their wrongdoing to the United States Congress.[63]

Ronald Kavanagh, PharmD, PhD, served as an FDA drug reviewer from 1998 to 2008. Kavanagh informed Martha Rosenberg with *Truthout* that the intimidation extends beyond the FDA's Center for Devices, stating:

> [t]here is also irrefutable evidence that managers at CDER [Center for Drug Evaluation and Research] have placed the nation at risk by corrupting the evaluation of drugs and by interfering with our ability to ensure the safety and efficacy of drugs. While I was at FDA, drug reviewers were clearly told not to question drug companies and that our job was to approve drugs. We were prevented, except in rare instances, from presenting findings at advisory committees. In 2007, formal policies were instituted so that speaking in any way that could reflect poorly on the agency could result in termination. If we asked questions that could delay or prevent a drug's approval—which of course was our job as drug reviewers—management would reprimand us, reassign us, hold secret meetings about us, and worse. Obviously in such an environment, people will self-censor.[64]

Kavanagh went on to explain the numerous tricks manufacturers use to create the illusion that their drugs are safe and effective. When savvy reviewers challenge the illusion, manufacturers report them to FDA management "and have the reviewer removed or overruled."[65] Kavanagh was replaced as the reviewer when he voiced opposition to the use of dangerous nerve agents that would eventually be used as weapons in the Gulf Wars. The whistleblower reported his concerns to Congress, which directed him to the Department of Justice. In the end, he doesn't believe his "complaints were taken seriously by the FBI or investigated."[66]

Corruption and collusion with industry is not a recent development. US Senator Abraham Ribicoff addressed the issue in a 1972 congressional hearing in which he listed "[t]he real problems" that "plague our regulatory programs." Some of the many problems Ribicoff mentioned were the

> day-to-day influence on regulators from outside the government . . . from representatives of the regulated industry; in which agencies with regulatory responsibilities also view themselves as advocates for a particular interest group; in which regulators move back and forth between jobs in government and executive positions in regulated industries; in which important decisions are made without input from a variety of affected interests.[67]

Ribicoff concluded, "We have to do better." Rather than doing better, the conflicts of interest are worse now than ever. In 1995, Congress established the CDC Foundation, which "connects the Centers for Disease Control and Prevention (CDC) with private-sector organizations and individuals to build public health programs that make our world healthier and safer."[68] Since then, pharmaceutical companies—companies that have paid billions in fines for criminal activities—have contributed millions of dollars to the Foundation, which makes the Foundation look very much like it's a front organization for criminals.[69] In 2015, Jeanne Lenzer, associate editor of the *British Medical Journal*, described a few of the problems with the CDC's profitable relationship with industry including the fact that the Foundation funnels money from industry to the CDC.[70]

One of the biggest conflicts of interest lies within the CDC itself because the agency is responsible for both vaccine safety and vaccine promotion. In 2004, Representative Dave Weldon addressed the matter with the supposedly independent Institute of Medicine. Weldon said,

> CDC is tasked with promoting vaccination, ensuring high vaccination rates, and monitoring the safety of vaccines. They serve as their own watchdog; neither common nor desirable when seeking unbiased research. This has been a recipe for disaster with other agencies.[71]

Five years before Weldon addressed the IOM, family practitioner Harold Buttram, MD, stated that the

. . . arbitrary decisions in the mandating of vaccines . . . made by the government bureaucracies, which are highly partisan to the pharmaceuticals, with no recourse open to parents . . . have all the potential ingredients for a tragedy of historical proportions.[72]

In 2009, the inspector general of the Department of Health and Human Services released a report on the conflicts of interest within the CDC. The *New York Times* covered the story by writing that

[m]ost of the experts who served on advisory panels in 2007 to evaluate vaccines for flu and cervical cancer had potential conflicts that were never resolved. . . . Some were legally barred from considering the issues but did so anyway.[73]

Robert F. Kennedy, Jr., documented extensive conflicts of interest in his book *Thimerosal: Let the Science Speak*. In 2015, Kennedy told former Minnesota governor and TV talk show host Jesse Ventura that 97% of the people who sit on vaccine panels have the same kinds of conflicts of interest that Paul Offit has. Kennedy asked,

So the American people have to wonder, are the . . . scheduled vaccines that CDC is advising them to take, which become mandatory under state law, are those being added . . . to advance public health or are they being added because . . . somebody is making a profit from them?[74]

It would appear that Brenda Fitzgerald is well qualified to answer Kennedy's question. Fitzgerald, stepped down from her position as director of the CDC in January 2018 shortly after Politico revealed that she had "purchased tobacco, drug company and food stock, along with other financial holdings in various health companies" only a month after assuming leadership of the agency in July of 2017. According to Politico,

. . . Fitzgerald participated in meetings related to the opioid crisis, hurricane response efforts, cancer and obesity, stroke prevention, polio, Zika and Ebola. . . .

Merck, whose stock Fitzgerald purchased on Aug. 9, has been working on developing an Ebola vaccine and also makes HIV medications. Bayer, whose stock she purchased on Aug. 10, has in the past partnered with the CDC Foundation, which works closely with the CDC, to prevent the spread of the Zika virus.[75]

Barbara Loe Fisher, mother of a vaccine-injured child, author, public speaker, and director of the National Vaccine Information Center, has spent much of her adult life advocating for transparency and safer vaccines. According to Fisher, she has "sat in rooms with these officials, both at scientific conferences and government meetings." In addition, she served for four years as "the token consumer representative" on the Vaccine Advisory Committee under HHS.[76]

Only five days after William Thompson "publicly admitted . . . that he and other CDC officials, including the current CDC's Director of Immunization Safety, . . . published a study about MMR vaccine safety in 2004 . . . that 'omitted statistically significant information' and 'did not follow the final study protocol,'" Fisher, speaking on behalf of the National Vaccine Information Center, renewed the organization's "call for oversight of vaccine safety to be removed from the Department of Health and Human Services (DHHS)." Fisher said in a highly referenced statement,

> It is a conflict of interest for DHHS to be in charge of vaccine safety and also license vaccines, . . . and take money from drug companies to fast track vaccines, . . . and partner with drug companies to develop and share profits from vaccine sales, . . . and make national vaccine policies . . . that get turned into state vaccine laws . . . while also deciding which children will and will not get a vaccine injury compensation award.[77]

The documentary *Vaxxed* also emphasizes the need to remove the charge of vaccine safety from the CDC.

In 2014, David Wright, the US Office of Research Integrity (ORI) director, "quit his job and issued a searing letter claiming pervasive scientific misconduct in biomedical research at the CDC, the National Institutes of Health (NIH), and the Public Health Service (PHS), all part of HHS, which he characterized as 'a remarkably dysfunctional bureaucracy.'"[78]

Wright's letter did not specifically address the problem of endemic conflicts of interest within HHS, but his summary statement to the HHS Assistant Secretary for Health regarding the "remarkably dysfunctional [HHS] bureaucracy" resonates with every American who is outraged that government has sacrificed its ethics as well as the health of American citizens on the altar of industry greed and corruption.

In the 1990s, the apostles of the vaccine industry, the medical establishment, and government greatly increased the size of their sacrificial altar, resulting in increased numbers of vaccine-injured and dead children. And in doing so, they introduced people around the world to a word that may have the potential to destroy both the Church and the entire vaccine program.

That word is autism.

Chapter Twelve

VACCINES CAUSE AUTISM: THE WORDS THAT SHALL NOT BE SPOKEN

Here is what I shoulder. I shoulder that the CDC has put the research ten years behind. Because the CDC has not been transparent, we've missed ten years of research because the CDC is so paralyzed right now by anything related to autism.[1]
—Dr. William Thompson, CDC senior scientist

You can never really say "MMR doesn't cause autism," but frankly when you get in front of the media you better get used to saying it because otherwise people will hear a door being left open when a door shouldn't be left open.[2]
—Paul Offit, vaccine developer

Representative Dan Burton, grandfather of a vaccine-injured autistic grandson, was the driving force behind the Mercury in Medicine Report submitted to the House of Representatives in 2003. The report was prepared by the staff of the Subcommittee on Human Rights and Wellness, Committee on Government Reform after a three-year investigation initiated in the Committee on Government Reform. It provided historical information about the use of mercury and a specialized mercuric formulation called thimerosal, which had been used as a preservative in vaccines and other biological and drug products since the 1930s. According to the report, "thimerosal is an organic compound made up of equal parts of thiosalicylic acid and ethylmercury. It is 49.6 percent ethylmercury by weight."[3]

John and Stephen Oller, coauthors of the book *Autism: The Diagnosis, Treatment, & Etiology of the Undeniable Epidemic*, provide additional information regarding the origins and intended use of thimerosal:

Research on the effects of ethyl mercury on animals and humans has always shown it to be extremely toxic, especially with respect to the brain, gut, and other vital organs. The form that this compound takes in thimerosal was not so much discovered as invented by Morris Selig Kharasch (1928). Thimerosal was intended to kill microbes (harmful bacteria and fungi) on or inside living plants, animals, and persons. Obviously, thimerosal had to be toxic to achieve its killing purpose. Thus it follows that thimerosal is and always was toxic. This characteristic was known from the work of Smithburn et al. (1930) as well as from Powell and Jamieson (1931) forward.[4]

Eli Lilly—the thimerosal patent holder—conducted the only safety study ever performed on thimerosal when it contracted with Dr. K.C. Smithburn— referred to by the Ollers in the previous paragraph—to test the concoction on his patients, all of whom had bacterial meningitis. In 1931, researchers H.M. Powell and W.A. Jamieson—Lilly employees—published a study in the *American Journal of Hygiene* based on Smithburn's experiment.[5, 6]

The FDA website cites the Powell and Jamieson report as evidence supporting the safety of thimerosal:

> Prior to its introduction in the 1930's, data were available in several animal species and humans providing evidence for its safety and effectiveness as a preservative (Powell and Jamieson 1931). Since then, thimerosal has been the subject of several studies . . . and has a long record of safe and effective use preventing bacterial and fungal contamination of vaccines, with no ill effects established other than minor local reactions at the site of injection.[7]

Later, on the same webpage, the FDA provides more details on the Smithburn study:

> The earliest published report of thimerosal use in humans was published in 1931 (Powell and Jamieson 1931). In this report, 22 individuals received 1% solution of thimerosal intravenously for unspecified therapeutic reasons. Subjects received up to 26 milligrams thimerosal/kg (1 milligrams equals 1,000 micrograms) with no reported toxic effects, although 2 subjects demonstrated phlebitis or sloughing of skin after local infiltration. Of note, this study was not specifically designed to examine toxicity; 7 of 22 subjects were observed for only one day, the specific clinical assessments were not described, and no laboratory studies were reported.[8]

The FDA's rendition of the 1931 report is fairly accurate. The original report, however, is a sham. All 22 of Smithburn's patients died after receiving thimerosal, seven within the first day and most by the end of the second day.[9] The fact that "7 of 22 subjects were observed for only one day" is probably true; it's hard to observe dead subjects.

The FDA learned the truth about Smithburn's study at least as early as 2002, when a whistleblower provided lawyers with internal Eli Lilly records documenting the study details.[10] That FDA would continue to make the claim that Dr. Smithburn's dead subjects experienced "no reported toxic effects" is reprehensible, just as reprehensible and just as mathematically irresponsible as St. Paul Offit's claim that babies can safely receive 100,000 jabs.

Congressman Burton's Mercury in Medicine Report is a scathing indictment of government's negligence and mismanagement of the use of thimerosal in vaccines. Among other things, the report demonstrated that the amount of thimerosal in vaccines far exceeds government recommendations.

In the course of regulating mercury, different government agencies have established different minimum risk levels for daily exposure to the toxicant. Exposure to less than the minimum risk level is believed to be safe, while exposure that exceeds that level is believed to increase the chances of injury. All of the levels apply specifically to ingested methylmercury.

The EPA established the most conservative level: 0.1 micrograms of mercury per kilogram of body weight per day. Under this standard, an 11-pound baby (roughly 5 kilograms) could be exposed to up to 0.5 micrograms of mercury per day and be considered safe. Yet this exposure standard level is only a tiny fraction of the 25 micrograms of mercury per vaccine that American children received in several vaccines in the 1990s and that children in many developing countries continue to receive.[11] By this standard, a baby would have to weigh 550 pounds (250 kilograms) to safely receive one vaccine containing 25 micrograms of thimerosal.

It's important to note that the EPA's safe exposure limit for methylmercury is based on adult exposure, not bolus doses (a quantity of fluid or medication given intravenously at a controlled, rapid rate) at birth and early childhood. And ". . . none of the Federal guidelines on mercury exposure have . . . included specific provisions for safe exposure limits for infants and children," this according to the Mercury in Medicine Report. "It is widely accepted that infants and young children would be five times more sensitive to the toxic effect of mercury or other neurotoxins than adults."[12]

Dr. Stephanie Cave's entire medical practice is the treatment of autistic children. She testified in the Subcommittee on Human Rights and Wellness hearing, stating that

[t]he bile production is minimal in infancy, making it more difficult for metals to be cleared from the body. When added to a vaccine, the

metals are even more dangerous because the vaccines trigger immune reactions that increase the permeability of the GI tract and the blood/brain barrier.[13]

Many people claim that the public has no cause for concern because methylmercury—the kind of mercury about which the public is warned when found in fish—is dangerous, while ethylmercury in vaccines is safe or at least not as dangerous. Scientists may quibble in their laboratories over which poison is more dangerous, but such quibbling is nonsense to parents. Poison is poison. And as stated previously, less poison does not equal safe, it equals less poisonous. Dr. George Lucier, the former director of the Environmental Toxicology Program at the National Institutes of Health, agrees with parents on this point. In 2001, he explained his position to the Institute of Medicine's Immunization Safety Review Committee, saying, "Ethylmercury is a neurotoxin. Infants may be more susceptible than adults. Ethylmercury should be considered equipotent to methylmercury as a developmental neurotoxin. This conclusion is clearly public health protective."[14]

In a 2002 Congressional hearing, Congressman Dave Weldon asked physician and researcher David Baskin, MD, about the relative toxicity of ethyl-versus methylmercury. Baskin replied,

> The cells that I showed you dying in cell culture are dying from ethylmercury. Those are human frontal brain cells. . . . most chemical compounds that are ethyl penetrate into cells better than methyl. . . . ethyl as a chemical compound pierces fat and penetrates fat much better than methyl.[15]

Boyd Haley, head of the chemistry department at the University of Kentucky and outspoken critic of government corruption, said,

> You couldn't even construct a study that shows thimerosal is safe. It's just too darn toxic. If you inject thimerosal into an animal, its brain will sicken. If you apply it to living tissue, the cells die. If you put it in a petri dish, the culture dies. Knowing these things, it would be shocking if one could inject it into an infant without causing damage.[16]

Haley adds his voice to several other researchers who have concluded that exposure to mercury in infancy reduces a child's intelligence, resulting in life-long diminished functioning as well as exorbitant costs to society.[17]

Which form of mercury is more toxic ignores the fact that public exposure to all forms of mercury is both toxic and virtually unavoidable. Dr. Jeffrey

Bradstreet testified in a 2002 Congressional hearing of his concern over "the almost complete absence of regard for compounding effect of thimerosal on preexisting mercury levels." Bradstreet added this disturbing statistic: "The NHANES [National Health and Nutrition Examination Survey] Study from the CDC had already established that perhaps one in ten children is born to mothers with elevated mercury burden."[18]

Scientists have been aware of the problems associated with thimerosal-containing vaccines for over 75 years. In 2014, Dr. Brian Hooker and Dr. Haley, together with five other researchers, published a paper that slammed the CDC for covering up the fact that thimerosal is toxic. The paper's abstract reads:

There are over 165 studies that have focused on thimerosal, an organic-mercury (Hg) based compound, used as a preservative in many child-hood vaccines, and found it to be harmful. Of these, 16 were conducted to specifically examine the effects of thimerosal on human infants or children with reported outcomes of death; acrodynia; poisoning; allergic reaction; malformations; auto-immune reaction; Well's syndrome; developmental delay; and neurodevelopmental disorders, including tics, speech delay, language delay, attention deficit disorder, and autism.[19]

The truth about thimerosal's toxicity began to emerge in 1935, when the Pitman-Moore Company tested the compound on dogs, leading to the conclusion that Lilly's safety claims about thimerosal "did not check with ours." They sent a letter to Lilly telling them that thimerosal "was unsuitable as a preservative in serum intended for use in dogs. . . ."[20]

Dr. Frank Engley discovered in 1948 that thimerosal is toxic down to "parts per billion." Decades later he would say,

Apparently the medical profession does not read the safety data sheets provided by Lilly and other chemical manufacturers made available to physicians, pharmacies, hospitals and health departments. It states for thimerosal: toxic, mutagen, allergen, hypersensitivity, alters genetic materials, may cause mild to severe mental retardation, may cause mild to severe motor coordination [impairment], all sounds a lot like autism.[21]

In 1973, Eli Lilly informed the FDA that thimerosal was nontoxic. Attorney Andy Waters filed papers in Texas alleging that Eli Lilly "lied to the FDA in a bid to avoid regulation." According to Waters, "[Eli Lilly] cited the fraudulent Jamieson and Powell study of 1930 [on dying meningitis patients] as its supporting scientific evidence. Despite knowledge to the contrary, Lilly continued to use the [study] to supports its conclusions that the product was safe and 'non-toxic.'"[22]

Emulating its corporate master, the FDA continues to deceive the American public and the world by citing the same fraudulent study that Eli Lilly cited in 1973 to deceive the FDA.[23] Evidently, the EPA doesn't buy the FDA's lies. According to the EPA's Toxicity Characteristic Leaching Procedure (TCLP) standard, many vaccines that are labeled preservative free still contain trace amounts of mercury—less than or equal to 1 microgram/0.5 mL—per dose. Even at this level, such vaccines exceed the TCLP standard; "therefore these vaccines, if deemed unusable, should be managed as hazardous waste as well."[24]

Robert F. Kennedy, Jr. writes of a 1977 Russian study that "found that the majority of adults who were exposed to much lower concentrations of ethyl mercury than those given to American children in vaccines were still suffering neurological injury and neuropathology several years after the exposure."[25]

In what looked like a rare moment of sanity, the FDA made a recommendation in 1982 that thimerosal be banned from topical over-the-counter products.[26] But it made no such recommendation for injected thimerosal in vaccines. It failed to finalize the ban on OTC use of thimerosal until 1998, nearly two decades after it had declared the neurotoxin as "not generally recognized as safe."[27]

So much for sanity!

In 1986, Congress created the National Childhood Vaccine Injury Act (NCVIA) to compensate victims of vaccine injury and to shield manufacturers from vaccine-related liability. The act was passed in good faith based on widespread belief in the dogma espoused by the Vaccine religion. Vaccine injury, according to believers, is an unfortunate and unavoidable sacrifice offered on behalf of the greater good. But properly indoctrinated members of the Church who believe propaganda like being injected with up to 100,000 vaccines is safe never could have anticipated the risk in adding half a dozen or so shots to the schedule. In their bamboozled state, in 1988 they added a newly reformulated Hib vaccine to the childhood schedule involving four jabs in the first year starting at two months of age. According to David Kirby, author of the *New York Times* bestseller *Evidence of Harm*, "Some, but not all, brands of Hib vaccine contained 25 micrograms of ethylmercury—each."[28]

In 1990, the World Health Organization met to discuss the problem of allergic reactions to thimerosal in vaccines. Internet blogger Jon Christian Ryter wrote,

> The concern expressed by WHO in 1990 with respect to methylmercury or ethylmercury, the metabolized form of thimerosal, was that there existed no international recommendations on the maximum allowable intake of this chemical in infants and small children.

Because standards did not exist, WHO was concerned that the accumulated [e]ffect of more than 200 [micrograms] of methylmercury in the system of a fetus or infant could cause moderate to severe brain damage that would result in a rise in learning impaired children.[29]

In 1991, the FDA showed more regard for pets than for newborn babies when it "considered banning thimerosal from animal vaccines"[30] and simultaneously licensed the hepatitis B vaccine, which also contained thimerosal. The schedule called for three jabs in the first year, each containing 12.5 micrograms of mercury, with the first administered at birth.[31]

The "birth dose" is an important part of the controversy surrounding the commercialization of the hepatitis B vaccine, but it begs the question, Why would the government add a vaccine to the schedule for hepatitis B—a disease predominantly found among intravenous drug users and the sexually promiscuous? When parents posed this question to Dr. Neal Halsey, "one of the architects of US vaccine policy," he replied, "Because we can."[32]

When Halsey says, "Because we can," it's important to know who the "we" are. The US House of Representatives' Committee on Government Reform provided the answer in 2000 in its "Conflicts of Interest in Vaccine Policy Making" report:

> Dr. Halsey serves on the advisory board to the Immunization Action Coalition, an advocacy group funded by vaccine makers including: Aventis Pasteur, Chiron Corporation, Glaxo Wellcome, Merck & Co., Nabi, North American Vaccine, SmithKline-Beecham, Wyeth-Lederle Vaccines.[33]

In addition, Halsey is employed at Johns Hopkins University, where he has sought out "start-up funds from most of the vaccine manufacturers for the establishment of an institute for vaccine safety. . . ." On top of that, he has "received $50,000 from Merck and was awaiting funds from Wyeth Lederle. He has received frequent reimbursements for travel expenses and honoraria from companies such as Merck."[34] But wait, there's more:

> Dr. Halsey also participated in the rotavirus working group of the ACIP [CDC's Advisory Committee on Immunization Practices]. Also, Dr. Halsey was the Chair of the [AAP] Committee on Infectious Diseases and representative of the American Academy of Pediatrics which, in conjunction with the CDC, sets and advertises the recommendations for schedules and dosages of immunizations.[35]

Halsey and associates could have also gone to the trouble to add up the total potential thimerosal exposure before turning a generation of children into what would later be called the thimerosal generation (1989–2003), but neither he nor anyone else in the government did so until 1997, and then only after outraged parents spurred Congress "to pass a law called the Food and Drug Administration (FDA) Modernization Act. The Act required the FDA to review the use of mercury in pediatric vaccine, foods, and other products."[36]

In Kirby's book *Evidence of Harm*, the investigative researcher provides the figures that the FDA didn't bother to add up:

> . . . The CDC's immunization advisory committee, by voting to add four Hib and three hep-B shots to the schedule, had saddled some kids with an additional 137.5 micrograms of ethylmercury during their first, most vulnerable year. Prior to 1988, only the DTP shot had mercury (four shots with 25 micrograms each). In just three years, total potential exposure leapt from 100 micrograms to 237.5 micrograms. And these figures did not account for additional maternal exposures from Rho(D) and the flu shot.[37]

Halsey told the *New York Times* in 2002 how he and others felt upon learning how much thimerosal babies had received for over a decade due to his influence in the national vaccine program:

> My first reaction was simply disbelief, which was the reaction of almost everybody involved in vaccines. In most vaccine containers, thimerosal is listed as a mercury derivative, a hundredth of a percent. And what I believed, and what everybody else believed, was that it was truly a trace, a biologically-insignificant amount. My honest belief is that if the labels had had the mercury content in micrograms, this would have been uncovered years ago. But the fact is, no one did the calculation.[38]

Halsey's admission that the amount of thimerosal used in vaccines was the result of belief—not science—sends a chilling message to the parents who participated in injuring their children due to their belief in the High Priests in the Vaccine religion. But Halsey's follow-up admission is far more chilling than the first: "My first concern was that it would harm the credibility of the immunization program. But gradually it came home to me that maybe there was some real risk to the children."

There it is in print in the *New York Times*: Halsey's first concern was harming the credibility of the immunization program. Harming millions of American children with toxic levels of thimerosal was a mere afterthought—an afterthought that the vaccine cartel could not allow to stand.

Four days after Halsey's statement hit the press, his employer, Johns Hopkins Bloomberg School of Public Health, issued a retraction on behalf of Halsey. The title of the press release included the recitation of the one of the most important doctrines in The Vaccinology Church: "Neal Halsey Reaffirms Vaccines Do Not Cause Autism." The press release spoke of Halsey in the third person. "Neal Halsey, MD, . . . does not and has not supported the belief that thimerosal or vaccines themselves cause autism in children, saying scientific evidence does not suggest any causal association between any vaccine and autism."[39]

Johns Hopkins stated that the *New York Times* misrepresented Halsey and called for a correction. The *Times* obliged the following day:

> An article and a subheading in *The Times Magazine* on Sunday about the possibility of a link between brain development in children and thimerosal, a preservative formerly used in vaccines, misstated the views of Dr. Neal Halsey, a Johns Hopkins researcher. Dr. Halsey says that when he described thimerosal injury as a possibility that "must be addressed," he was referring to developmental delay, not to autism. Thus the subheading—under the title "The Not-So-Crackpot Autism Theory" — erred in saying of a possible autism link that Dr. Halsey "thinks it's an issue worth investigating."[40]

Halsey undoubtedly learned from his masters that honest statements to the press would not be tolerated. And the public—the vaccine informed public, that is—learned the same thing. They also learned that behind naïve vaccine believers are vaccine sociopaths whose primary interest is the health of the vaccine program, not the health of the public. Representative Burton's Mercury in Medicine Report summarized as much by declaring:

> It is clear that the guiding principal for FDA policymakers has been to avoid shaking the public's confidence in the safety of vaccines. For this reason, many FDA officials have stubbornly denied that thimerosal may cause adverse reactions. Ironically, the FDA's unwillingness to address this issue more forcefully, and remove thimerosal from vaccines earlier, may have done more long-term damage to the public's trust in vaccines than confronting the problem head-on. Given the serious concerns about the safety of thimerosal, the FDA should have acted years earlier to remove this preservative from vaccines and other medicines.[41]

In summary, government scientists have known for decades that thimerosal is a potent neurotoxin and claims to the contrary are motivated by the mandate "to avoid shaking the public's confidence in the safety of vaccines." That mandate continues today as evidenced by the following lies on a CDC webpage titled "Frequently Asked Questions about thimerosal":

Is thimerosal safe?

Yes. thimerosal has been used safely in vaccines for a long time (since the 1930s).

Scientists have been studying the use of thimerosal in vaccines for many years. They haven't found any evidence that thimerosal causes harm.

Is thimerosal still used in vaccines for children?

No. Thimerosal hasn't been used in vaccines for children since 2001.

However, thimerosal is still used in some flu vaccines. Yearly flu vaccines are recommended for all children. If you are worried about thimerosal, you can ask for a flu vaccine without it.

Does thimerosal cause autism?

No. Research does not show any link between thimerosal and autism.[42]

The webpage would be been more accurately titled, "Phony Answers to Frequently Asked Questions About Thimerosal," but apparently the CDC is allergic to accuracy.

Many European countries banned the use of thimerosal in the early 1990s. In 2009, the US Congress failed to implement even a partial ban when it "considered, but did not pass, legislation (H.R. 2617) that would have banned the administration of mercury containing vaccines to pregnant women and children under age six with certain exceptions."[43]

That didn't stop six states—California, Delaware, Illinois, Missouri, New York, and Washington—from issuing their own bans on thimerosal in vaccines for use on pregnant women and children. The details vary from state to state. At first glance, they appear to protect their citizens from thimerosal-containing vaccines, but if public health officials declare that they're short on thimerosal-free vaccines, they can petition the appropriate authority, receive permission, and inject children and pregnant women with thimerosal-containing vaccines just as they did before the laws were passed.[44]

This scenario played out in California in the fall of 2015 when Kris E. Calvin, executive director of the American Academy of Pediatrics-CA, Susan Hogeland, the CAE executive vice president of the California Academy of Family Physicians, and Erika Jenssen, MPH, the president of the California Immunization Coalition, sent a letter to Diana Dooley, the secretary of Health and Human Services Agency in California, requesting a "temporary exemption for use of thimerosal-containing vaccine."[45]

The letter addressed the shortage and included a dramatic plea that might have made vaccine believers cry and the vaccine informed vomit:

Physicians across California are reporting that delays of preservative-free flu vaccine are resulting in significant missed opportunities for vaccination and protection of vulnerable members of our community—hundreds of parents who desire the flu vaccine for their infants and toddlers are being turned away. Many young children and pregnant women may be at risk for serious disease and even death if providers are legally prohibited from administering flu vaccine that contains thimerosal, which is safe and effective for these groups.[46]

Of course, Ms. Dooley granted her approval with attendant pomp and drama. State laws banning the use of thimerosal-containing vaccines provide citizens with only the illusion of protection against thimerosal and governmental collusion with industry, yet they provide vaccine sociopaths with the means to profit from the poisoning of America's most vulnerable citizens.[47]

With thimerosal levels far above EPA safety guidelines, it is no surprise that the autism epidemic exploded in the 1990s. Ever-increasing numbers of American parents watched their children "regress" after routine childhood vaccinations. "They were fine until they got their shots, and then they just faded away" became a story heard again and again across the country. Paul Thomas, MD, author of the 2016 book *The Vaccine Friendly Plan*, described the story from his perspective as a pediatrician:

I saw it once a year from 2004 to 2008 where a one-year-old was totally normal at one, good eye contact, starting to talk, starting to walk, and then after their one-year-old vaccines which included the MMR, either immediately or within weeks, sometimes a few times within months they lost all eye contact, all speech, and to look into the eyes of a little one who's gone blank, it's heartbreaking.[48]

Parents of vaccine-injured children eventually connected with one another and connected the dots: no matter what their doctors or the CDC told them, they knew it was the vaccines, and many believed that thimerosal was to blame. Needless to say, they were outraged. They had trusted their government. They had vaccinated their children to protect them, not to destroy their minds and their lives. It was at this stage that many parents first discovered that the government had taken away their right to sue vaccine manufacturers and had left them with the National Vaccine Injury Compensation Program or "Vaccine Court" as it is commonly called.

Originally designed to be a salve to a few unfortunate victims of vaccine injury, the Vaccine Injury Compensation Program morphed into yet another jab from the government that had betrayed its citizenry. Attorney Robert Krakow described that betrayal in a 2010 Chicago gathering:

> [The Department of Justice] will deny your reality. They'll deny your word. They'll say you're lying. They'll say you made it up. They'll say you're mistaken. They'll say you're very well-educated so you know how to game the system. And then you'll come up against the full weight of their authority—expert witnesses with unlimited funds who will say that your child's injury is genetic, genetic, genetic. You'll find obstruction in the Department of Justice. You'll find resistance. You'll find scorn.[49]

In 1996, the problems with the Vaccine Court gained increased public attention when *Money Magazine* published an article written by Andrea Rock titled "The Lethal Dangers of the Billion-Dollar Vaccine Business." According to Rock:

> A 1986 law promoted by the drug industry dramatically limits vaccine manufacturers' legal liability in cases where their products cause injury or death. . . . the reform effectively removed one of the drug industry's most compelling incentives to ensure that its products are as safe as possible. . . . the damages awarded are not paid by drug companies; they are paid by you—in the form of a user tax tacked onto the price of each vaccination.[50]

Alan Phillips, an attorney who represents parents of vaccine injured children, summed up the entire vaccine program as a racket:

> The federal government subsidizes vaccine research and development to the tune of billions of dollars each year. The federal government passed laws removing the vaccine manufacturers liability from the death and disability caused by their products. State and federal governments mandate vaccines. State and federal governments purchase vaccines, and the federal government compensates those who manage to successfully get through the Vaccine Injury Compensation Program. This is the biggest racket anywhere on the planet.[51]

Barbara Loe Fisher, director of the National Vaccine Information Center, played a part in the creation of the Vaccine Court, and she was hopeful that it would fulfill its intended purpose. According to the testimony Fisher shared before the California State Senate Committee on Health and Human Services in 2002, it did nothing of the kind:

I worked with Congress in the early 1980s on that [vaccine compensation] law and watched it be turned into a cruel joke as 2 out of 3 vaccine injured children are denied federal compensation for their often catastrophic vaccine injuries because HHS [Department of Health and Human Services] and the Department of Justice officials fight every claim, viewing every award to a vaccine injured child as admission that vaccines can and do cause harm.[52]

Many parents, however, won their cases in the adversarial "court" proceedings, including dozens of parents whose children regressed into autism after receiving their shots. The Elizabeth Birt Center for Autism Law & Advocacy (EBCALA) ferreted out such cases by interviewing parents who had filed claims with the Vaccine Injury Compensation Program. The report, published in a peer-reviewed law journal, examined "claims that the VICP compensated for vaccine-induced encephalopathy and seizure disorder." EBCALA posted an article on its website describing the findings in their report:

This study found 83 cases of acknowledged vaccine-induced brain damage that include autism, a disorder that affects speech, social communication and behavior. In 21 published cases of the Court of Federal Claims, which administers the VICP, the Court stated that the petitioners had autism or described autism unambiguously. In 62 remaining cases, the authors identified settlement agreements where Health and Human Services (HHS) compensated children with vaccine-induced brain damage, who also have autism or an autism spectrum disorder.[53]

Members of the medical cartel, mainstream media, and astroturf bloggers specialize in confusing the public with word games regarding vaccine-induced autism. Here is one of many examples:

Ryan [a boy whose parents received compensation from the NVIC] did not have autism. He had encephalitis (inflammation of the brain) which caused brain injury. This can cause symptoms which superficially might resemble autism (to a non-expert), but it's not autism.[54]

Investigative reporter Jon Rappoport has little tolerance with the games adults play to obfuscate the reality of vaccine-induced injury including autism:

Whether you call vaccine damage autism or encephalopathy or developmental delay or some other cooked-up name, the central event is the same: a child was vaccinated; the child was severely injured. The child's brain and nervous system took a heavy, heavy blow.

There are no mitigating circumstances or clever terms to cover up the fact.

The children and the parents are the living evidence of harm.

Don't let this go. Don't let the truth slip away.[55]

It's important to note that autism is only one of many disorders linked to thimerosal. Reverend Lisa K. Sykes, a proponent for safer vaccines, writes,

Published studies have shown that thimerosal and its mercury break-down product contribute to: Alzheimer's, Cancer, Autism Spectrum Disorders, Attention Deficit Disorders, Bipolar Disorder, Asthma, Sudden Infant Death Syndrome, Arthritis, Food Allergies, Premature Puberty, and Infertility.[56]

In addition, vaccines are associated with over 200 known medical issues, symptoms, conditions, and diseases, but autism is the condition that strikes the greatest fear in most parents. Therefore, autism is the condition that most scares the vaccine industry. When parents started beating on the doors of the Vaccine Court in the 1990s, the industry and the government knew it had a crisis on their hands, not the crisis of angry parents or vaccine-injured children, but the crisis of an increasingly savvy and informed public—a public that couldn't be allowed to abandon the sacred cow of public health and kill the cash cow of vaccine industry profiteers. But thimerosal was just the beginning. The Church of Vaccinology was about to run head-on into a doctor who would soon threaten the entire vaccine paradigm. The threat originated in the unorthodox and dangerous behavior the physician exhibited with parents of vaccine injured children: he listened to them.

Chapter Thirteen

DR. ANDREW WAKEFIELD: THE VACCINE INDUSTRY'S WORST NIGHTMARE

You do not become a "dissident" just because you decide one day to take up this most unusual career. You are thrown into it by your personal sense of responsibility, combined with a complex set of external circumstances. You are cast out of the existing structures and placed in a position of conflict with them. It begins as an attempt to do your work well, and ends with being branded an enemy of society.[1]

—Václav Havel

Dr. Andrew Wakefield received his medical degree from St. Mary's Hospital Medical School (part of the University of London) in 1981 and pursued a career in gastrointestinal surgery with a particular interest in inflammatory bowel disease. He has published over 130 original scientific articles, book chapters, and invited scientific commentaries.

With such credentials, Wakefield was a High Priest among Priests in the church of modern medicine. Yet, even High Priests sometimes go astray. His undoing started in the early 1990s, when his research into a possible cause of Crohn's disease led him to an unlikely suspect: the measles virus. He published a 1993 study titled "Evidence of persistent measles virus infection in Crohn's disease" and coauthored a 1995 article published in *The Lancet*. Did he know at the time that even the title of the article—"Is measles vaccine a risk factor for inflammatory bowel disease?"—bordered on vaccine heresy?[2, 3]

Wakefield's paper resonated with parents of autistic children, some of whom believed that the MMR vaccine was the catalyst for their children's regression into autism. When the first of such parents approached Wakefield, he said that he was a gastroenterologist and as such was not particularly informed about autism. The parent persisted, saying that her child suffered from gastrointestinal problems and that she believed those issues merited medical attention just as they would for any other child. Wakefield listened and learned from her and from the parents who followed.

By listening, Wakefield and his colleagues proved to be an anomaly in their profession. Parents had grown accustomed to dismissive or hostile reactions from professionals for having the audacity to suggest that the sacred cow of the Vaccine religion had gone rogue and stomped on their children. Wakefield learned from one couple long after he had examined their son that they had initially omitted the MMR-autism connection with Wakefield because:

> . . . the reaction of successive doctors to the suggestion that MMR might have been involved ranged from patronizingly dismissive to outright hostile. Mentioning the vaccine was beginning to negatively impact their ability to get help for their son. By the time they came to the Royal Free Hospital, the father had urged his wife not to mention the MMR again in order to avoid discrimination by doctors who considered her to be crazy.[4]

Anything but crazy, Wakefield believed the parents had stumbled onto something significant. He consulted with his colleagues, and together they decided to investigate the potential relationship between the MMR vaccine, autism, and what looked to be like a novel form of bowel disease. They studied 12 children with a similar array of symptoms. The parents of 8 of the 12 associated their children's regression and bowel disease with the triple jab. Wakefield—a vaccine believer—was alarmed at what he and his team were observing. Thirsting for additional knowledge, he scoured the available literature and wrote a 250-page manuscript on the documented risks associated with the MMR vaccine. He concluded that the triple-valent jab was unnecessarily unsafe and that children would be better served by receiving the three antigens—measles, mumps, and rubella—delivered in separate injections.

Wakefield's colleagues—also vaccine believers—expressed concern over the potential fallout from merely mentioning the possible role the MMR vaccine might play in the development of autism or bowel disease. Wakefield questioned if they would have the same reservation if the wild measles virus were implicated in their research. They concluded that truth must prevail, come what may.

The question Wakefield posed to his colleagues bears consideration. If their research had implicated the wild type measles virus instead of the triple jab, vaccine crusaders would have proclaimed Wakefield and his team as Prophets in The Church of Vaccinology. Viruses would be more frightening than ever and vaccines would be more powerful than ever. But it was not to be; the sacred cow of the church and the antivirus talisman might not be what the crusaders proclaimed it to be. Furthermore, Wakefield's research led him to conclude that the Church itself was nothing more than a house of cards.

The Royal Free Hospital organized a press conference to announce the results of the soon-to-be published paper. Wakefield thought it wise to inform his colleagues that, if asked, he would tell the press that he recommended the monovalent vaccines over the three-in-one MMR combination. That recommendation alone was surely enough to provoke retaliation from the UK's vaccine politburo. However, as seen in a few highlights from a letter Wakefield sent to his colleagues five weeks before their paper was to be published, the intrepid doctor was prepared not only to defend his position, but to attack the integrity and character of those who profess to serve the public good:

> . . . [I]f my opinion is sought, I cannot support the continued use of the polyvalent MMR vaccine.

> . . . [A]ttempts to sustain credence in MMR safety by quoting data from a surveillance scheme that is widely recognized to be inadequate and to dismiss parents' claims of a link between their child's disorder and MMR without due investigation, in breach of the most fundamental rules of clinical medicine is unacceptable. The failure of the regulatory authorities to honour their commitments to MMR vaccine safety has created a House-of-Cards that threatens all vaccine policies.

> . . . Doctors such as us, perceive a pattern to the disease and its links with the MMR that becomes self-evident. When the data are presented, the anger of many parents boils over, the press has a field day, and the House of Cards crashes to the ground.

> Loss of trust in the regulatory authorities is inevitable and vaccination compliance, across the board, is affected—a difficult and dangerous situation. There is no doubt in my mind that responsibility for this volatile state of affairs rests, not with us, but firmly upon the shoulders of the policy makers; that is, the JCVI [Joint Committee on Vaccination and Immunisation] and the Department of Health . . . . Any drug, and especially one that involves 3 live viruses, must be considered dangerous until proven otherwise; this has never been proven and, therefore, all claims of adverse events should have been thoroughly investigated. They have failed to honour this obligation.

> In an attempt to avert the House-of-Cards collapsing, I will strongly recommend the use of monovalent vaccines as opposed to the polyvalent vaccines.[5]

Wakefield was one of 13 prominent physicians and researchers who were about to sign off on *The Lancet* paper. These were not "just some mothers" to be dismissed. They were medical professionals who refused to dismiss the parents and affected children who had come into their offices, and these professionals were about to expose and potentially bring down the UK's vaccine program.

It is doubtful that Wakefield had any inkling at the time of the penalty he would pay for challenging the multibillion-dollar vaccine industry. If he had known, he probably would not have acted any differently. Just as he had argued with his colleagues, the truth must prevail, come what may. And just as he had promised his colleagues, when the press asked him about the MMR vaccine, he recommended the monovalent vaccines as the safer choice.

That pronouncement set in motion a chain of events that would eventually lead to the retraction of the ill-fated paper and the delicensing of Wakefield and his colleague, Professor John Walker-Smith, a man described as one of the world's leading pediatric gastroenterologists. Contrary to what highly placed individuals later claimed, the paper did not state that the case series proved that the MMR vaccine causes autism. It stated the opposite. "We did not prove an association between measles, mumps and rubella vaccine and the syndrome described. Virological studies are underway that may help to resolve this issue."[6]

Ironically, the British government responded to Wakefield's recommendation for using monovalent vaccines by removing them from the market, forcing parents to choose either to receive the triple jab or to abstain from the vaccine altogether. Predictably, measles vaccination rates declined. However, Wakefield, and not the British government, was blamed for later disease outbreaks.[7]

In 2004, Dr. Richard Horton, editor of *The Lancet*, held a news conference and announced that the 1998 paper was "fatally flawed," not because the information presented in the case series was incorrect, but because Wakefield had failed to disclose alleged conflicts of interest. British reporter Brian Deer detailed those alleged conflicts in the *Sunday Times*. Deer also informed the British General Medical Council of the alleged conflicts. The GMC then initiated a multiyear, multimillion-dollar show trial, which climaxed in written findings announced in January and in April of 2010, followed by a written decision on May 24, 2010, concluding "that Dr. Wakefield and Professor Walker-Smith were guilty of serious professional misconduct. . . . It ordered that the names of Dr. Wakefield and Professor Walker-Smith be erased from the register of medical practitioners."[8]

On February 6, 2010, *The Lancet* retracted the offending article because "the claims in the original paper that children were 'consecutively referred' and that investigations were 'approved' by the local ethics committee have been proven to be false."[9] The global media machine dutifully reported both the GMC ruling and *The Lancet*'s retraction. Wakefield was a huckster, and his claim that the

MMR triple jab caused autism (a claim neither Wakefield nor his colleagues ever made) was false. Vaccines are safe and effective. Wash. Rinse. Repeat.

Dr. Wakefield shared the story the media refused to tell in his 2010 book, *Callous Disregard: Autism and Vaccines—the Truth Behind a Tragedy*. Not light reading, Wakefield detailed the minutiae of these events, both defending his honor and exposing the fraudsters who accused him of fraud.

The opening paragraph from the book's prologue essentially summarized the contents of the book:

> If autism does not affect your family now, it will. If something does not change—and change soon—this is almost a mathematical certainty. This book affects you also. It is not a parochial look at a trivial medical spat in the UK, but dispatches from the battlefront in a major confrontation—a struggle against compromise in medicine, corruption of science, and a real and present threat to children in the interests of policy and profit. It is a story of how "the system" deals with dissent among its doctors and scientists.[10]

Wakefield declares that the great vaccine crusaders—those who place vaccine compliance above vaccine safety—are anti-vaccine. "Those who are a threat to public confidence, those who do not mandate a safety first agenda, are the greatest threat to the vaccine program; they are ultimately anti-vaccine."[11]

In the book's afterword, written by Wakefield and attorney James Moody, the two men make a final plea and a final denunciation of the increasingly corrupt vaccine system:

> Politicians, regulators, manufacturers, attorneys, bloggers, and hangers-on: Act now to protect children. Act now to protect the benefits of the vaccine program. Put **safety first** above any other consideration. Insist on this, Mr. and Mrs. Gates.

> There is no place for indulging futile displacement activity, sanctimonious posturing, and self-protectionism. In the battle for the hearts and minds of the public, you have already lost. Why? Because the parents are right; their stories are true; their children's brains are damaged; there is a major, major problem. In the US, increasingly coercive vaccine mandates and fear-mongering advertising campaigns are a measure of your failure—vaccine uptake is not a reflection of public confidence, but of these coercive measures, and without public confidence, you have nothing [emphasis in original].[12]

Professor Walker-Smith appealed the GMC's ruling to the British High Court, giving the judiciary the opportunity to rule on his integrity, but financial considerations prevented Wakefield from following through with his own appeal. This was the first time the case had been heard in a proper legal setting. Inasmuch as the GMC had charged Walker-Smith and Wakefield with nearly identical charges, one may rightly assume that the court's findings on Walker-Smith also apply to Wakefield. What took the GMC years to deliberate took Justice Mitting just five days to quash. He summarized that:

> . . . the panel's overall conclusion that Professor Walker-Smith was guilty of serious professional misconduct was flawed, in two respects: inadequate and superficial reasoning and, in a number of instances, a wrong conclusion. . . .

> The panel's determination cannot stand. I therefore quash it. . . . The end result is that the finding of serious professional misconduct and the sanction of erasure are both quashed.[13]

The great media machine, including the *Sunday Times*, failed to report the judge's decision. *The Lancet* also failed to reverse its retraction of the Wakefield et al. paper.

In the perfect world, people and personalities would play but a minor role in science. The focus would lie almost exclusively on hypotheses, transparent studies, and empirical conclusions. But, as Wakefield discovered, the world of science and medicine in which he functioned for so many years is far from perfect. There are commandments that are not to be broken. There are penalties for breaking those commandments, and they increase based on one's position in the Church.

Wakefield, a High Priest, broke three primary commandments:

1. Thou shalt not question the safety of a vaccine or impugn the integrity of the chief vaccine crusaders.
2. Thou shalt not suggest that a particular vaccine might be linked to autism.
3. Thou shalt not suggest that parents have a right to choose which vaccines they will and will not allow their children to receive.

By breaking these commandments, the medical pharisees turned Wakefield into a latter-day scapegoat. The ruling elite imbued his name and character with evil. Less man and more symbol, his opprobrium provided reassurance to vaccine believers around the world. Vaccines do not cause autism. And the only man who ever said differently was a fraud. Germs are bad. Vaccines are good. Vaccines save lives. In vaccines we trust. All is well in The Church of Vaccinology.

Never mind that in the USA, the Vaccine Injury Compensation Program has been compensating parents of vaccine-injured autistic children for more than twenty years.[14] Never mind that several peer-reviewed, published studies corroborate the findings of Wakefield and his twelve colleagues.[15] Never mind that thousands of parents have witnessed in helpless horror the harm done to their children by the MMR and other vaccines. Never mind that in worshipping the vaccine golden calf, humanity has exchanged childhood diseases that strengthen the immune system for chronic diseases, disabilities, and unnecessary deaths.

Wakefield's inquisition resulted in three major legacies:

1. It gave a temporary reprieve to the inevitable fall of the house of cards Wakefield sought to bring down, giving credence to the deception that vaccines are equally safe and equally effective, and strengthening the myth that vaccines do not cause autism.
2. It sent a warning message to vaccinators around the world: dissidents will be punished. Wakefield and James Moody describe in detail the hostile political climate medical professionals face if they so much as question the vaccine paradigm.

Doctors just won't take the risk of a protracted investigation that may be for collateral purposes such as the settling of scores, much less of losing their license, and will settle in to the safe mediocrity of doling out medicine "by the books." Medicine will no longer be a learned profession, but just a series of rote steps performed mechanically and utterly without inspiration. Patients' care will suffer, which is exactly the opposite of GMC's supposed mission. Although all of medicine will suffer, the impact will be most immediately borne by the most severely ill autistic children. They will continue to be denied the diagnosis and care that is their basic human and ethical right.[16]

3. It bolstered the idea that autism is a brain disease best treated by psychotropic medications, and by so doing it consigned suffering children and their suffering parents to medical providers who are blinded to the medical components of autism. More important, these benighted professionals also fail to see autism, autoimmune disorders, endocrine disorders, neurological disorders, gastrointestinal disorders, nervous disorders, etc., for what they are in far too many cases: iatrogenic conditions delivered through ever-increasing numbers of vaccines. The third legacy encourages

intolerant doctors to amp up their intolerance, pitting parents of vaccine injured children against arrogant white-coated fools.

The day the GMC stripped Wakefield of his license was also the day the GMC verified and cemented its corrupt relationship with the global vaccine industry. Elite members of the PharMafia cheered at the news of Wakefield's modern-day witch-burning ritual. Attorney James Moody was present and documented one of the celebrations:

. . . [T]he announcement of the retraction of *The Lancet* paper following the January 28, 2010, GMC findings was proclaimed at the February 4, 2010, meeting of the National Vaccine Advisory Committee (which advises the Secretary of Health and Human Services on vaccine policy). This was greeted with cheers and "high fives" from the federal and public health elite in attendance. My public comment at the end of the meeting simply pointed out that this Orwellian effort to erase history and the contributions made to science by these 12 children [in the original study] will not succeed.[17]

In the long run, Moody is right. The GMC's show trial will go down in history as a farce. But in the short run, the farce is also a tragedy. Countless numbers of children and their parents suffer needlessly, and far too often they encounter indifference, accusations, hostility, and grossly inappropriate care for their vaccine-injured autistic children.

Alex Spourdalakis was one such child. His mother and godmother dragged their nonverbal son from doctor to doctor and hospital to hospital begging for help with Alex, who they believed was suffering from severe and painful gastrointestinal issues. The professionals prescribed dozens of pharmaceuticals for diseases the boy did not have, they strapped him to his bed for several days, and in the end, they threatened to remove him from his mother's care and have him institutionalized. But they refused to treat the cause of his pain. When professionals fail in such situations, desperate parents—the people who love their children the most—sometimes resort to desperate means to alleviate their children's suffering.

Wakefield—stronger and more determined than ever to bring down the house of cards—produced the documentary film *Who Killed Alex Spourdalakis?*[18] Viewers are left with no doubt: the failure of medical professionals to recognize and treat what Wakefield and his colleagues had discovered in 1998, the failure to even consider the medical components of autism, and the failure of medical professionals to listen to their patients resulted in an unnecessary catastrophe. That catastrophe is now playing out to one degree or another in virtually every clinic and hospital around the world. And it will continue to play out until sufficient numbers of vaccine-informed people join with Wakefield to protect children, families, freedom, and democracy from vaccine sociopaths and their vaccine mandates. Wakefield doesn't mince words when he speaks of industry corruption and autism:

> This is the most important issue in America today. Forget foreign policy, forget everything else. If this is going to continue, there is no economy, there is no foreign policy. And the irony is that even without a standing army, no one is going to want to invade this country because it is a country of damaged people.[19]

As long as vaccine believers believe the lies told about Wakefield, they will be powerless to stand up to the corrupt Church in which they worship. The Church elite—not Wakefield—are guilty of perfidy. Also guilty of perfidy are Wakefield's colleagues who ran for cover, leaving him to face the farce of the General Medical Council's show trial. Also perfidious are those in the medical profession who know that the vaccine paradigm is built upon fraud and corruption, who, even in their knowledge, vaccinate pregnant women, premature infants, babies, toddlers, teens, and the aged.

In the world of vaccines, Andrew Wakefield is a litmus test. Vaccine believers despise him. The vaccine informed hold him in high regard. Vaccine sociopaths fear him, and their fear is well founded. Wakefield is on a mission to protect children, which means he is on a mission to bring the vaccine industry to its knees. But when the GMC wrongfully stripped him of his license and media "presstitutes" churned out lies regarding his case, millions of minds closed and millions of hearts hardened against anything Wakefield had to say or do. To open their minds and their hearts, the message of industry corruption would have to come from another source. It would have to come from the inside, it would have to come from what most people believe is the heart of the vaccine program: the Centers for Disease Control and Prevention.

That day would not come until 2014, but in 1998 the CDC had other battles to fight. The MMR vaccine and thimerosal had united as a two-headed monster threatening to destroy the vaccine program and vaccine profits. Were the CDC power brokers powerful enough to overcome the threats? Were they cunning enough to pull off what Wakefield would later describe as ". . . the greatest medical fraud in the history of the world"?[20]

They were up for the fight. Other than the health of the children they profess to protect, their careers and reputations, their freedom and possibly their lives, they had nothing to lose.

Chapter Fourteen

CRISIS AND DAMAGE CONTROL

I'm so ticked off about my grandson, and to think that the public-health people have been circling the wagons to cover up the facts!
Why, it just makes me want to vomit![1]
—Representative Dan Burton, Congressional Hearing, June 2002

By 1999, the link between thimerosal and autism as well as non-thimerosal containing vaccines and autism was not new information to vaccine insiders. As previously mentioned, the Vaccine Court had awarded compensation to dozens of parents whose children had regressed into autism following vaccinations. Original MMR and DTaP package inserts included autism as a possible side effect. (Autism magically disappeared as a side effect in subsequent package inserts as well as from various government and other industry-influenced websites.)[2, 3, 4, 5]

The problem for the vaccine industry was not that vaccines cause autism; the problem was that the industry was losing control of the vaccine story. People were connecting to the Internet, connecting with one another, and learning that the pretty public story of vaccines was really an ugly illusion.

The magicians might have been able to maintain the deception if they had maintained a vaccine schedule from a former era. Paralyzing children with the polio vaccine made sense to people still paralyzed with the fear of polio, but injuring and killing children with the highly reactive DTP vaccine made less sense. Giving newborn babies the neurotoxin thimerosal on the day of birth for the unnecessary Hepatitis B vaccine made no sense at all. And when The Church launched its crusade against chickenpox in 1995, it further trivialized its salvational role. In addition to chickenpox, the government saw fit to add the Hepatitis A vaccine to the schedule in 1995 as well as the rotavirus vaccine in 1998. With chickenpox, people at least knew about the disease, and many could therefore be convinced of the utility of the vaccine. But how many children in the neighborhood were suffering from Hepatitis A, and what the hell is rotavirus? A

Department of Health official from Oregon answered that question in 2009 and explained why the Beaver State didn't include it on its list of mandated vaccines: "Rotavirus is just some diarrhea for a day or two. It's just not a big deal. That one will never be on our list."[6] It was, however, a big deal when the original rotavirus vaccine was pulled from the schedule a few months after it was introduced because it had injured and killed too many babies even for the CDC.

Congress was not impressed. In 1999, legislators held hearings on the hepatitis B vaccine, vaccine safety, and the National Vaccine Injury Compensation Program (VICP). Questions multiplied. Charges of incompetence, ignorance, conflicts of interest, and greed became part of the dialogue in Washington, DC, and among the growing numbers of vaccine informed scientists, medical professionals, parents, and patients.

A war was brewing. Lined up on one side were the causalities of the vaccine program—former believers whose children's lives had been forever altered or lost entirely. A smattering of supporters stepped forward from every social class and from every profession: common folk as well as doctors, lawyers, scientists, clergy, professors, politicians, reporters, and celebrities.

Lined up on the other side was a multibillion-dollar industry that had created for itself unlimited growth potential with virtually zero accountability or liability. Supporters included a similar cast of lay individuals and professionals. Their numbers were enormous, their power limitless, and their influence endless.

Or so it seemed.

Public health officials—the Church proselytizers—had successfully maintained the façade of unity in their fight against infectious disease. But when the fight against disease turned into a fight against vaccine-injured children, dissension broke out among the Church elite.

For many, perhaps most, protecting the vaccine program was paramount. Never mind the fact that Church healers had ignorantly injected millions of babies with a potent neurotoxin in excess of every governmental guideline. Never mind the fact that parents of vaccine-injured children were overwhelming the Vaccine Court. Proponents of the Protect-The-Program-And-The-Public-Be-Damned paradigm knew that removing thimerosal from vaccines would be an admission of error and culpability, would reduce vaccination compliance, and, most important, would reduce profit margins.

The European Medicines Evaluation Agency (EMEA) met in London on April 19, 1999, to address the thimerosal issue. The EMEA is responsible for establishing guidelines for the use of drugs and biologics in the European Union.[7] The FDA's Dr. Norman Baylor was present. (Baylor is the man with the cheesy slide show from Chapter 5 who glosses over the issue of vaccine ingredients.) Two months later, the EMEA issued a statement that, no doubt, displeased the majority of American public health policy makers:

Vaccines: The fact that the target population for vaccines in primary immunization schedules is a healthy one, and in view of the demonstrated risks of thiomersal [*sic*] and other mercurial containing preservatives, precautionary measures (as outlined below) could be considered.

For vaccination in infants and toddlers, the use of vaccines without thimerosal . . . and other mercurial preservatives should be encouraged.[8]

The CDC's Advisory Committee on Immunization Practices (ACIP) met in Atlanta for two days starting on June 20, 1999. Guided by CDC officials, the committee concluded that it would maintain its no preference policy on the issue of thimerosal in vaccines. This in spite of the fact that manufacturers assured the CDC that they had the capacity to switch to thimerosal-free vaccines with little interruption in supply. Dr. Neal Halsey argued for at least a reduction in the amount of thimerosal a child should receive in one day. No serious consideration was given to his suggestion. In the end, financial considerations trumped the safety of American children as evidenced by CDC's Dr. Roger Bernier's repeated statements:

We think that having this type of a more staged transition reduces the potential for financial losses of existing inventories, and this is somewhat akin to what was done in the transition from oral polio to inactivated polio . . .

It could entail financial losses of inventory if current vaccine inventory is wasted. It could harm one or more manufacturers and may then decrease the number of suppliers. . . .

The evidence justifying this kind of abrupt policy change does not appear to exist, and it could entail financial losses for all existing stocks of vaccines that contain thimerosal.[9]

Representative Dan Burton may well have been thinking of his own vaccine-injured grandchild when he and his committee later castigated Bernier and the CDC for their disgraceful priorities:

The financial health of the industry should never have been a factor in this decision. The financial health of vaccine manufacturers certainly should never have been more important to the Federal health officials than the health and well being [of] the nation's children. . . . If there were any doubts about the neurological effects of ethylmercury in vaccines on children—and there were substantial doubts—the prevailing consideration should have been how best to protect children from potential harm. However, it appears that protecting the industry's profits took precedent [*sic*] over protecting children from mercury damage.[10]

On June 22nd, Dr. Halsey participated in an FDA meeting in which the topic of thimerosal in vaccines was discussed. The following day, Halsey wrote a letter to the members of the American Academy of Pediatrics Committee on Infectious Diseases, which he chaired:

In the past few days, I have become aware that the amount of thimerosal in most hepatitis B, DTaP, and Hib vaccines that we administer to infants results in a total dose of mercury that exceeds the maximum exposure recommended by the EPA, the FDA, CDC and WHO . . . .[11]

A former FDA official, Dr. Peter Patriarca, described in an email message to Martin Meyers, Acting Director of the National Vaccine Program Office at the CDC, the potential fallout from removing thimerosal from vaccines, stating that it would

. . . raise questions about FDA being "asleep at the switch" for decades by allowing a potentially hazardous compound to remain in many childhood vaccines, and not forcing manufacturers to exclude it from new products. It will also raise questions about various advisory bodies regarding aggressive recommendations for use. (We must keep in mind that the dose of ethylmercury was not generated by "rocket science". Conversion of the percentage thimerosal to actual micrograms of mercury involves ninth grade algebra. What took the FDA so long to do the calculations? Why didn't the CDC and the advisory bodies do these calculations when they rapidly expanded the childhood immunization schedule?)[12]

Dr. Elain Esber sent an email message to Linda Suydam, her colleague in the FDA, describing the Public Health Service's fear that stating a recommendation for thimerosal-free vaccines might ". . . result in unwarranted loss of confidence in immunization programs in the US and internationally, shortages of childhood vaccines might ensue, and other potential far-reaching ramifications are envisioned."[13]

Esber's use of the word "unwarranted" in this context demonstrates the profound bias of the majority of public health professionals in favor of vaccination over protecting the minds and bodies of American children from poisoning.

Dr. Ruth Enzel of the Department of Agriculture noted the same bias in a letter to three members of the American Academy of Pediatrics:

As you know, the Public Health Service informed us yesterday that they were planning to conduct business as usual, and would probably indicate no preference for either product. While the Public Health Service may think that their "product" is immunizations, I think their "product" is their recommendations. If the public loses faith in the PHS recommendations, then the immunization battle will falter. To keep faith, we must be open and honest now and move forward quickly to replace these products.[14]

On July 7, 1999, the AAP issued a joint statement with the US Public Health Service. The statement represented a compromise between those who wanted to remove thimerosal from vaccines and those who didn't. Representative Burton and committee summarized the statement with the following points:

- Acknowledged that some children may have been exposed to levels of mercury that exceed one Federal guideline on methylmercury during the first six months of life;
- Asserted that there is no evidence of any harm caused by thimerosal in vaccines;
- Called on vaccine manufacturers to make a clear commitment to reduce as expeditiously as possible the mercury content of their vaccines;
- Urged doctors and parents to immunize all children even if thimerosal-free vaccines are not available; and
- Encouraged doctors and parents to postpone the Hepatitis B vaccine (which contained thimerosal at the time and was generally given immediately after birth) until the child is two to six months old unless the mother tested positive for Hepatitis B.[15]

In August 1999, the National Vaccine Advisory Group and the Interagency Working Group on Vaccines met at Bethesda in the Lister Auditorium to discuss the thimerosal issue. As a result, thimerosal was banned from the hepatitis B vaccine, but American children continued to receive the neurotoxin until supplies were exhausted, approximately two to three years.[16]

The joint statement issued by the American Academy of Pediatrics and the Public Health Service put pressure on the CDC to announce its position on thimerosal. Accordingly, the CDC's Advisory Committee on Immunization Practices met on October 20th to review the situation. The committee concluded:

The risk, if any, to infants from exposure to thimerosal is believed to be slight. The demonstrated risks for not vaccinating children far outweigh the theoretical risk for exposure to thimerosal-containing vaccines during the first 6 months of life.

Given the availability of vaccines that do not contain thimerosal as a preservative, the progress in developing such additional vaccines, and the absence of any recognized harm from exposure to thimerosal in vaccines, hepatitis B, DTaP, and Hib vaccines that contain thimerosal as a preservative can continue to be used in the routine infant schedule beginning at age 2 months along with monovalent or combination vaccines that do not contain thimerosal as a preservative.[17]

The committee also warned against "failure to vaccinate newborns at high risk for perinatal hepatitis B virus . . ." and advised health care professionals to vaccinate all newborns—regardless of risk—with the hep B vaccine, whether or not the vaccine contained thimerosal.[18]

Russell Blaylock, MD, a harsh critic of CDC corruption, dressed down the ACIP for its ongoing allegiance to the pharmaceutical industry:

Now, we need to stop and think about what has transpired here. We have an important group here; the ACIP that . . . plays a role in vaccine policy that affects tens of millions of children every year. And, we have evidence from the thimerosal meeting in 1999 that the potential for serious injury to the infant's brain is so serious that a recommendation for removal becomes policy. In addition, they are all fully aware that tiny babies are receiving mercury doses that exceed even EPA safety limits, yet all they can say is that we must "try to remove thimerosal as soon as possible." Do they not worry about the tens of millions of babies that will continue receiving thimerosal-containing vaccines until they can get around to stopping the use of thimerosal?[19]

Congressman Burton also took a swing at the lackluster response from Federal officials:

Given the information that the Federal agencies had at the time, the plan of action laid out in the joint statement was inadequate.

They could have, but did not, acknowledge that the amount of thimerosal in vaccines exceeded every Federal guideline for exposure to methylmercury for the majority of infants. They could have, but did not, require vaccine manufacturers to remove thimerosal from vaccines by a specific date. They could have, but did not, urge pediatricians to choose thimerosal-free vaccines when both thimerosal-containing and thimerosal-free vaccines were available.

As a result of the limited steps taken in 1999, vaccines containing thimerosal remained on the market for nearly two years. GlaxoSmithKline's Hepatitis B vaccine did not become thimerosal-free until March of 2000, and Aventis Pasteur's DTaP vaccine did not become thimerosal-free until March 2001. In addition, thimerosal-containing vaccines on the shelves in doctor's offices around the country continued to be used in spite of the fact that thimerosal-free versions were available. The fact that more forceful action to remove thimerosal from the vaccine marketplace was not taken in 1999 is disappointing. Just as disappointing, and even more difficult to understand, is the fact that the CDC, on two separate occasions, refused to publicly state a preference for thimerosal-free vaccines.[20]

During the same time period, the *Journal of the American Medical Association* published an article in which the CDC advocated for restrictions against philosophical and/or religious exemptions to mandatory vaccinations, a position that that has since grown stronger.[21] Clearly, the government's long-term goal is mandatory vaccination regardless of vaccine contents.

In August, Burton and the Committee on Government Reform initiated an investigation into the Federal vaccine policy, starting at the top of the Department of Health and Human Services. Burton wrote to HHS Secretary Donna E. Shalala requesting detailed personnel and financial records "on every staff employee within DHHS (the Department of Health and Human Services) who is involved with vaccines at any level." Some two months later he followed up with a second request giving "Shalala one week to produce the records or face a subpoena."

His request struck heavily at the CDC, where scores of staff members work on vaccine matters.

The CDC sent the records to Washington, where they were screened by DHHS lawyers and then forwarded to Burton's committee in mid-October. Included in the records were emails, correspondence, résumés, financial disclosure forms, records of outside activities, and travel documents for the previous three years.

The FDA, NIH, HRSA officials, and members of the CDC's Advisory Committee on Immunization Practices (ACIP) also were required to supply their information.[22]

The following year, the committee's investigation resulted in the release of yet another scathing indictment against Federal vaccine players.[23] In the fall of 1999, the CDC initiated a plan to counter the growing numbers of claims linking thimerosal to autism by mining its Vaccine Safety Datalink to prove that there is no relationship between the neurotoxin and the disorder. According to the CDC,

> The Vaccine Safety Datalink (VSD) is a collaborative project between CDC's Immunization Safety Office and nine health care organizations. The VSD started in 1990 and continues today in order to monitor safety of vaccines and conduct studies about rare and serious adverse events following immunization.[24]

Barbara Lardy with America's Health Insurance Plans states that the VSD is a "crucial part of the federal government's systematic effort to monitor the safety of vaccines commonly used in the United States and to reassure public confidence in vaccines."[25] The CDC had already researched the database and published an article in the June 1997 issue of *Pediatrics* touting the power of the VSD to identify problems in vaccine safety. Among other things, Robert Chen, then-chief of CDC/Immunization Safety Branch, and more than a dozen other researchers noted that the risk of seizures more than doubled on the same day the DTP vaccine was administered. They also found that the risk of seizures for the MMR vaccine increased by 300% "8 to 14 days after receipt of MMR. . . ."[26]

Chen was confident that the VSD would exonerate thimerosal from any relationship with autism and thus legitimize the agency's ongoing love affair with it. Thomas Verstraeten, a young CDC epidemiologist, was assigned to crunch the numbers, and he completed his initial findings in November and December of 1999. Far from reassuring, Verstraeten discovered that when he compared one-month-old babies with no thimerosal exposure to one-month-old babies with exposure levels at or above 25 micrograms of thimerosal, the relative risk of autism increased from 7.62 times (November results) to 11.35 times (December results).[27]

Verstraeten's November analysis also revealed the following increases in relative risk: ADHD (8.29), ADD w/o hyperactivity (6.38), Tics (5.65), Sleep disorders (4.98), and Speech/language (2.08).[28]

Verstraeten first alluded to his findings on November 29 in an email message he sent to his supervisors Robert Davis and Frank DeStefano.

From: Verstraeten, Thomas

Sent: Monday, November 29, 1999 11:45 AM

To: 'Robert Davis'

Cc: 'Frank Destefano'

Subject: thimerosal analysis

Hi Bob,

After running, re-thinking, re-running, re-thinking . . . for about two weeks now I should touch base with you, I think, to see whether you can agree with what I came up with so far. I'll attach the SAS programs hoping you or one of your statisticians can detect major flaws before I jump to conclusions. I'll try to structure my findings . . .

Thomas Verstraeten, M.D.[29]

On December 17, the researcher followed up with another email message to the same individuals. The subject of the message was "It just won't go away. . . ." Further analyses of the data had led the epidemiologist to the conclusion that ". . . except for epilepsy, all the harm is done in the first month." He further wrote, ". . . some of the RRs [relative risks] increase over the categories and I haven't yet found an alternative explanation. . . . Please let me know if you can think of one." Verstraeten signed off with a cheery "Happy holidays!"[30]

Thus began the saga of the now-infamous "Verstraeten Study"—one of several fraudulent studies the Institute of Medicine would cite four years later to justify its claim that thimerosal does not cause autism. Of course, the IOM never saw the figures that Verstraeten, Davis, DeStefano, and other CDC vaccine sociopaths saw. Neither did the 60 vaccine industry insiders who met at the CDC's invitation in June 2000 in Norcross, Georgia, at the Simpsonwood Retreat Center. But what they saw there was still enough to destroy the public's blind faith in the mystical power of the vaccine paradigm.

They could never allow that to happen.

Chapter Fifteen

SIMPSONWOOD AND OTHER BULL

The right to search for truth implies also a duty; one must not conceal any part of what one has recognized to be true.[1]

—Albert Einstein

Sixty vaccine program insiders held a secret meeting on June 7th and 8th, 2000. This gathering would one day give the vaccine-informed public a rare glimpse at the inner machinations of those who profess to represent public health. The CDC's National Immunization Program had convened at the Simpsonwood Conference & Retreat Center outside of Atlanta, Georgia, under the false pretense of discussing Thomas Verstraeten's findings in his thimerosal-related Vaccine Safety Datalink research. But the CDC had no intention of sharing Verstraeten's original findings with this body of so-called "experts" or with anyone else. Lest the participants forget the sensitive nature of the meeting, meeting handouts were stamped in bold letters "DO NOT COPY OR RELEASE" and "CONFIDENTIAL" [emphasis in original].[2]

Only later did the public find out about the massaged data and the Simpsonwood meeting following a Freedom of Information Act (FOIA) request. The parents who made the discovery named the initial CDC findings "Generation Zero" to separate them from the later published versions of Verstraeten's study. According to the website Put Children First, in the months leading up to the secret meeting, the CDC had

> . . . used many techniques to dumb-down the numbers including removing comparisons to children who had received no thimerosal, lowering the age of children available for the analysis, and including a bankrupt HMO that had notoriously faulty data systems in their final round of analysis. The inclusion HMO helped neutralize the findings reviewed at Simpsonwood.[3]

The parents reported, "The general drift of their design changes was clear, to reduce the statistical power through conscious manipulation of statistical methods, data classifications, and samples."[4]

Meeting participants were under the false assumption that the database that included the records of 100,000 children was not large enough to analyze the relative risk of neurological disorders among children who had received no thimerosal. Verstraeten, Bob Davis, and Frank DeStefano knew very well that was not the case, but they played along in the deception to keep the truth from the meeting's participants. By means of such statistical chicanery, Verstraeten and his coconspirators had managed to drive the relative risk of autism from 7.62 down to 1.69.[5] A relative risk of 1.69 might not have awakened public interest if applied to ADHD or tics, but vaccine insiders knew that the public would not tolerate any increased risk of vaccine-induced autism.

In all likelihood, the representatives from the various vaccine-producing drug companies had done their own research and also knew that the 1.69 figure was a lie, but, if they did, they played along in the charade with the invited "experts," many of whom knew next to nothing about the effects of thimerosal, including the self-proclaimed "vaccinologists."

Dr. Walter Orenstein opened the meeting with his self-introduction as the Director of the National Immunization Program at the CDC. Following Orenstein, all other participants stated their names and positions. There were five voting members on the Advisory Committee on Immunization Practices (ACIP), the committee that makes recommendations to the CDC. There were also representatives from the FDA, the National Vaccine Program Office, state agencies, World Health Organization, American Academy of Pediatrics, American Academy of Family Physicians, and various universities. Also present were representatives from GlaxoSmithKline, Merck, Wyeth, and Aventis Pasteur.

After the introductions, Orenstein turned the meeting over to Dr. Roger Bernier, the associate director for science in the National Immunization Program. Bernier provided a brief summary of recent events related to thimerosal in vaccines. "In the United States there was a growing recognition that cumulative exposure may exceed some of the guidelines." Bernier was referring to the guidelines set by the Agency for Toxic Substances and Disease Registry (ATSDR), the Food and Drug Administration (FDA), and the Environmental Protection Agency (EPA).

Bernier then discussed some of the events reviewed in the previous chapter including the joint statement from the Public Health Service and the American Academy of Pediatrics, the August meeting that resulted in the eventual removal of thimerosal from the hepatitis B vaccine, and the October ACIP meeting that "looked this situation over again and did not express a preference for any of the vaccines that were thimerosal free."

Bernier then turned the meeting over to Dr. Dick Johnston, the meeting chairperson and immunologist and pediatrician at the University of

Colorado School of Medicine and National Jewish Center for Immunology and Respiratory Medicine.

The entire 258-page Simpsonwood transcript is available online as are several excellent commentaries.[6, 7, 8, 9] For the purposes of this book—demonstrating how the vaccine industry, medical establishment, and government stick it to you and your family—a few quotations and comments will suffice.

Dr. Dick Johnston, pediatrician and meeting chair, described himself as a "vaccinologist" and then went on to describe some of the characteristics shared by his peers:

> As an aside, we found a cultural difference between vaccinologists and environmental health people in that many of us in the vaccine arena have never thought about uncertainty factors before. We tend to be relatively concrete in our thinking. Probably one of the big cultural events in that meeting, at least for me, was when Dr. Clarkson repetitively pointed out to us that we just didn't get it about uncertainty, and he was actually quite right. It took us a couple of days to understand the factor of uncertainty in assessing environmental exposure, particularly to metals.

Johnston identifies "vaccinologists" as people who tend to be "relatively concrete in [their] thinking," who "have never thought about uncertainty factors before." This admission is obviously true, but the fact that a pediatrician, immunologist, and meeting chair—in a brief moment of enlightenment—recognized and gave voice to that truth demonstrates the paucity of rational thought and science among vaccine program elites and raises yet another red flag for the vaccine-informed public. Russell Blaylock, MD, skewers Johnston and his fellow "vaccinologists" for their collective blindness:

> First, what is a vaccinologist? Do you go to school to learn to be one? How many years of residency training are required to be a vaccinologist? Are there board exams? It's a stupid term used to describe people who are obsessed with vaccines, not that they actually study the effects of the vaccines, as we shall see throughout this meeting. Most important is the admission by Dr. Johnson [sic] that he and his fellow "vaccinologists" are so blinded by their obsession with forcing vaccines on society that they never even considered that there might be factors involved that could greatly affect human health, the so-called "uncertainties". Further, that he and his fellow "vaccinologists" like to think in concrete terms—that is, they are very narrow in their thinking and wear blinders that prevent them from seeing the numerous problems occurring with large numbers

of vaccinations in infants and children. Their goal in life is to vaccinate as many people as possible with an ever-growing number of vaccines.[10]

By the second day of the meeting, Dr. Johnston's awareness of the risks associated with thimerosal in vaccines was growing. Like millions of parents and patients around the world, he was becoming vaccine informed. The conversation moved from theoretical to personal when the vaccinologist described the following event:

> Forgive this personal comment, but I got called out at eight o'clock for an emergency call and my daughter-in-law delivered a son by C-section. Our first male in the line of the next generation, and I do not want that grandson to get a thimerosal containing vaccine until we know better what is going on. It will probably take a long time. In the meantime, and I know there are probably implications for this internationally, but in the meanwhile I think I want that grandson to only be given thimerosal-free vaccines.

There it is. The meeting chair, immunologist, and pediatrician expressed a preference for thimerosal-free vaccines . . . sort of. His preference extends only to his family members but does not include the family members of the people he serves or humanity in general. The elite versus The Herd value system is a common trait among vaccine insiders. Dr. Isabelle Rapin, a neurologist for children at Albert Einstein College of Medicine, echoed Johnston's position when she told the group of her concerns with the potential risk of thimerosal to decrease her grandchildren's IQs. "Even in my grandchildren, one IQ point I am going to fight about."

There is no way that vaccine-informed program administrators or people of influence would allow their loved ones to receive vaccines laced with thimerosal. Years after Simpsonwood, Kathleen Stratton with the Institute of Medicine refused to answer the question "Would you give thimerosal to your own children?"[11]

The more informed people become in general, the less likely they are to vaccinate. As previously cited, that would explain why in 2015 less than 30% of Congress admitted to vaccinating their own children.[12]

The difference between the vaccine informed among the general public and vaccine program sociopaths is that the public wants to extend information and choice to everyone, while program sociopaths manipulate, distort, bury, and destroy information so the public will continue to receive vaccines that the sociopaths would never allow their loved ones to receive.

Program elites tend to come from powerful, rich countries. Their allegiance lies primarily with their families and secondarily with the program. People of conscience include all of humanity in their sphere of compassion. Sociopaths draw lines demonstrating a clear "us versus them" mentality that continues to corrupt vaccine policy today. Dr. Johnston, the meeting chair, essentially stated at Simpsonwood that the participants in the 1999 meeting he attended at Bethesda were fine with administering thimerosal to poor people of color in developing countries (the people least able to tolerate its toxic effects) while advocating for the removal of thimerosal from vaccines in the USA:

> We agreed that it would be desirable to remove mercury from US licensed vaccines, but we did not agree that this was a universal recommendation that we would make because of the issue concerning preservatives for delivering vaccines to other countries, particularly developing countries, in the absence of hard data that implied that there was in fact a problem.

Mary Holland, JD, delivered a passionate speech at the United Nations in April 2016. When she told the panel and audience that "mercury should never be a preservative in any vaccine anywhere in the world because there are better and safer alternatives," she got a round of applause from the audience and a grimace from a public health official on the panel.[13] It would seem that vaccine-informed people in developing countries are no fonder of damaging their children's brains with thimerosal than are the vaccine informed in wealthier nations.

Considerable discussion at Simpsonwood focused on how to manipulate the data to reduce the evidence of thimerosal's toxic effects upon the minds and bodies of newborn babies and toddlers. Dr. William Weil with the American Academy of Pediatrics cut through the statistical gimmicks when he said near the end of the meeting, "The number of dose-related relationships [between mercury and autism] are linear and statistically significant. You can play with this all you want. They are linear. They are statistically significant."

Dr. Robert Chen, Chief of Vaccine Safety and Development at the National Immunization Program, made a couple of statements that must be considered side by side to appreciate their significance:

> . . . [T]he issue is that it is impossible, unethical to leave kids unimmunized, so you will never, ever resolve that issue [studying health outcomes with unvaccinated children]. . . .

> We have been privileged so far that given the sensitivity of information, we have been able to manage to keep it out of, lets [sic] say, less responsible hands. . . .

Chen, apparently a true believer, believes that it would be unethical to conduct a study in which children are intentionally left unvaccinated. It's likely that Chen also believes that allowing parents not to vaccinate their children is unethical. Such a belief is commonplace among concrete thinking "vaccinologists" and associates. Chen's second statement confirms the secret nature of the meeting. What was said at Simpsonwood was meant to stay at Simpsonwood. Dr. Bernier, associate director for science in the National Immunization Program, stated more on that subject: "This information has been held fairly tightly." Later he called it "embargoed information" and "very highly protected information." When "public servants" speak of "protected information," it becomes clear that such people are unworthy to be called public servants. Such servants are little more than servants of industry and their own personal interests. As the meeting was drawing to a close, Dr. John Clements with the World Health Organization summarized the thinking of a global vaccine sociopath:

> I am really concerned that we have taken off like a boat going down one arm of the mangrove swamp at high speed, when in fact there was not enough discussion really early on about which way the boat should go at all. And I really want to risk offending everyone in the room by saying that perhaps this study should not have been done at all, because the outcome of it could have, to some extent, been predicted and we have all reached this point now where we are left hanging, even though I hear the majority of the consultants say to the Board that they are not convinced there is a causality direct link between Thimerosal and various neurological outcomes.

Several times during the meeting, the "experts" used "the-studies-haven't-been-done" argument to justify the ongoing use of thimerosal in vaccines. And if Clements were running the vaccine show, he would make sure studies such as the Verstraeten CDC study would never be done. The position of Clements and people of his ilk is that scientific information about the risks of vaccines leaves vaccine elites hanging, an image that's not altogether inappropriate considering the combined atrocities they commit. If Clements hoped to offend his colleagues by arguing for the perpetuation of institutional ignorance to advance a global vaccine agenda, he likely failed. He did, however, successfully offend the sensibilities of every vaccine-informed person who has since read his statement.

The fact that "the majority of the consultants" were "not convinced there is a causality direct link between thimerosal and various neurological outcomes" says nothing about thimerosal and says everything about the power of the human mind to believe nonsense in its own self-interest. Similar groups have concluded that it's unethical to deprive dark-skinned races of the benefits of slavery.

The Simpsonwood deck was stacked from the beginning. The conclusion was planned and preordained. If their intention had been to learn about the toxic effects of thimerosal, the CDC would have invited the scientific experts who had long since proven that thimerosal is toxic at single digit parts per billion.

Clements continued:

> I know how we handle it from here is extremely problematic. The ACIP is going to depend on comments from this group in order to move forward into policy, and I have been advised that whatever I say should not move into the policy area because that is not the point of this meeting. . . . But there is now the point at which the research results have to be handled, and even if this committee decides that there is no association and that information gets out, the work has been done and through freedom of information that will be taken by others and will be used in other ways beyond the control of this group. And I am very concerned about that as I suspect it is already too late to do anything regardless of any professional body and what they say. . . .

> So I leave you with the challenge that I am very concerned that this has gotten this far, and that having got this far, how you present in a concerted voice the information to the ACIP in a way they will be able to handle it and not get exposed to the traps which are out there in public relations.

Once again, Clements expressed the outrageous idea that scientific information is not an aid to vaccine elites, it's a problem that must be "handled" before it is presented to the advisory committees such as the ACIP in order to minimize "traps which are out there in public relations." Of course, handling "extremely problematic" information is what the vaccine industry does best. The irony in this particular situation, however, is beyond the pale. The CDC "handled" the information before it was even presented at Simpsonwood. It "handled" the conversation at Simpsonwood by excluding legitimate thimerosal experts from participation. And now Clements is calling for the already "handled" information to be "handled" yet again before passing it along to the ACIP, where committee members will undoubtedly "handle" it before they complete the loop by handing it back to the original handlers, the CDC. Had Clements forgotten that five voting members of the ACIP were present at Simpsonwood? Was it the job of those members to "handle" the information before presenting it to the other committee members? More from Clements:

> My mandate as I sit here in this group is to make sure at the end of the day that 100,000,000 are immunized with DTP, Hepatitis B and if possible Hib, this year, next year and for many years to come, and that will

have to be with thimerosal containing vaccines unless a miracle occurs and an alternative is found quickly and is tried and found to be safe.

Thus the truth is revealed. No matter what was discussed at Simpsonwood, no matter what the science had or would reveal, Clements was under mandate to vaccinate 100,000,000 children. Not vaccinating was, and will never be an option. When the representatives from Merck and the other drug cartels heard Clements declare his mandate, they probably wet themselves with excitement. As powerful as Clements and cohorts may be as vaccine program insiders, they're little more than pawns among pawns being moved about by those in charge of the global vaccine game—a game that the master players intend to execute regardless of the science and regardless of the casualties.

The importance of Simpsonwood cannot be overstated. The elite gathering provided the world with a brief glimpse of deluded deceivers deceiving one another and strategizing to further deceive the public. It reinforced what vaccine-informed people have long since known: the vaccine paradigm is a grand illusion foisted on the public by gullible "public servants" and ruthless vaccine fascists. If Simpsonwood taught the world anything, it taught that one of the most dangerous epidemics of all is the infection of greed and power that transforms well-meaning people into vaccine sociopaths—causing them to sacrifice scientific advancement and people for profit.

Thomas Verstraeten walked away from Simpsonwood disillusioned. The case against thimerosal was compelling, and he was disturbed that his colleagues failed to share his concern. On July 14, the researcher sent a message to Philippe Grandjean and cc'ed the same to Robert Chen, Frank DeStefano, Robert Pless, Roger Bernier, Tom Clarkson, and Pal Weihe. With the exception of Grandjean and Weihe, all had participated in the Simpsonwood meeting. Grandjean, CDC consultant and researcher, was well versed on the effects of chemicals on developing brains. Among other things, Verstraeten wrote,

Unfortunately I have witnessed how many experts, looking at this thimerosal issue, do not seem bothered to compare apples to pears and insist that if nothing is happening in these studies [two studies on mercury toxicity from the consumption of fish] then nothing should be feared of thimerosal. I do not wish to be the advocate of the anti-vaccine lobby and sound like being convinced that thimerosal is or was harmful, but at least I feel we should use sound scientific argumentation and not let our standards be dictated by our desire to disprove an unpleasant theory.

Sincerely,

Tom Verstraeten.[14]

Verstraeten's call for "sound scientific argumentation" demonstrates profound naïveté in the nature of the vaccine paradigm. Apparently, even after Simpsonwood, the researcher still believed that the paradigm was based on science. The vaccine-informed public has known since the 1800s that the vaccine paradigm is based on faith and not on scientific principles. And like many faith-based organizations, The Church of Vaccinology is led by a corrupt clergy that hides real vaccine-induced injuries and deaths while manipulating data, science, politicians, parents, and patients with lies.

Evidently, unbeknownst even to Verstraeten, the purpose of Simpsonwood was not how to apply sound scientific principles for the betterment of the vaccine program. It was how to "handle" the fact that behind Verstraeten's numbers were living and breathing people who were experiencing pain, suffering, and loss.

Clements, representing the WHO, castigated the CDC for shining a spotlight on vaccine casualties. He knew—even if Verstraeten didn't—that science is the enemy to the vaccine paradigm. He knew that the door to the Vaccine Safety Datalink never should have been opened. He knew that belief in vaccines can only thrive in darkness.

The House of Representatives' Government Reform Committee faced that darkness in the spring of 2000 when Congressmen Burton and Henry Waxman wrote to HHS Secretary Shalala asking her to examine the "possible connections between autism and the MMR vaccine."[15] As of July 18, 2000, Shalala had failed to respond. It was Burton's turn to castigate vaccine insiders—not in a secret meeting like Simpsonwood, but before the world in a House Committee meeting:

> We both asked [Secretary Shalala] to put together a panel of the best experts in the field to look at this issue. That was May 16—2 months ago. No response.
>
> That's intolerable. If your position is that we should base our policies on good science and good research, then fine. I agree with you 100 percent. But if you are not willing to do the research, if you're not willing to ask the questions, then we have a real problem on our hands.[16]

William Egan, acting office director, Office of Vaccine Research and Review (OVRR) with the FDA and Simpsonwood participant, had been assigned the unenviable task of lying to Burton on behalf of the FDA. He did so by reciting the standard trance-inducing testimonial as to the mystical power of vaccines and then added, "FDA considers all vaccines currently available to be safe and effective. It is essential that children continue to receive all vaccines according to currently recommended schedules."[17]

All vaccines. Safe and effective. Essential. No question. No discussion. No exception. Blessed be the name of our golden calf and sacred cow. Amen and

Hallelujah. Congressman Burton—no longer a member of Egan's church—chopped up Egan's bull and grilled it over a high flame. Although Egan was visibly shaken by Burton's common-sense questions, Egan maintained the Simpsonwood oath of secrecy. His statement is recorded on the FDA website with the following statements in bold print:

> **There are no convincing data or evidence of any harm caused by the low levels of thimerosal that some children may have encountered in following the existing immunization schedule . . . .**
>
> **No children or infants were receiving toxic levels of mercury from vaccines, but FDA still believed it appropriate to pursue alternatives to using thimerosal as a preservative in vaccines. . . .**
>
> **The amounts [of thimerosal children receive in the childhood vaccination schedule] . . . do not exceed the recommended guidelines set by FDA, the Agency for Toxic Substances and Disease Registry, and the World Health Organization.**[18]

A few weeks prior to the hearing, Lyn Redwood, cofounder of the Coalition for SafeMinds, had submitted a paper with four others to the journal *Medical Hypotheses*.[19] The title of the paper, "Autism: a novel form of mercury poisoning," was both bold and provocative. As one of the first speakers in the July 18 hearing, Redwood acted as a true prophet in her testimony which preceded Egan's testimony:

> You may hear today from some officials that the mercury exposure from medicinal sources is insignificant. The fact is that neurological damage is documented to occur in infants at these levels of exposure. You may also hear that these levels of exposure only exceed EPA guidelines the first 6 months of life. That is because the data was inaccurately averaged over a 6-month period of time. As any independent toxicologist will tell you, mercury has a long half-life and its inherent pharmacokinetics you cannot legitimately calculate the effect of a bolus dose as though it were ingested in small amounts over a long period of time. To make a simple analogy, what FDA is trying to assert is that giving someone two Tylenol a day for 30 days has the same effect of giving them 60 Tylenol all at once in 1 day. This defies common sense, much less sound medical practice.
>
> The truth is vaccines are the single largest source of mercury exposure postnatally in infants, but nowhere in the mercury literature of EPA, FDA, ATSDR are these products even identified as being a source of exposure.[20]

Representative Helen Chenoweth-Hage grew up on an Idaho farm. She had undoubtedly mucked through plenty of manure, and, based on her testimony, she was clearly not in the mood to muck through the crap spewing out of the mouths of government witnesses:

> . . . [Y]ou are willing to, with a straight face, tell us that you are eventually going to phase [thimerosal] out after we know that a small baby's body is slammed with 62 times the amount of mercury that it is supposed to have. . . . It doesn't make sense. No wonder people are losing faith in their government. And to have one of the witnesses tell us it is because mothers eat too much fish? Come on. We expect you to get real.
>
> We heard devastating testimony in this hearing today, and we heard it last April. And this is the kind of response we get from our government agencies?
>
> I am sorry.
>
> I recommend that you read this. Side by side, page after page of analysis of the symptoms of people who are affected with mercury poisoning compared to autism, . . . and you folks are trying to tell us that you can't take this off the market when 8,000 children are going to be injected tomorrow; 80 children may be coming down, beginning tomorrow, with autism? What if there was an E. coli scare? What if there was a problem with an automobile? The recall would be like that.
>
> . . . This case could dwarf the tobacco case.[21]

The Congresswoman was right on the money . . . vaccine industry money. A wave of vaccine injury court cases was building. Yes, the court cases would gut industry profits, but more important, it would destroy the fragile faith of vaccine believers, which would kill the Church's sacred cow.

As discussed previously, the industry would later attempt to fight the wave of court cases with the shady introduction of the Eli Lilly Rider into the Homeland Security Bill, but it needed to go beyond that. Vaccine sociopaths needed to create the illusion that science had once and for all "debunked" the damning relationship among thimerosal, the MMR vaccine, and autism. If they could pull off that trick, then the court cases would magically disappear. Some of the magicians were willing to give science a shot at the task, but in the end, the people running the vaccine scam would never let a little thing like science stop them from poisoning billions of people in exchange for billions in profit.

Chapter Sixteen

VACCINES DO NOT CAUSE AUTISM: THE GREATEST FRAUD IN THE HISTORY OF MEDICAL SCIENCE

*It is very risky, if not perilous, to assume that those in positions of
responsibility are responsible.*[1]

—David McCullough

*Autism is just a bullshit name that they give our children because they can't admit
that they're vaccine injured.*[2]

—Polly Tommey

Top-ranking vaccine insiders—believers and sociopaths alike—devised a
plan to pull off the illusion that vaccines do not cause autism. The plan
included the following elements:

1. Direct the "independent" Institute of Medicine to make a statement
   declaring that vaccines do not cause autism and that no further research
   funds should be spent to prove otherwise,
2. Gin up several "outside" studies designed to reach the preordained conclusion that thimerosal does not cause autism,
3. Conduct internal epidemiological studies designed to reach the preordained conclusion that the MMR vaccine does not cause autism,
4. Hide and/or destroy evidence that substantiates the link between vaccines
   and autism,
5. Hinder or block public access to government data including the Vaccine
   Safety Datalink and the data used to create the fraudulent 2004 CDC
   paper that concluded that the MMR vaccine does not cause autism,

6. Take the focus off of vaccines by funding research into non-vaccine-related causes of autism,
7. Deny funding for vaccine-induced autism research and biomedical treatment of autism,
8. Intimidate scientists who research the relationship between vaccines and autism, and
9. Have Department of Justice lawyers lie in the Vaccine Court about the known and proven link between vaccines and autism.

The plan hit pay dirt in 2009 when a government-funded "special master" with the National Vaccine Injury Compensation Program ruled in favor of government-funded lawyers, throwing out more than 5,000 claims filed by parents who had watched their children regress into autism following vaccination.[3]

The aggregate frauds committed from 2000 to 2010 (the year the General Medical Council stripped Dr. Andrew Wakefield and Professor John Walker-Smith of their medical licenses) have without doubt impacted the lives of more people than any other frauds perpetrated in the history of medical science. Every person on the planet is affected to a lesser or greater degree. The details of this crime against humanity fill volumes and will yet fill many more. A brief telling of the story follows:

On January 12th, 2001, the Institute of Medicine's Immunization Safety Review Committee held a closed meeting. Dr. Marie McCormick, committee chair, laid out the ground rules at the meeting's start assuring participants that the "closed session transcripts will never be shared with anybody outside the committee and the staff."[4] The transcripts were later leaked, revealing both the IOM's master and its mandate. It's important to note that Dr. Dick Johnston, the concrete thinking "vaccinologist" who chaired the Simpsonwood meeting and who would never inject a thimerosal-containing vaccine into his own grandchildren, was present at this meeting, as well. Following are a few quotations from McCormick and Dr. Kathleen Stratton, a member of IOM staff and study director of the committee:

DR. MCCORMICK: [The CDC] wants us to declare, well, these things are pretty safe on a population basis [p. 33].

DR. STRATTON: The point of no return, the line we will not cross in public policy is pull the vaccine, change the schedule. We could say it is time to revisit this, but we would never recommend that level. Even recommending research is recommendations for policy. We wouldn't say compensate, we wouldn't say pull the vaccine, we wouldn't say stop the program. [p. 74]

DR. MCCORMICK: We wouldn't talk about the policy of exemptions, but we could certainly talk about the implications of not immunizing, for whatever reason. [p. 74]

DR. MCCORMICK: . . . we are not ever going to come down that [autism] is a true side effect . . . . [p. 97][5]

The IOM held a second closed door meeting on March 10, 2001, which included the following exchange between committee member Dr. Gerald Medoff and McCormick:

DR. MEDOFF: You just want us to say the evidence favors rejection of the hypothesis?

DR. MCCORMICK: Yes, that's what they want to say.[6]

True to McCormick's word, the IOM committee later issued the following "Causality Conclusions": "The committee concludes that the evidence favors rejection of a causal relationship between thimerosal-containing vaccines and autism. The committee concludes that the evidence favors rejection of a causal relationship between MMR vaccine and autism."[7]

The committee also recommended that "available funding for autism research be channeled to the most promising areas," while recommending against further investigation into the relationship between vaccines and autism:

At this time, the committee does not recommend a policy review of the licensure of MMR vaccine or of the current schedule and recommendations for the administration of the MMR vaccine.

At this time, the committee does not recommend a policy review of the current schedule and recommendations for the administration of routine childhood vaccines based on hypotheses regarding thimerosal and autism.

Given the lack of direct evidence for a biological mechanism and the fact that all well-designed epidemiological studies provide evidence of no association between thimerosal and autism, the committee recommends that cost-benefit assessments regarding the use of thimerosal-containing versus thimerosal-free vaccines and other biological or pharmaceutical products, whether in the United States or other countries, should not include autism as a potential risk.[8]

Surely, the committee's final recommendation earned the approval of the vaccine sociopath John Clements with the World Health Organization who told his Simpsonwood peers that the Verstraeten study never should have been done.

In 2005, key members of both the Senate and the House reviewed a 55-page document titled "Conflicts of Interest: How the CDC Exerted Influence over the 5 Epidemiological Studies Used to Dismiss the thimerosal-Autism Link."[9, 10] The document highlighted pervasive conflicts of interest in five European-based studies the IOM used to support its conclusion that vaccines do not cause autism, including the CDC's relationship with one of the major players in the studies, Poul Thorsen, who later played the CDC when he absconded with almost two million dollars earmarked for vaccine research.[11] According to Dr. William Thompson, Thorsen continues to share his loot and his love in Denmark with Diana Schendel, a former CDC researcher.[12] Thorsen's story gets full book coverage in James Ottar Grundvig's 2016 publication of *Master Manipulator: The Explosive True Story of Fraud, Embezzlement, and Government Betrayal at the CDC.*[13]

In addition to the European studies, the government presentation notes that the IOM also reviewed the 2003 Verstraeten et al. study, which, after five revisions, had managed to erase the association between thimerosal and autism. The document exposed the tangled web of relationships and crooked methodologies that led to the IOM's faulty if not fraudulent report. The conclusions follow:

- The CDC NIP [National Immunization Program] is both vaccine advocate and vaccine safety watchdog for the United States, which constitutes a huge conflict of interest.
- The CDC funded the IOM VSR [Vaccine Safety Review] Committee and all associated activities.
- The CDC had both monetary and personnel connections to all five epidemiology studies used as the basis of the final IOM VSR Committee Reports conclusions on causality between thimerosal and autism.
- Coauthors on all five epidemiological studies used as the basis for the IOM VSR Committee 5/14/04 report final conclusion have direct ties to vaccine manufacturers.[14]

As previously cited, the vaccine-informed public gained additional information regarding the CDC fraud that influenced the IOM's incorrect 2004 conclusion when Dr. William Thompson passed thousands of documents to Representative Bill Posey in 2014. Dr. Brian Hooker, the scientist who recorded four of numerous conversations with Thompson, coauthored a complaint dated October 14, 2014, with Dr. Andrew Wakefield and James Moody, JD. Addressed to Dr. Harold Jaffee, MD, MA, CDC's associate director for science, and Dr. Don Wright, MD, MPH, acting director of the HHS's Office of Research Integrity, the three men identify the key players and the far-reaching consequences in what Thompson described as CDC fraud. Following are a few excerpts:

> We write to report apparent research misconduct by senior investigators within the National Immunization Program (NIP), Battelle Memorial Institute at the Centers for Public Health Evaluation (CPHE), and the National Center on Birth Defects and Developmental Disabilities (NCBDDD), and to request an immediate investigation.
>
> The Analysis Plan dated September 5, 2001 [Exhibit 2] set forth the objective of the research reported in the above-titled article, to compare ages at first MMR vaccination between children with autism and children who did not have autism, and to test the hypothesis that age of first MMR vaccination is associated with autism risk.
>
> The research team . . . found statistically significant associations between the age of first MMR and autism in (a) the entire autism cohort, (b) African-American children, and (c) children with "isolated" autism, a subset defined by The Group as those with autism and without comorbid developmental disabilities.
>
> However, valid results pertaining to the latter groups (b) and (c), crucial to resolving the debate over MMR and autism causality, obtained according to the Analysis Plan, were omitted from The Paper. The concealed results rendered The Paper's conclusion false and misleading: "we found that, overall, the age at time of first MMR administration was similar among case and control children." . . .
>
> This false and misleading report contributed to the CDC's conclusion that MMR vaccine did and does not cause autism, to rejection of a causal association by the Institute of Medicine (IOM), and to denial of compensation mandated by Congress in the National Vaccine Injury Compensation Program (NVICP).[15]

Thompson was assigned to present the CDC's fraudulent findings to the IOM in its Vaccine Safety Review scheduled for February 9, 2004. "As the date approached he became more and more uneasy about the prospect of presenting false and misleading findings."[16] Breaking protocol, the conflicted researcher wrote directly to CDC Director Dr. Julie Gerberding, informing her, "I will have to present several problematic results relating to statistical associations between receipt of the MMR vaccine and autism."[17] Thompson's job was threatened, he was replaced at the IOM meeting by the serial liar, Dr. Frank DeStefano, and he signed off on the fraudulent paper. More than 10 years later, treating Hooker as a friend, confidant, and priest, Thompson confessed,

> . . . I was basically telling this guy [Thompson's whistleblower lawyer] I was complicit, and I went along with this, we did not report significant findings. . . . I'm not proud of that . . . it's the lowest point in my career that I went along with that paper. . . . When I talk to you [Dr. Hooker], you have a son with autism. I have great shame now when I meet families with kids with autism because I have been part of the problem. . . . Here's what I shoulder. I shoulder that the CDC has put the research ten years behind. Because the CDC has not been transparent, we've missed ten years of research because the CDC is so paralyzed right now by anything related to autism. They're not doing what they should be doing because they're afraid to look for things that might be associated.[18]

As previously cited, Congressman Bill Posey quoted Thompson on the floor of the House in July 2015, describing the MMR vaccine's particularly devastating effects on black children.[19]

Representative Dave Weldon, MD, scolded the IOM in its February 2004 meeting for taking part in a culture that persecutes scientists who pursue the link between vaccines and autism:

> I must begin by sharing how disappointed I am by the number of reports I continue to receive from researchers regarding their difficulties in pursuing answers to these questions. It is past time that individuals are persecuted for asking questions about vaccine safety; we have recognized error before in the case of live polio, whole-cell pertussis, and rotavirus.
>
> I am repeatedly informed by researchers who encounter apathy from government officials charged with investigating these matters, difficulty in getting their papers published, and the loss of research grants. Some report overt discouragement, intimidation and threats, and have abandoned this field of research. Some have had their clinical privileges revoked and others have been hounded out of their institutions. . . .
>
> This atmosphere of intimidation even surrounds today's hearing. I received numerous complaints that this event is not a further attempt to get at the facts but rather a desire to sweep these issues under the rug.[20]

Considering the abundant evidence, it's apparent to honest investigators that when the CDC trashed damning evidence that contributed to the IOM's flawed findings and antiscientific recommendations, it also trashed the lives of millions of people who would fall victim to their treachery. Further treachery occurred when the CDC lost or destroyed the original data sets Verstraeten used to calculate his original, never-published findings.[21] If that were not enough, in 2002, the CDC paid the American Association of Health Plans (AAHP) to hide the Vaccine Safety Datalink from public access, preventing independent researchers from uncovering its secrets.[22]

In spite of the IOM's recommendation that no further vaccine-autism research be done, the CDC just can't seem to leave it alone. The AAP's journal *Pediatrics* published one of the more recent and more absurd CDC studies in 2013. The first name attached to the paper is none other than Frank DeStefano, the man who played a major role in erasing the autism signal in both Verstraeten's study and the CDC's fraudulent MMR study. The researchers found that "Increasing Exposure to Antibody-Stimulating Proteins and Polysaccharides in Vaccines Is Not Associated with Risk of Autism," leading them to conclude that vaccines are not associated with autism.[23] The late Dr. Mayer Eisenstein got such a laugh out of the paper that he posted an April Fools' Day critique:

> The following study must have been prepared especially for April Fools Day. It appeared in the March 29th issue of *The Journal of Pediatrics*. . . . What a nonsensical study! And the best response to that was in the Philadelphia newspaper. . . . "You have to be kidding me! Did I read this right? Children with autism and those without have the same total exposure to vaccine antigens. That is like saying, because I smoked as much as the guy down the street and he got cancer and I did not, smoking does not cause cancer. The one with cancer and the one without were both exposed to the same amount of smoke."
>
> You know, the real study is finding unvaccinated children and I'm blessed to have over 50,000 of them in my 40 years of practice. Virtually no autism! Virtually none! And I've made this statement now for more than 10 years. And yet we've had virtually no one come forth and say, "I have no vaccines in my children and they have autism." But it's more than autism. It's autism, ADD, ADHD, peanut allergy. All these things have some kind of link to vaccines.[24]

Dr. Brian Hooker trashed the paper for its lack of new data, meaningless antigen correlation, selection bias due to high participant refusal rate, overmatching statistical error, lack of an unvaccinated control group, autism variances from neurotypical children not studied, and CDC conflicts of interest. Hooker concluded,

Of all of the papers I have reviewed over my 26-year career as a research scientist, this is perhaps the most flawed and disingenuous study I have encountered. The DeStefano et al. 2013 study is to science what the movie *Ishtar* was to cinema.[25]

In spite of the government's efforts to convince parents that their children's regression into autism was not related to vaccines, parents didn't buy it. They knew what their kids were like prior to vaccinating; they were with their kids through the fevers, the lethargy, and the high-pitched screams. They grieved as their children faded away right before their eyes. The Department of Justice lumped over 5,000 of the parents' claims together in a process that was anything but just. "Special magistrates" heard six cases and applied their findings to all the other cases. George Hastings, Jr., the special magistrate in the Cedillo case, expressed "deep sympathy and admiration" for the family and expressed contempt for doctors who mislead parents into believing that vaccines cause autism, which is, in Hastings's opinion, "gross medical misjudgment."[26]

Hannah Poling, one of the original six case subjects in the Omnibus Autism Proceeding (OAP), was removed, and her case was heard prior to the OAP. Dr. Andrew Zimmerman, a senior pediatric neurologist from Johns Hopkins, served as the government's expert witness in the Poling case. In 2006, Zimmerman coauthored a paper with Hannah Poling's father, John Poling, and two other researchers.[27]

The paper concluded that not only did vaccines cause Hannah's autism, it also described the mechanism by which the injury occurred:

The cause for regressive encephalopathy in Hannah at age 19 months was underlying mitochondrial dysfunction, exacerbated by vaccine-induced fever and immune stimulation that exceeded metabolic energy reserves. This acute expenditure of metabolic reserves led to permanent irreversible brain injury.[28]

On a side note, Hannah's mitochondrial disorder is not rare. Her mother has the same disorder with no clinical manifestations. Dr. Wakefield wrote that approximately 20% of autistic children have mitochondrial disorder and "as many as 1 in 50 to 1 in 200 children might carry the DNA mutation that predisposes them to vaccine-induced mitochondrial disorder."[29]

The two Department of Justice lawyers in the Poling hearing, Lynn Ricciardella and Vincent Matonoski, concurred with the court's ruling to award money to Hannah's parents for their daughter's injury, and they conceded the mechanism of injury as explained by their expert witness, Dr. Zimmerman. The case was closed and the records were sealed.

When Ricciardella and Matonoski argued on behalf of the government and against the parents in the OAP, Zimmerman provided the lawyers with a different report that claimed, "There is no scientific basis for a connection between measles, mumps, and rubella (MMR) vaccine or mercury (Hg) intoxication and autism." Matonoski quoted Zimmerman in his closing arguments saying, "We know [Dr. Zimmerman's] views on this." He and his partner in crime did indeed know Zimmerman's "views on this." They knew that Zimmerman was lying. They knew because they had conceded the Hannah Poling case based on Zimmerman's previous report, which clearly implicated vaccines in Hannah's regression into autism. Based on the lawyers' presentation of Zimmerman's deceptive report, the court threw out the six test cases and with them 5,000 similar cases.

Rolf Hazlehurst, assistant district attorney general for the State of Tennessee, is the father of Yates Hazlehurst, one of the six test cases that were thrown out due to Ricciardella and Matonoski's use of Zimmerman's second report. Hazlehurst appealed the case. Ricciardella represented the government in the appeal. The judge asked if perhaps the burden of proof on parents was too high. Surely there was some evidence that vaccines can cause autism in some cases. Ricciardella replied, ". . . [W]e are not even at a stage where [a link] is medically or scientifically possible." Ricciardella's statement was a lie. She had Zimmerman's original report in her possession.

There is great irony in the fact that Matonoski and Ricciardella were representing the Department of Justice when their actions, combined with Zimmerman's false report, resulted in the obstruction of justice, which in fact denied justice to the families in the Omnibus Autism Proceeding as well as to the families who would later appeal for help from the corrupted court system.

In opposition to Hazlehurst and tens of thousands of other parents around the world, Dr. Michael T. Brady, a pediatrician and spokesman for the American Academy of Pediatrics, said the academy was "obviously very satisfied" with the omnibus ruling. He was hopeful "that pediatricians would meet less resistance from parents over vaccinating children."[30] Would the Academy be equally satisfied knowing that the omnibus rulings were the result of industry influence over government and obstruction of justice?

As an attorney, Hazlehurst is well qualified to make the following accusation:

The bottom line is that during the autism omnibus proceedings, the United States Department of Justice, representing the United States Department of Health and Human Services, willfully and intentionally concealed critical material evidence about how vaccines cause autism. . . .

Let me put that in perspective for you. If I did to a criminal, in a United States court of law, what the Department of Justice did to vaccine injured children in the so-called vaccine court, I would be disbarred and I would be facing criminal charges.[31]

Hazlehurst spoke of his experience in a 2013 congressional briefing, saying, "The Vaccine Injury Compensation Program is an absolute invitation for an abuse of power. That's what I witnessed—a level of deceit, dishonesty and abuse of power which I would not have believed if I had not witnessed it for myself."[32]

It is interesting to note that Zimmerman was never called as a witness in the omnibus cases. Why? Dr. Wakefield provides the probable answer: "I would speculate because under cross-examination that previous report might have emerged. But if he wasn't there and there was no compulsion for him . . . in this court system to come forward, then it never happened and the case was denied."[33]

The vaccine autism cover-up surely ranks among the greatest cover-ups in US and world history. The Age of Autism website summarized the situation in a blog titled "The Vaccine Autism Link":

Autism is the defining disorder of our Age and points to the terrible state of health care in America, the suppression of free speech and the triumph of a kind of political correctness that is essentially a smiling mask for good old-fashioned bullying.[34]

One only needs to examine what the Unholy Trinity has added to the US schedule since the year 2000 to see why the worst of the autism epidemic as well as a host of other disorders is likely yet to come:

- 2000 – Pneumococcal conjugate vaccine
- 2003 – Intranasal influenza vaccine – trivalent
- 2005 – Meningococcal conjugate vaccine for adolescents
- 2005 – Tdap vaccine for adolescents
- 2006 – HPV vaccine for adolescent girls
- 2006 – Rotavirus vaccine (RotaTeq®)
- 2006 – Shingles vaccine (60 yrs & older)
- 2008 – Rotavirus vaccine (RotaRix®)
- 2009 – HPV vaccine for adolescent boys
- 2013 – Inactivated and intranasal influenza vaccine – quadrivalent
- 2014 – Meningococcal B vaccine licensed
- 2015 – 9vHPV (Merck's Gardasil 9 replaced the prior 4-valent version)
- 2015 – FDA approved Quadracel, a new combination DTaP+IPV vaccine for use in children age 4–6 years.

- 2015 – FDA approved new injectable influenza vaccine, Fluad, for use in people age 65 years and older.
- 2015 – FDA expanded Gardasil 9 licensure to include males age 16–26 years.
- 2016 – FDA approved Hiberix for full Hib vaccine series.
- 2016 – ACIP voted that live attenuated influenza vaccine (LAIV) should not be used during the 2016–2017 flu season.
- 2016 – FDA extended the age indication for PCV13 (Prevnar 13) to include adults age 18 through 49 years.
- 2016 – FDA approved extending the age range for use of FluLaval Quadrivalent to include children 6 to 35 months of age.
- 2017 – AAP issued policy stating that newborns should routinely receive hepatitis B vaccine within 24 hours of birth.
- 2017 – FDA expanded licensure of Afluria quadrivalent (Seqirus) to include people age 5 years and older.
- 2017 – FDA licensed Shingrix, the new shingles vaccine from Glaxo-SmithKline, for use in adults age 50 and older.
- 2018 – ACIP recommended Heplisav-B vaccine against hepatitis B virus.
- 2018 – ACIP recommended the live attenuated influenza vaccine (LAIV) (with no evidence that it's more effective than the LAIV it advised against using in 2016). [35] [36] [37] [38]

The flu jab, added to the childhood schedule in 2003, and the HPV vaccine merit special attention in the following chapters.

Chapter Seventeen

FLU JABS, PRETERM JABS, AND OTHER ATROCITIES

*Speak out on behalf of the voiceless and for the rights of
all who are vulnerable.*
—Proverbs 31:8

*A nation's greatness is measured by how it
treats its weakest members.*
—Mahatma Gandhi

*The mad vehemence of Modern Medicine is nowhere more evident
than in the yearly influenza vaccine farce.*[1]
—Robert S. Mendelsohn, MD

Humans are injected with more influenza vaccines than all other shots combined. In that sense, the flu jab represents the Unholy Trinity's greatest success. So far, it's the only vaccine that adults routinely submit to. FiercePharma, a pro-pharma, pro-business website, stated in 2012, "A big part of the growth in vaccine sales has been in the adult influenza market with the big focus on flu prevention and an acceptance of adult vaccines."[2]

The industry uses the flu vaccine in adults and children down to the age of six months just as it uses the birth dose of the hepatitis B vaccine: both serve as tools to modify thought and behaviors. Year after year, the CDC recycles the lies about the numbers of people killed by the flu and then follows up with its unsupported claim that the flu vaccine is "the first and best way to protect against influenza."[3]

The same people who fall for the trick are the people most likely to roll up their and their kids' sleeves for anything and everything the CDC promotes. The CDC pulls off the exaggerated body bag count by combining influenza and pneumonia deaths.[4] When the CDC tells the public that the flu kills 36,000 per year, the real number ranges from 257 to 3,006. That means that pneumonia deaths comprise from 90% to 99% of the deaths the CDC attributes to the flu.[5] Some may argue that the flu is a precursor to pneumonia and pneumonia deaths, so the number of deaths due to pneumonia would be higher were it not for the protective effect of the flu vaccine. Further reading will show that even *that* argument doesn't hold water.

A cursory study of the literature reveals that the flu vaccine is definitely not the best way to protect against influenza. Further research into the matter reveals that the jab does more than harm than good. Even the CDC, which is famous for putting out propaganda about vaccine efficacy, occasionally slips up and tells the truth as documented on FiercePharma's website:

> The Centers for Disease Control and Prevention (CDC) recently noted that only 56% of people who received the jab were protected from influenza, on the very low end of effectiveness spectrum. It was particularly ineffective among the elderly, one of the key target groups. The results led CDC Director Dr. Thomas Frieden to lament, "We simply need a better vaccine against influenza, one that works better and lasts longer."[6]

The package insert for FLUVIRIN®, manufactured by Novartis Vaccines, discusses the efficacy under the "Limitations of Vaccine Effectiveness" heading. The total information provided in this section is: "Vaccination with FLUVIRIN® may not protect all individuals."[7]

That's an understatement. Under the "Indications and Usage" heading, it reads: "FLUVIRIN® is not indicated for children less than 4 years of age because there is evidence of diminished immune response in this age group. . . ." In other words, even biased researchers failed to create the impression that the shot actually provides some level of benefit in young children.

The flu vaccine got a lot of bad press in the 2017–2018 flu vaccine season because the viruses in the vaccine did not match the viruses in the environment, making it virtually worthless. However, the news reporting that season perpetuated the illusion that a bad year is an anomaly and that the vaccine normally protects about 60% of vaccinees from getting the flu. A closer look at the numbers reveals the truth.

GlaxoSmithKline manufactures the Fluarix Quadrivalent vaccine. Keeping in mind that GSK profits from the sale of vaccines, the Fluarix package insert should be read with a grain a salt, but it should still be read. According to the insert, ". . . antibody titer post-vaccination with inactivated influenza virus vaccines have not been correlated with protection from influenza illness but the . . . antibody titers have been used as a measure of vaccine activity." The insert further states that antibody titers above a specific count "have been associated with protection from influenza illness in up to 50% of subjects."[8]

In other words, a protection level of 50% of subjects is as good as it gets, and that's only for subjects with the specified antibody titer count. But what exactly does 50% mean? Does it mean that if 100 people get the Fluarix vaccine, 50 of them will be protected from getting the flu? No, it means nothing of the sort.

GSK tested Fluarix in 2 European countries during the 2006–2007 influenza season and found that 3.2 percent of the unvaxxed subjects came down with the flu or an "influenza-like illness" (ILI), while 1.2 percent of the subjects in the Fluarix group contracted the flu or an influenza-like illness. This equates to a 62.5% efficacy rate.

The math used to obtain 62.5% is as follows: Divide 3.2 into 1.2 to get .375 or a 37.5% reduced incidence of flu in the treatment group. Subtract 37.5 from 100 to get an efficacy rate of 62.5%. This figure is not technically a lie, but it is absolutely deceptive. It gives the impression that Fluarix prevents the flu in 62.5% of people who get the jab. GSK knows full well that according to its own efficacy test, for every 100 people who are vaccinated with Fluarix, only 2 people derive any benefit (3.2 minus 1.2 equals 2). Two out of 100 equals an absolute risk reduction or vaccine efficacy rate of 2% with a corresponding vaccine worthless rate of 98%.

According to the 2015 meta-analysis conducted by the Cochrane Collaboration, the 98% worthless rate is fairly consistent among flu vaccine recipients. The Collaboration reviewed 90 reports and found that on average, flu jabs prevent 2.5% of people from coming down with an influenza-like illness and only 1.4% of people from contracting the flu. In other words, the flu jab is from 97.5% to 98.6% worthless.[9]

As worthless as standard flu vaccines tend to be, they look like superstars compared to the live attenuated influenza vaccine (LAIV) marketed as FluMist. In June 2016, the CDC and the AAP announced that pediatricians should trash their FluMist supply because it is only 3% effective.[10, 11] That doesn't mean that the FluMist prevents 3% of recipients from getting the flu. It means that the FluMist prevents somewhere in the neighborhood of 0.1% of people or 1 in 1,000 people from getting the flu. So the "effective" flu vaccine is about 98% worthless, while the ineffective FluMist is 99.9% worthless.

Speaking of worthless, in February 2018, the CDC's Advisory Committee on Immunization Practices (ACIP) voted 12-2 to bring back a reformulated Flumist vaccine as "an option for influenza vaccination for persons for whom it is appropriate" in the 2018–2019 influenza season. Lisa Grohskoph, MD, of the CDC admitted that the new formulation's vaccine efficacy is unknown and will remain unknown until The Herd tests it out. David Stephens, MD, one of two people who voted against the recommendation, said, "I'm really concerned about what message this [approval] sends."[12]

Even if the snorted and injected flu vaccines were 100% effective against the A and B strains of influenza, those particular strains represent only about 10% of the more than 200 viruses that cause influenza and flu-like symptoms.[13]

However, those figures fail to include the numbers of people who get sick *because* of the flu vaccine.

Vaccine manufacturers and the CDC state emphatically, "Flu vaccines CANNOT cause the flu" because they "are made with either killed or weakened viruses" [emphasis in original]. The CDC further claims:

> Flu vaccines are safe. Serious problems from the flu vaccine are very rare. The most common side effect that a person is likely to experience is either soreness where the injection was given, or runny nose in the case of nasal spray. These side effects are generally mild and usually go away after a day or two.[14]

The FLUARIX package insert tells a different story. Sixteen percent of adult test subjects experienced muscle aches, headache, and fatigue up to seven days after receiving the jab.[15]

Children fared worse than adults:

- In children aged 3 through 17 years, the injection site adverse reactions were pain (44%), redness (23%), and swelling (19%). . . .
- In children aged 3 through 5 years, the most common (≥10%) systemic adverse events were drowsiness (17%), irritability (17%), and loss of appetite (16%); in children aged 6 through 17 years, the most common systemic adverse events were fatigue (20%), muscle aches (18%), headache (16%), arthralgia (10%), and gastrointestinal symptoms (10%). . . .[16]

Arthralgia is defined as pain in joints, and gastrointestinal symptoms are defined as "nausea, vomiting, diarrhea, and/or abdominal pain." The CDC shares the following information about the flu and typical flu symptoms:

> Influenza (also known as the flu) is a contagious respiratory illness caused by flu viruses. It can cause mild to severe illness, and at times can lead to death. . . . People who have the flu often feel some or all of these symptoms:
>
> Fever* or feeling feverish/chills
>
> Cough
>
> Sore throat
>
> Runny or stuffy nose
>
> Muscle or body aches

Headaches

Fatigue (tiredness)

Some people may have vomiting and diarrhea, though this is more common in children than adults.

It's important to note that not everyone with flu will have a fever.[17]

In summary, the flu vaccine cannot (CDC's word) give vaccinees the flu, but it can and does give up to 20% of flu vaccine victims one or more symptoms of the flu. Not to belabor the obvious, but the CDC's attempt to minimize the adverse effects of the vaccine is a blatant misrepresentation of fact, and medical professionals routinely pass such nonsense on to their patients by telling recently vaccinated individuals that they were going to get sick anyway and that the vaccine did not cause their illness.[18]

So, if the flu vaccine sickens up to 20% of the population, how did Novartis get away with its claim that the FLUARIX vaccine reduced the incidence of influenza-like illness in its efficacy trial? First they "monitored for influenza-like illnesses (ILI) starting 2 weeks post-vaccination and lasting for approximately 7 months." That statement is informative, but it's also a lie. The monitoring began the moment the vaccines were administered. The side effects mentioned above were the result of the monitoring in the 7-day period following vaccination. Those data were intentionally excluded from the efficacy trial because they would have demonstrated that for every two people the vaccine helps, there are up to 20 others who get a flu-like illness from the vaccine. In short, the flu jab is 10 times more likely to harm than to help the public. That ratio is even more damning among young children and the elderly, who derive even less benefit and even more harm from the ubiquitous jab.

These and other disturbing facts are not unknown to high-ranking officials, as illustrated by the speech Congressman Bill Posey made on the floor of the House in 2013:

In 2000 there was near universal agreement that mercury should be removed as a preservative for vaccines. Yet, today, nearly half of all annual flu vaccines, which are recommended for children and pregnant women, still contain mercury as a preservative—not simply trace amounts of mercury. It's 2013! Why are we still injecting ethylmercury into babies and pregnant women?[19]

Dr. William Thompson rhetorically asked Dr. Brian Hooker a similar question in a recorded telephone conversation after explaining the fact that the CDC knows that vaccinating pregnant women results in an increased risk of tics in their babies. "Do you think a pregnant mother would take a vaccine that they knew caused tics?" Thompson then answered his own question. "Absolutely not! I would never give my wife a vaccine that I thought caused tics."[20] Nor would Alexander Langmuir, former head of the CDC. James S. Turner, Esq. quoted Langmuir when he said,

> I would not take the flu vaccine. My wife does not take the flu vaccine. No one should take the flu vaccine. And in fact when I was head of CDC, I wanted to make that as a public statement and I refused to say that you should take the flu vaccine. That's why I'm now professor at Harvard.

Turner clarified Langmuir's statement by adding, "He got fired for that. That was what he told me."[21]

Russell Blaylock, MD, an expert in brain damage caused by vaccinologists, said, "I cannot think of anything more insane than vaccinating pregnant women."[22]

Clearly, people of influence realize that the flu vaccine is a hoax. Medical journals routinely publish papers exposing various aspects of the hoax. Following are a few of many examples:

The Lancet, 2005:
We recorded no convincing evidence that vaccines can reduce mortality, admissions, serious complications, and community transmission of influenza.[23]

Allergy and Asthma Proceedings, 2012:
Trivalent inactivated influenza vaccine did not provide any protection against hospitalization in pediatric subjects, especially children with asthma. On the contrary, we found a threefold increased risk of hospitalization in subjects who did get trivalent inactivated influenza vaccine.[24]

PLOS Medicine, 2010:
We report findings from four epidemiologic studies in Canada showing that prior receipt of 2008-09 trivalent inactivated influenza vaccine was associated with increased risk of medically attended pandemic H1N1 illness during the spring-summer 2009.[25]

Journal of Virology, 2011:
. . . long-term annual vaccination using inactivated vaccines may hamper the induction of cross-reactive CD8+ T cell responses by natural infections and thus may affect the induction of heterosubtypic immunity.

This may render young children who have not previously been infected with an influenza virus more susceptible to infection with a pandemic influenza virus of a novel subtype.[26]

Clinical Infectious Diseases, 2012:
We randomized 115 children to trivalent inactivated influenza vaccine (TIV) or placebo. Over the following 9 months, TIV recipients had an increased risk of virologically-confirmed non-influenza infections (relative risk: 4.40; 95% confidence interval: 1.31-14.8). Being protected against influenza, TIV recipients may lack temporary non-specific immunity that protected against other respiratory viruses. . . . We identified a statistically significant increased risk of non-influenza respiratory virus infection among trivalent inactivated influenza vaccine recipients, including significant increases in the risk of rhinovirus and coxsackie/echovirus infection.[27]

Clinical Infectious Diseases, 2013:
In vaccinated subjects with no evidence of prior season vaccination, significant protection (62%) against community-acquired influenza was demonstrated. Substantially lower effectiveness was noted among subjects who were vaccinated in both the current and prior season.[28]

British Medical Journal, 2009:
The disparity in effectiveness between the high profile of influenza vaccines and antivirals and the low profile of physical interventions is striking. Public health recommendations are almost completely based on the use of vaccines and antivirals despite a lack of strong evidence.[29]

Archives of Internal Medicine, 2005:
We could not correlate increasing vaccination coverage after 1980 with declining mortality rates in any age group. We conclude that observational studies substantially overestimate vaccination benefit.[30]

Vaccine, 2009:
Cohort studies have consistently reported that vaccination reduces all-cause winter mortality by about 50%—an astonishing claim given that only about 5% of all winter deaths are attributable to influenza. This vaccine efficacy overestimation has now been attributed to profound confounding frailty selection bias.[31]

According to the vaccine researcher and author Neil Miller, the *Vaccine* paper found that "During the 1980s and 1990s, the percentage of seniors who received influenza vaccines increased fourfold yet CDC epidemiologists found that national influenza-related death rates actually increased."[32]

International Journal of Family Medicine, 2012:
The studies aiming to prove the widespread belief that staff vaccination has a substantial effect on patient morbidity and mortality are heavily flawed. No reliable evidence shows that healthcare worker vaccination has noteworthy advantage to their patients—not in reducing patient morbidity or mortality, not in increasing patient vaccination, and not in decreasing [healthcare worker] work absenteeism.[33]

British Medical Journal, 2009:
Most of our studies (70%) were of poor quality with overoptimistic conclusions—that is, not supported by the data presented. Those sponsored by industry had greater visibility as they were more likely to be published by high impact factor journals and were likely to be given higher prominence by the international scientific and lay media, despite their apparent equivalent methodological quality and size compared with studies with other funders.[34]

JAMA Internal Medicine, 2013:
The evidence that influenza represents a threat of public health proportions is questionable, the evidence that influenza vaccines reduce important patient-centered outcomes such as mortality is unreliable, the assumption that past influenza vaccine safety is predictive of future experience is unsound, and nonpharmaceutical interventions to manage influenza-like illness exist.[35]

British Medical Journal, 2013:
Closer inspection of influenza vaccine policies shows that although proponents employ the rhetoric of science, the studies underlying the policy are often of low quality and do not substantiate officials' claims. The vaccine might be less beneficial and less safe than has been claimed, and the threat of influenza appears overstated.[36]

Cochrane Database of Systematic Reviews, 2013:
Vaccinating healthcare workers who care for those aged 60 or over in long-term care institutions showed no effect on laboratory-proven influenza or complications (lower respiratory tract infections, hospitalization or death due to lower respiratory tract illness) in those aged 60 or over resident in long-term care institutions.[37]

Cochrane Database of Systematic Reviews, 2014:
The real impact of biases could not be determined for about 70% of the included [influenza vaccine] studies. . . . Just under 10% had good methodological quality.[38]

Public Library of Science, 2017:
More realistic recalibration based on actual patient data instead shows that at least 6000 to 32,000 hospital workers would need to be vaccinated [with influenza vaccines] before a single patient death could potentially be averted. . . . The impression that unvaccinated HCWs [health care workers] place their patients at great influenza peril is exaggerated.[39]

Cochrane Database of Systematic Reviews, 2018:
The evidence for a lower risk of influenza and ILI with vaccination is limited by biases in the design or conduct of the studies. Lack of detail regarding the methods used to confirm the diagnosis of influenza limits the applicability of this result. The available evidence relating to complications is of poor quality, insufficient, or old and provides no clear guidance for public health regarding the safety, efficacy, or effectiveness of influenza vaccines for people aged 65 years or older. Society should invest in research on a new generation of influenza vaccines for the elderly.[40]

Proceedings of the National Academy of Sciences in the United States of America, 2018:
Self-reported vaccination for the current season was associated with a trend ($P < 0.10$) toward higher viral shedding in fine-aerosol samples; vaccination with both the current and previous year's seasonal vaccines, however, was significantly associated with greater fine-aerosol shedding in unadjusted and adjusted models ($P < 0.01$). In adjusted models, we observed 6.3 (95% CI 1.9–21.5) times more aerosol shedding among cases with vaccination in the current and previous season compared with having no vaccination in those two seasons.[41]

But wait. There's more. The FLUARIX package insert provides an additional list of adverse events that occurred in vaccine victims. These include: lymphadenopathy, tachycardia, vertigo, conjunctivitis, eye irritation, eye pain, eye redness, eye swelling, eyelid swelling, abdominal pain or discomfort, swelling of the mouth, throat, and/or tongue, asthenia, chest pain, feeling hot, injection site mass, injection site reaction, injection site warmth, body aches, anaphylactic reaction including shock, anaphylactoid reaction, hypersensitivity, serum sickness, injection site abscess, injection site cellulitis, pharyngitis, rhinitis, tonsillitis, convulsion, encephalomyelitis, facial palsy, facial paresis, Guillain-Barré syndrome, hypoesthesia, myelitis, neuritis, neuropathy, paresthesia, syncope, asthma, bronchospasm, dyspnea, respiratory distress, stridor, angioedema, erythema, erythema multiforme, facial swelling, pruritus, Stevens-Johnson syndrome, sweating, urticarial, Henoch-Schönlein purpura, and vasculitis.[42]

Some of the more tragic aspects of the flu vaccine atrocity occurred between the years of 1997 and 2004. In 1997, the Advisory Committee on Immunization Practices "recommended the trivalent inactivated flu vaccine to pregnant women after the first trimester."[43] In 2003, the CDC added the jab to the recommended childhood schedule.[44] And then in 2004, in the words of Kelly Brogan, MD, author of *A Mind of Your Own*, the ACIP expanded its flu vaccine recommendation "to encompass all pregnant women (and every human over 6 months of age), regardless of personal risk factors, immune determinants, diet, regional exposures, and timing of injection."[45]

The blanket recommendation that pregnant women receive the flu shot was a slap in the face to the House Committee on Government Reform's 2003 Mercury in Medicine Report, which documented the problems associated with the use of thimerosal in vaccines. According to the report,

> The research is explicit that fetal brains are more sensitive than the adult brains to the adverse effects of methylmercury, which include:
> - Severe brain damage
> - Delayed achievement of developmental milestones
> - Neurological abnormalities such as brisk tendon reflexes
> - Widespread damage to all areas of the fetal brain, as opposed to focal lesions seen in adult tissue
> - Microcephaly
> - Purkinje [neuron] cells failed to migrate to the cerebellum
> - Inhibition of both cell division and migration, affecting the most (extraneous return)
> - basic process in brain development.[46]

The Mercury in Medicine Report was far from the first report to document the risks of thimerosal to pregnant mothers and their developing fetuses. The FDA prepared an internal Point Paper in 1998 for the Maternal Immunization Working Group. The paper advised against the use of multidose vials to avoid "the potential neurotoxic effect of mercury especially when considering cumulative doses of this component in early infancy. . . ."[47] FDA officials addressed those concerns in 1999 in the HHS's National Vaccine Advisory Committee, where Dr. Bernard Schwetz, the Director of the FDA's toxicology center, said,

> . . . the sensitivity of the fetus versus the neonate is very important, and for some of you who have forgotten about the sensitive windows during fetal development, the nervous system develops post-natally. So it isn't unreasonable to expect that there would be particular windows of sensitivity. So it isn't the matter of averaging the dose over the whole

neonatal period—it's what's the week or what's the day or what's the series of hours that represent a particular event in the development of the nervous system when this whole thing might be dangerous. There may be weeks surrounding that when there isn't a major problem. We don't have that information.[48]

In 2000, a "leading researcher" made the following statement to the House Committee on Government Reform:

There's no question that mercury does not belong in vaccines. There are other compounds that could be used as preservatives. And everything we know about childhood susceptibility, neurotoxicity of mercury at the fetus and at the infant level, points out that we should not have these fetuses and infants exposed to mercury. There's no need of it in the vaccines.[49]

In July 2001, the AAP published an internal study that concluded, "Mercury in all of its forms is toxic to the fetus and children and efforts should be made to reduce exposure to the extent possible to pregnant women and children as well as the general population."[50]

As previously cited, one of the adverse effects of mercury on "fetal brains" described in The Mercury In Medicine Report is microcephaly, a disorder vaccine elites blame on the mosquito-borne Zika virus. The same people who parrot the phrase "correlation does not equal causation" to dismiss the link between vaccines and autism or vaccines and infant deaths misdiagnosed as SIDS are now convinced that the Zika virus causes microcephaly based on a virtual lack of correlation.[51]

Mercury, however, is not the exclusive vaccine-related cause of microcephaly. The Institute of Medicine published a report in 1991 titled "Adverse Effects of Pertussis and Rubella Vaccines."[52] The report details numerous adverse effects from the pertussis and rubella vaccines that occur pre-, peri-, or postnatally, including microcephaly.[53] According to Indian researcher Jagannath Chatterjee, in recent years Brazilian children have experienced high rates of birth defects due to "rampant malnutrition" combined with "pesticide and herbicide poisoning" from Monsanto and other global poisoners.[54]

In October 2014, ten months before microcephaly hit the news, the Brazilian health authorities increased the risk of microcephaly by recommending up to three doses of the TDap (tetanus toxoid, reduced diphtheria toxoid, and acellular pertussis vaccine) vaccine during pregnancy, the same vaccine the ACIP has recommended for pregnant American women since 2011.[55, 56, 57] It is interesting to note that since that time Brazilian authorities have apparently done their best to erase any record of the original document, but it can still be found using historical web search engines.[58] When the supply of TDap ran low in Brazil, the vaccinators switched over to the "highly reactive DTP vaccine." The Latin American country also exposes pregnant women to thimerosal with its aggressive flu vaccine campaign.[59]

In addition, some pregnant women receive the MMR vaccine. Again, it is no surprise that pregnant women who were jabbed with jabs known to cause microcephaly gave birth to babies with microcephaly. It is also no surprise that the World Health Organization would blame the benign Zika virus, not the vaccines, for the birth defects.[60] Blaming vaccines would greatly reduce the profits WHO makes from its global vaccination program. Blaming the Zika virus creates yet another source of vaccine revenue with a Zika vaccine. The CDC capitalized on the likely false connection between the Zika virus and microcephaly when its 2016 prediction of the imminent Zika apocalypse resulted in a $1.8 billion Zika award from the US Congress.[61] Part of that money was used to spray US citizens in a few select locations with fear and neurotoxic poisons.[62] Since that time, the CDC's prediction of the Zika apocalypse has been largely forgotten because it failed to materialize. Regardless, as of 2018 the US government continues to support the development of a Zika vaccine, the irony of which cannot be overstated: the Zika vaccine will owe its existence to microcephaly, a condition that is likely a vaccine-induced disorder.[63]

It's important to remember that microcephaly is only one disaster attributed to the vaccination of pregnant women. Dr. Stephanie Seneff, MIT researcher, has written extensively on aluminum toxicity in the brain. The TDap vaccine contains aluminum. Seneff also documented the synergistic toxicity that occurs when aluminum is combined with glyphosate, the "active ingredient" in Monsanto's Roundup. Virtually all people have glyphosate in their bodies. Women living in the agrochemical-intensive regions of Brazil undoubtedly carry high levels of glyphosate. Glyphosate is a powerful metal chelator. Chelators bind to metals and minerals and then release them in acidic environments. Blood becomes more acidic before returning to the lungs. The pineal gland, positioned outside the blood-brain barrier, is near the end of the circulation system. "So," stated Seneff in a 2016 interview, "it's the perfect opportunity for glyphosate to carry aluminum that's in the vaccine to the pineal gland and ruin the pineal gland," resulting in sleep disorders, Alzheimer's, Parkinson's, as well as other neurological diseases.[64]

It's also important to remember that the damage caused by aluminum in vaccines extends beyond the brain. Dr. Suzanne Humphries, a nephrologist, eventually left her lucrative practice due to her employer's refusal to stop injuring her kidney-impaired patients with required vaccinations. Humphries stated,

We're very careful as nephrologists when treating babies because the kidney functions of babies isn't the same as adults—it's vastly reduced. But when it comes to vaccines, this reduced kidney function in infants is always left out of the discussion.[65]

Christopher Exley, a professor with the UK's Keele University, wrote a chapter in the 2008 book *Molecular and Supramolecular Bioinorganic Chemistry*. According to Exley, "Human diseases which have been linked to exposure to aluminium" include: Alzheimer's Disease, Parkinson's Disease, Motor Neuron Disease (MND/ALS), Dialysis Encephalopathy, Multiple Sclerosis, Epilepsy, Osteomalacia, Osteoporosis, Arthritis, Anemia, Calciphylaxis, Asthma, Chronic Obstructive Pulmonary Disease, Vaccine-related Macrophagic Myofasciitis, Vaccine-related Cutaneous Lymphoid Hyperplasia, Vaccine-related Hypersensitivity to Aluminum, Immunotherapy-related Hypersensitivity, Cancer, Diabetes, Sarcoidosis, Down's Syndrome, Muscular Dystrophy, Cholestasis, Obesity, Hyperactivity, Autism, Chronic Fatigue Syndrome, Gulf War Illness, Aluminosis, Crohn's Disease, Vascular Disease/Stroke.[66] The researcher concludes,

> There is no evidence that human physiology is prepared for the challenge of biologically-reactive aluminium and it is naïve to assume that aluminium is a benign presence in the body. Aluminium is contributing to human disease and will continue to do so if its accumulation in the body is not checked or reversed.[67]

Some ten years later, Exley provided hard evidence that aluminum is indeed contributing to human disease when he and his fellow researchers documented record levels of aluminum in the brains of deceased teenagers with autism. The *Journal of Trace Elements in Medicine and Biology* published their paper titled "Aluminium in brain tissue in autism." Their conclusion reads as follows:

> We have made the first measurements of aluminium in brain tissue in ASD and we have shown that the brain aluminium content is extraordinarily high. We have identified aluminium in brain tissue as both extracellular and intracellular with the latter involving both neurones and non-neuronal cells. The presence of aluminium in inflammatory cells in the meninges, vasculature, grey and white matter is a standout observation and could implicate aluminium in the aetiology of ASD.[68]

Following the publication of the paper, Exley stated in an interview,

> I was not prepared for the vitriol, largely anonymous, which accompanied our publication. I have been elucidating upon the potential dangers

of the aluminium age for 34 years now but I have never before had my life threatened openly. I can only assume that our research has weighed very heavily on the toes of those who will not counter the possibility that not all vaccines are 100% safe. . . .

Our research on aluminium and autism took two years of extremely hard and dedicated work to complete. While the response to it through social media in the main has been gratifying, the vitriol of some individuals has been difficult, as have the decisions by mainstream media and the scientific establishment to ignore the findings. The silence in this case has not been 'golden' it has been deafening and it has only served to reinforce that which is of burgeoning realisation that we are already suffering the consequences of the tyranny of the aluminium age.[69]

Returning to the topic of thimerosal, 2003 was about the year when the last of the remaining stocks of thimerosal-containing vaccines were injected into American children. (No thimerosal-containing vaccines were ever recalled in spite of Representative Dan Burton's repeated requests for a recall.[70]) Nearly 50% of flu vaccines, however, still contained thimerosal; and the CDC refused, as it has always done, to state a preference for thimerosal-free flu vaccines.[71]

From that moment onward, fully vaccinated 5-year-old children would receive 53% of the mercury children received during the peak years of the thimerosal generation,[72] and medical professionals advised pregnant women to get the flu shot, regardless of the gestational age of their unborn babies, with nary a word of warning about the risks of mercury. This, in spite of the fact that Eli Lilly, a manufacturer of thimerosal, included the following information in its own 1999 Material Safety Data Sheet for Thimerosal:

Primary Physical and Health Hazards: Skin Permeable. Toxic. Mutagen. Irritant (eyes). Allergen. Nervous System and Reproductive Effects.

Caution Statement: Thimerosal may enter the body through the skin, is toxic, alters genetic material, may be irritating to the eyes, and causes allergic reactions. Effects of exposure may include numbness of extremities, fetal changes, decreased offspring survival, and lung tissue changes . . . .

Effects of Overexposure: . . . Thimerosal contains mercury. Mercury poisoning may occur and topical hypersensitivity reactions may be seen. . . . Exposure to mercury in utero and in children may cause mild to severe mental retardation and mild to severe motor coordination impairment. . . .

Reproduction: Thimerosal—Decreased offspring survival.

Mercury—Changes in sperm production, decreased offspring survival, and offspring nervous system effects including mild to severe mental retardation and motor coordination impairment. . . .

Mutagenicity: Thimerosal - Mutagenic in mammalian cells.[73]

Adding to the insanity, with the exception of the birth dose of the hepatitis B vaccine, the ACIP advises medical professionals to vaccinate preterm infants on the same schedule as babies born full term. Furthermore, "The full recommended dose of each vaccine should be used. Divided or reduced doses are not recommended."[74]

It's important to note that the FDA categorizes both influenza and Tdap vaccines as Pregnancy Category B because in the words of Barbara Loe Fisher, President of the National Vaccine Information Center, "it is not known whether the vaccines are genotoxic and can cause fetal harm or can affect maternal fertility and reproduction. . . ." Therefore, ". . . administering influenza and Tdap vaccines to pregnant women is an off-label use of these vaccines."[75]

As demonstrated by the aforementioned evidence, scientists have long known that vaccinating pregnant women results in severe fetal harm. For government regulators to claim otherwise is a crime against humanity.

After acknowledging the risks associated with the Fluzone vaccine, the manufacturer provides the following warning: "Fluzone should be given to a pregnant woman only if clearly needed."[76] If doctors heeded that one tidbit of sane advice in a world of insane vaccine indoctrination, no pregnant woman—or any other person for that matter—would ever be jabbed with another flu shot.

On October 1, 2001, the Institute of Medicine's Immunization Safety Review Committee released a report titled "Thimerosal Containing Vaccines and Neurodevelopmental Outcomes." The "independent" body downplayed the risk of thimerosal but still recommended "the use of thimerosal-free DTaP, HIB, hepatitis B vaccines in the United States, despite the fact that there might be remaining supplies of thimerosal-containing vaccine available." It further recommended "that full consideration be given by appropriate professional societies and government agencies to removing thimerosal from vaccines administered to infants, or pregnant women in the United States."[77]

Two years after the ACIP recommended the flu jab for all pregnant women, Researchers David Ayoub and Edward Yazbak published a paper titled "Influenza vaccination during pregnancy: a critical assessment of the recommendations of the Advisory Committee on Immunization Practices (ACIP)." Among other things, they concluded:

The [CDC] recommendation of influenza vaccination during pregnancy is not supported by citations in its own policy paper or in current medical literature. Considering the potential risks of maternal and fetal mercury exposure, the administration of thimerosal during pregnancy is both unjustified and unwise.[78]

In 2014, Dr. William Thompson, the CDC whistleblower, confided in a recorded telephone conversation with Dr. Brian Hooker his thoughts on why "they" still give mercury to pregnant women. "My theory on that is that the drug companies think that if it is in at least that one vaccine then no one could argue that it should be out of other vaccines outside of the US." Almost as an afterthought, the CDC scientist added, "So I don't know why they still give it [the flu shot] to pregnant women, like that's the last person I would give mercury to."[79]

Thompson's statement is of special interest because it destroys the notion that the CDC and the Advisory Committee on Immunization Practices are the gatekeepers of the US vaccine program. If it is true as Thompson suggests that "the drug companies" keep thimerosal on the US market just to assuage the fears of concerned people on foreign soil, that would confirm the findings detailed in the "Conflicts of Interest in Vaccine Policy Making" report that was submitted to the US House of Representatives in 2000: the FDA's Vaccines and Related Biological Products Advisory Committee (VRBPAC) and the CDC's Advisory Committee on Immunizations Practices (ACIP) are nothing more than front organizations for the pharmaceutical industry. Kelly Brogan, MD, reveals her disdain for the ACIP with the following statement:

> This group of "thought leaders" is charged with the task of determining what vaccines will be pushed upon you during your doctor's check-ups and wellness visits. It consists of heads of pharmaceutical companies such as Novartis and Sanofi Pasteur, and is a prime example of the enmeshment between the Center for Disease Control (CDC) and industry.[80]

Referring specifically to the policy and practice of vaccinating pregnant women, Brogan wrote, ". . .the guiding authorities you have been led to believe are acting in your best interest are guilty of some pretty heinous crimes of abuse and neglect, and never more so than in the pregnant population."[81]

As if to prove Brogan's point, *Vaccine* published a CDC study in 2017 titled "Association of spontaneous abortion with receipt of inactivated influenza vaccine containing H1N1pdm09 in 2010–11 and 2011–12." Analyzing data from the Vaccine Safety Datalink, the researchers found that the risk of spontaneous abortion (miscarriage) increased by 670% in women who had received the pH1N1-containing vaccine for two consecutive seasons, demonstrating once again that vaccine risk increases with vaccine exposure.[82]

Following is the CDC's heinous response:

CDC and its Advisory Committee on Immunization Practices (ACIP) are aware of these data, which were first presented to ACIP at a public meeting in June 2015. At this time, CDC and ACIP have not changed the recommendation for influenza vaccination of pregnant women. It is recommended that pregnant women get a flu vaccine during any trimester of their pregnancy because flu poses a danger to pregnant women and a flu vaccine can prevent influenza in pregnant women.[83]

In a relatively enlightened era where pregnant women know they should avoid all alcohol, it is more than evident that vaccinating pregnant women with any vaccine, let alone thimerosal-containing vaccines and aluminum-containing vaccines, is a throwback to a former era when doctors delivered babies with the blood of cadavers still on their hands.

Speaking of blood on their hands, vaccinating preterm infants, especially low-weight preterm infants, surely ranks as one of the most senseless and most egregious crimes committed against some of the most vulnerable people on the planet. Neal Halsey, "one of the architects of US vaccine policy,"[84] delivered a presentation in an FDA-sponsored workshop in August 1999 in which he reviewed multiple issues stemming from the vaccination of babies—risks that increase in preterm infants. The presentation came shortly after the FDA had finally done the math and figured out that the smallest infants receive 240 times the EPA's daily allowance for mercury.[85] Halsey was reportedly seen crying when he first learned how much mercury children were receiving in the vaccines he believed to be "safe and effective."[86]

In the ensuing years, researchers have repeatedly documented the dangers of vaccinating preterm infants. Following are a few of their findings:

Journal of Pediatrics, 2007:
Our study revealed that some vaccines, including DTaP, even if administered alone, were associated with cardiorespiratory adverse events and abnormal CRP values in premature infants in the NICU. However, the incidence of these events was higher following simultaneous administration of multiple vaccines compared with administration of a single vaccine.[87]

Vaccine, 2007:
Hexavalent (DTaP, inactivated polio, Hib and hepatitis B) immunization can cause apnea/bradycardia/desaturation in premature babies with chronic disease.[88]

According to vaccine researcher Neil Miller, the scientists involved in this study found that "[n]early 22% of vaccinated premature newborns with chronic disease had adverse reactions."[89] Miller also commented on a 2008 paper published in *The Journal of Pediatrics* on the

> . . . recurrence of cardiorespiratory events following repeat DTaP-based combined immunization in very low birth weight premature infants, saying, "More than half (51.5) of all vaccinated premature infants had an adverse cardiorespiratory reaction after their first vaccination, and 18% of these had a recurrence after their second vaccination."[90, 91]

Two other teams of researchers have also documented "adverse cardiorespiratory events" in low birth weight babies.[92, 93] As common sense would suggest, "Adverse reactions were more common in younger and lower weight infants."[94]

A 2015 paper published in *JAMA Pediatrics* added to the overwhelming weight of evidence against jabbing preterm infants: "Immunization of extremely low-birth-weight (ELBW) infants in the neonatal intensive care unit (NICU) is associated with adverse events, including fever and apnea or bradycardia, in the immediate postimmunization period." The six authors follow up with a jaw-dropping statement: "These adverse events present a diagnostic dilemma for physicians, leading to the potential for immunization delay and sepsis evaluations."[95]

Rest assured that no vaccine-informed parent would share this "diagnostic dilemma" with the doctors they trust to "First do no harm."

The authors then settle the issue for conflicted doctors with the following conclusion:

> **All ELBW infants in the NICU had an increased incidence of sepsis evaluations and increased respiratory support and intubation after routine immunization. Our findings provide no evidence to suggest that physicians should not use combination vaccines in ELBW infants.** Further studies are needed to determine whether timing or spacing of immunization administrations confers risk for the developing adverse events and whether a prior history of sepsis confers risk for an altered immune response in ELBW infants [emphasis added].[96]

The conclusion drawn by these researchers, published in what is considered to be one of most reputable medical journals, demonstrates in stunning clarity the power of the vaccine paradigm over the hearts and minds of medical professionals.

Michelle Rowton, a whistleblower nurse, grew tired of working with such people in Neonatal Intensive Care Units. As the founding member of Nurses Against Mandatory Vaccines,[97] Rowton routinely speaks out against the cavalier manner in which professionals prepare for the expected adverse events following vaccination of preterm infants:

I've sat in a room with our on-call staff of physicians and practitioners [when they say] "Oh wow, this is so embarrassing this 25 weeker never actually required a breathing tube and going on the vent after he was born, he was so strong. But we gave him his two month vaccinations and he got intubated last night ha ha, oops how embarrassing." The step-down units are calling the NICU's and saying "Hey, we're going to go ahead and give these four babies their two month shots today; make sure you have beds ready because we all know they're going to have increased breathing difficulties, feeding and digestion difficulties, apnea, and bradycardia."[98]

Make no mistake; the vaccination of pregnant women, infants, and preterm babies is fundamentally misogynistic. It's a full-on assault against a mother's instincts to protect her children against harm. The media's portrayal of vaccine-informed mothers as hysterical women is also misogynistic, demeaning, and blatantly sexist. In a speech delivered on the grounds of the California State Capitol in April 2015, Robert F. Kennedy, Jr. blasted those who abuse vaccine-informed mothers:

This movement that calls you anti-vax is the most misogynistic movement that I have seen in my lifetime. It is a movement that is anti-mother and it is anti-woman. The names that I hear coming out of people's mouths about hysterics, and "refrigerator moms," and all of this in our major newspapers like the *New York Times*, is extraordinary. And I want to say something about these women before I stand down. I was raised around extraordinary women. My grandmother, Rose Kennedy, was mother of three senators, and the mother of a president. My aunt Eunice Shriver started the Special Olympics. But I have never met women like the ones that I have met in this movement. They are articulate. They're eloquent. They're pharmacists. They're doctors. They're lawyers. They have read the science. They know what the science says. And they can destroy any of these politicians if they were given the ability to debate.[99]

Kennedy then shared in detail the difficulties faced by women and parents who are traumatized by a system that injured their children and further traumatized by the denial of injury from medical professionals and the hateful rhetoric from the press. He concludes,

. . . all of the barriers that are meant to protect our children: the government, the lawyers, the regulatory agency, and the press, the checks and balances in our democratic system that are supposed to stand between corporate power and our little children have been removed. There's only one barrier left, and that's the parents. We need to keep that in the equation.[100]

Standing in direct opposition to misogynistic professionals, Andrew Wakefield listened to the parents who believed their children were injured by the MMR vaccine. Since that time he has said countless times, "The parents were right." Wakefield addresses parents and honors mothers in the introduction to his book *Callous Disregard*:

To the parents I would say, trust your instincts above all else. When considering how to vaccinate your children, read, get educated, and demand fully informed consent and answers to your questions. When you are stonewalled or those answers are not to your satisfaction, trust your instinct. I say this as someone who has studied and engaged in the science and who has become aware of the limitations of our knowledge and understanding of vaccine safety issues. Maternal instinct, in contrast, has been a steady hand upon the tiller of evolution; we would not be here without it.[101]

Finally, Dr. Frank B. Engley, the scientist who since the 1940s has researched, spoken out, and published papers on the toxicity of thimerosal, addressed a Chicago audience in 2008, shortly before he passed away at the age of 88. He, perhaps more than any other person alive at the time, had witnessed the failure of the medical establishment and government to protect the public from the rapacious pharmaceutical industry. His words stand as an eternal indictment against that system and an eternal testament to the power and wisdom of mothers:

May I say that industry and the pediatricians and the obstetricians and NIH and CDC and their ilk don't realize what they're up against: they're up against the greatest force on this Earth, and that's Mother love.[102]

Chapter Eighteen

HPV VACCINE: ONE MORE CON JOB

The public equally needs life-saving drugs as it needs protection from potentially hazardous ones.[1]

—Lucija Tomljenovic, PhD

Human papillomavirus (HPV) is a sexually transmitted infection caused by more of 150 related viruses. According to a CDC webpage, "HPV is named for the warts (papillomas) some HPV types can cause. Some other HPV types can lead to cancer, especially cervical cancer. There are more than 40 HPV types that can infect the genital areas of males and females."[2]

In 2006, the FDA licensed Merck's human papillomavirus (HPV) vaccine Gardasil. Three weeks later, the Advisory Committee on Immunization Practices (ACIP) of the Centers for Disease Control and Prevention (CDC) recommended the jab for girls and women from nine to twenty-six years of age.[3] The same recommendation followed for boys and young men in 2009.[4]

It was billed as an anti-cancer vaccine, and Merck lobbied extensively from the beginning not only for its approval and commercialization, but also for nationwide mandatory vaccination.[5] The pharmaceutical giant targeted mothers, teen, and preteen girls with trauma-based advertising campaigns, assuring them that the vaccine would make them "one less" cervical cancer statistic. Since that time, elementary-aged school children are often told by well-meaning vaccine believers that they will get cancer if they don't submit to all three doses of Gardasil. In some states, children as young as 12 years old can give legal consent to the jabs without informing their parents.[6]

If a vaccine's success is measured in dollars, Gardasil and, to a lesser degree, GlaxoSmithKline's Cervarix are blockbusters. Gardasil revenue reached nearly $1.5 billion in 2007 and Cervarix brought GSK $292 million by 2009.[7] Merck's "one less" campaign was so successful that the trade magazine *Pharmaceutical Executive* named Gardasil the pharmaceutical "brand of the year" in 2006 for building "a market out of thin air."[8]

The market was not the only thing Merck built out of thin air. And Merck was far from alone in the chain of events that brought Gardasil into being. In fact, when all the players are brought into view, Merck's contribution appears almost insignificant. Mark Blaxill, editor of the website Age of Autism and coauthor of *The Age of Autism: Mercury, Medicine, and a Manmade Epidemic*, provided a detailed analysis in three 2010 blogs of what will likely be the template for future vaccine development, manufacturing, licensing, recommendation, and limiting liability.[9, 10, 11]

Two government scientists employed by the National Cancer Institute, one of the largest of the NIH institutes, invented a technological process that was patented and licensed to Merck and GSK for use in their HPV vaccines. Profits from vaccines using the patented technology would be shared with the Department of Health and Human Services. The two NCI scientists were also eligible to receive royalty payments of up to $150,000 per year. By 2009, HPV vaccines brought in more revenue from royalties to the National Institutes of Health than any other product.[12] NIH refuses to disclose the exact amount, citing legal protection even from FOIA requests.[13]

The financial success of Gardasil is partially based on Merck's success at getting the FDA to ignore the fact that their clinical trials were not based on sound scientific methodology. Rather than use double-blind randomized controlled trials (RCT), long considered the gold standard of the scientific method of learning, Merck cooked up a bizarre experiment that would have gotten a failing grade in a middle school science fair. Three test groups were divided unequally by number, age, and gender, creating confounding variables from the beginning. The reference group received Gardasil with most of the subjects receiving all the shots. One of the two "placebo" groups received "amorphous aluminium hydroxyphosphate sulfate adjuvant . . . and was visually indistinguishable from vaccine." The second "placebo" group, a much smaller and younger group, received a vaccine described as a "non-alum placebo" or a "saline placebo," which contained "identical components to those in the vaccine, with the exception of HPV L1 VLPs [the antigen] and aluminum adjuvant, in a total carrier volume of 0.5 mL."[14] The adverse event profile resulting from this "experiment" demonstrated similar risks of harm in the Gardasil and the aluminum containing "placebo" groups with little risk of harm in the third group, which included fewer than 600 children.[15]

Blaxill crunched the numbers and concluded, "Gardasil was not safe."[16] The FDA did the same and concluded otherwise. However, Merck convinced the FDA that Gardasil was not only safe, but that the jab also met the criteria for fast-track approval. Researchers Lucija Tomljenovic and Christopher A. Shaw authored a lengthy paper published in the *Journal of Law, Medicine & Ethics* in 2012. The scientists argued that Gardasil did not meet any of the criteria required to fast-track a product to market.[17]

As has been cited by many others, Tomljenovic and Shaw stated that HPV vaccines provide no additional benefit to the public beyond the routine use of Pap smear screens. Largely because of such screens, the incidence of cervical cancer deaths in developed countries occur 1.4 to 2.3 times per 100,000 women.[18] The Gardasil package insert essentially acknowledges this point with the following statement: "GARDASIL does not eliminate the necessity for women to continue to undergo recommended cervical cancer screening."[19]

Diane Harper, MD, MPH, MS, was one of the lead researchers on the Gardasil vaccine trials. She appeared in the documentary film *The Greater Good*, where she made the following observation:

> The FDA has a particular process that's called Fast Tracking when there is a promising drug that comes forward. [Merck] had scheduled a four-year trial [for Gardasil], but after 15 months they went to the FDA and said, "There is nothing like this vaccine on the market. Would you please consider this for Fast Track?" And the FDA said yes. So within six months they approved it and as soon as they had it approved, Merck said, "We will no longer continue our trial. We're gonna stop our trial because our drug is now approved."[20]

When asked why Harper was raining on the Gardasil parade, the whistle-blower responded, "I want to be able to sleep with myself when I go to bed at night."[21] There is no evidence to suggest that FDA officials lost any sleep over their Fast Track approval of Gardasil even though final safety and efficacy data would not be available for another year.[22]

Three weeks after the FDA licensed Gardasil, the CDC's Advisory Committee on Immunization Practices (ACIP) provided its nod of approval, as well. Vaccine safety advocates who were present on the occasion noted, "After the vote the place erupted in applause. There was hand-shaking and back-slapping. It seemed kind of odd and inappropriate to us." One observer stated, " . . . they were so clearly cheering the recommendation. It was clear and absolutely a celebratory reaction."[23]

Yes, the committee's response to the vote would be "odd and inappropriate" to people who believe that HHS, the FDA, and the CDC exist to protect public health. Less than four years later, the National Vaccine Advisory Committee would respond with "cheers and 'high fives'" to news that the UK's General Medical Council had stripped Dr. Wakefield of his medical license and *The Lancet* had retracted the paper written by Wakefield and 12 colleagues.[24]

If nothing else, such behavior demonstrates profound bias in favor of an ever-expanding vaccine program, which happens to be the same bias held by the criminally run pharmaceutical industry. It would appear that sleeping with one's self has fallen out of fashion among vaccine industry regulators.

The name Gardasil is a stroke of marketing genius, but shortly after the jab was brought to market, vaccine-injured girls and boys soon realized the government had failed to guard against Merck, in much the same way it had failed to protect the public against the known risks of Merck's blockbuster drug Vioxx that resulted in strokes and heart attacks to an estimated 100,000 Americans before it was taken off the market.[25]

Dr. David Graham, the FDA associate director in the Office of Drug Safety, essentially foretold the coming Gardasil catastrophe when he testified at the US senate hearings, stating that the FDA "as currently configured is incapable of protecting America against another Vioxx."[26] Nor is the FDA capable of protecting children who are being subjected to the HPV vaccine, sometimes without parental knowledge or consent.[27]

Even if given the chance, these children wouldn't be able to read or understand the relative lack of benefit when weighed against the very real risk of adverse events as listed in the Gardasil package insert, including: autoimmune hemolytic anemia, idiopathic thrombocytopenic purpura, lymphadenopathy, pulmonary embolus, nausea, pancreatitis, vomiting, asthenia, chills, death, fatigue, malaise, autoimmune diseases, hypersensitivity reactions including anaphylactic/anaphylactoid reactions, bronchospasm, and urticarial, arthralgia, myalgia, acute disseminated encephalomyelitis, dizziness, Guillain-Barré syndrome, headache, motor neuron disease, paralysis, seizures, syncope (including syncope associated with tonic-clonic movements and other seizure-like activity) sometimes resulting in falling with injury, transverse myelitis, cellulitis, and deep venous thrombosis.[28]

Such events occur far more than the "one in a million" cases often quoted by rigid-thinking "vaccinologists." They're also more than one in a thousand and even more one in a hundred. A 2008 FDA clinical review reported that 73.3% of subjects developed "new medical history" after one day in HPV safety studies. Subsets of the injured include "Blood and Lymphatic system disorders" (2.9%), "Gastrointestinal disorders" (13.4%), "Pregnancy, puerperium, and perinatal conditions" (2.0%), "Reproductive and Breast Disorders" (24.8%), "Respiratory, thoracic, and mediastinal disorders" (5.5%), "Skin and subcutaneous tissue disorders" (7.4%), and "Surgical Procedures" (10.2%). A whopping 52.9% developed "Infections and Infestations" including "UTI" (8.5%), "Vaginal candidiasis" (10.9%), "Vaginitis bacterial" (9.8%), and "Vulvovaginal infections" (5.7%).[29] Considering the previous FDA statistics, it's surprising that only 10% of Canadian female HPV vaccine recipients received emergency hospital services up to 42 days after receiving the jab.[30] It is not surprising, however, that after interviewing 170 parents of HPV recipients, Concordia University's Genevieve Rail "condemned the vaccine and called for a moratorium on its use."[31]

In December 2015, the FDA approved Merck's *Gardasil 9*, so named because Merck claims it protects against 9 human papillomaviruses. The new and improved shot not only added antigens to the mix, it more than doubled the shot's aluminum content, giving children 500 mcg per dose, 1,500 mcg per 3-shot series.[32] The synergistic toxicity of aluminum and mercury is well documented. In addition, several researchers have studied aluminum's neurotoxic effects in the absence of mercury.[33]

The CDC's response to the public's growing awareness of the dangers of mercury was to deny those dangers and then to gin up studies giving thimerosal a free pass. In 2015, the CDC used the same playbook when seven CDC scientists authored a paper making the ridiculous claim that girls and women who were pregnant or became pregnant after receiving the HPV vaccine had no cause for concern.[34]

Pronouncing something unclean as clean proves yet again that vaccine safety needs to be removed from the bloody hands of CDC automatons. Their efforts have resulted in carnage around the world. Gardasil injured so many young people in Japan that it took only three months for the Japanese government to withdraw its approval of the vaccine in 2013.[35] Denmark's mainstream news channel TV2 broadcast a documentary on the lives of women that have been destroyed by the HPV jab.[36] The Irish Senator Paschal Mooney stood on the floor of the House of Oireachtas and condemned the medical profession for "protecting the pharmaceutical companies by denying that there are any adverse side effects," and also by denying patient access to HPV "information leaflets" prior to signing consent forms.[37]

According to investigative journalist Jefferey Jaxen, Ireland's National Immunization Office

> . . . scrambled to pull all their information and damning evidence offline that showed orders coming directly from the top. A slide deck given to schools and nurses performing the HPV vaccine immunizations specifically stated and instructed that "packs should not include a patient information leaflet."[38]

In 2017, India's National Technical Advisory Group on Immunization (NTAGI), the country's top immunization advisory body, severed all financial ties with the Bill and Melinda Gates Foundation.[39] Among other concerns, the Foundation had funded an unethical experiment in which illiterate parents were given £10 in exchange for their thumbprint on the consent form's signature line, unaware that their children were "unwitting human guinea pigs for a new multi-billion-pound anticervical cancer drug [Gardasil 9]." Neither were the children given accurate information about the purpose of the vaccine trial: "BMGF says the vaccines were licensed and therefore already established to be safe and efficacious."[40]

Is it possible that Gates really harbors the naïve belief that slapping a license on vaccines cleanses them from industry fraud and greed? If so, perhaps he should have attended the funerals of the dead subjects and informed the mourners that the timing of the vaccine with their children's deaths was just a coincidence. That's the line the CDC uses to explain away the growing number of injured and dead American girls.[41]

Merck inferred as much in its Gardasil 9 package insert, in which it acknowledged that 2.5% (185 people) of Gardasil victims "reported a serious adverse event" and 2.3% (354 people) of Gardasil 9 victims reported the same. Those figures add up to 539 human beings. Merck concluded, "Four GARDASIL 9 recipients each reported at least one serious adverse event that was determined to be vaccine-related. The vaccine-related serious adverse reactions were pyrexia, allergy to vaccine, asthmatic crisis, and headache."[42]

Dr. Bernard Dalbergue doesn't buy the coincidence argument. The former pharmaceutical industry physician with Merck stated in a 2014 interview with the French magazine *Principes de Santé* (Principles of Health), ". . . everyone knew when this vaccine was released on the American market that it would prove to be worthless!" Dalbergue also said,

> I predict that Gardasil will become the greatest medical scandal of all times because at some point in time, the evidence will add up to prove that this vaccine, technical and scientific feat that it may be, has absolutely no effect on cervical cancer and that all the very many adverse effects which destroy lives and even kill, serve no other purpose than to generate profit for the manufacturers.[43]

Evidently, Dalbergue was unaware that the journal *Annals of Medicine* had already reported in 2013 that "clinical trials show no evidence that HPV vaccination can protect against cervical cancer," which is "a rare disease with mortality rates that are several times lower than the rate of reported serious adverse reactions (including deaths) from HPV vaccine."[44]

Dalbergue's claim as a former insider that "decision-makers at all levels are aware of . . . the fraud and scam of it all" confirms what the vaccine-informed public knows all too well: sociopaths are—"at all levels"—running the scam.

Dr. Sin Hang Lee, director of the Milford Molecular Diagnostics Laboratory in Connecticut, corroborated Dalbergue's allegation when he identified in an "open-letter of complaint to the Director-General of the World Health Organization, Dr. Margaret Chan" the organizations and the names of the sociopathic HPV related decision makers.[45]

The pathologist placed the following statement in bold print at the top of the 16-page letter: **"Allegations of Scientific Misconduct by GACVS/WHO/CDC Representatives et al"** [emphasis in original]. GACVS stands for the Global Advisory Committee on Vaccine Safety, the committee that advises the World Health Organization "on vaccine safety," the same committee that played in a role in the 2009 H1N1 flu vaccine scam.[46]

Lee explained to Dr. Chan that he had obtained a series of email exchanges involving highly placed GACVS, WHO, and CDC representatives who "deliberately set out to mislead Japanese authorities regarding the safety of the human papillomavirus (HPV) vaccines, Gardasil® and Cervarix®, which were being promoted at that time."

He named several government officials and university researchers and alleges that they "may have been actively involved in a scheme to deliberately mislead the Japanese Expert Inquiry on human papillomavirus (HPV) vaccine safety before, during and after the February 26, 2014 public hearing in Tokyo."

According to Lee, the email messages reveal that among other things the experts knew and hid the "scientific evidence that HPV vaccination does increase cytokines, including tumor necrosis factor (TNF), particularly at the injection site compared to other vaccines." Lee goes on to explain the process by which aluminum salts in vaccines ". . . boost immune responses of the host to the protein antigens. . . ." The letter continues:

> ". . . [T]he mechanism of the adjuvant effects of aluminum salts has only been recently investigated at the molecular level. It is now generally agreed in . . . the scientific community that aluminum salts used as adjuvants are toxic and always damage the cells of the host at the site of injection, causing a localized inflammation at the vaccination site."

By the letter's end, Lee dispenses with tentative allegations, instead calling for disciplinary action against the wrongdoers:

> It is my opinion that Dr Pless, those whose names appeared in the emails attached to this complaint, and all who blindly dismiss the potential toxicity of the newly created HPV L1 gene DNA/AAHS compound in order to continue to promote HPV vaccinations should be held accountable for their actions. There is no excuse for intentionally ignoring the scientific evidence. There is no excuse for misleading global vaccination policy makers at the expense of public interest.

It is my contention these people have not only violated the Terms of Reference of the WHO Global Advisory Committee on Vaccine Safety (GACVS); they have violated the public trust. Immediate, independent and thorough investigations into their actions with appropriate disciplinary action is the only option available that might restore the public's confidence in worldwide health authorities.[47]

On another occasion, Dr. Lee provided a big-picture perspective on the HPV vaccine, a jab that global decision makers want to inject into every child with or without parental content. According to the scientist:

HPV vaccination is unnecessary and potentially dangerous to some recipients. This is the first vaccine invented by the government, patented by the government, approved by the government, regulated by the government and promoted by the government to prevent an already preventable disease (cervical cancer) 30 years down the road based on using a poorly demarcated, self-reversible surrogate end-point (CIN2/CIN3 lesions) for evaluation of vaccine efficacy, a big scientific fraud. There are no cervical cancer epidemics in any developed countries.[48]

There is, however, an epidemic of greed—an epidemic that has long since proven to be one of the most destructive epidemics of all time. Merck and greed are synonymous terms. Vioxx proved it. Its fraudulent mumps vaccine proved it. And Gardasil proved it yet again. Quoting the trade magazine *Pharmaceutical Executive*: " . . . Gardasil is Merck at its best."[49]

However, when it comes to greed, Gardasil is Merck at its worst.

Chapter Nineteen

RACISM AND THE VACCINE PROGRAM: IT'S A BLACK-AND-WHITE ISSUE

You may choose to look the other way,
but you can never say again that you did not know.
—William Wilberforce

Of all the forms of inequality, injustice in health is the most shocking and the most inhumane.[1]
—Martin Luther King, Jr.

Early American slave traders and owners justified their cruel treatment of fellow human beings by classifying them as subhuman or even nonhuman. Not surprisingly, such a belief leant itself to the practice of racially based medical experiments. Researcher Harriet A. Washington treats the subject in her book *Medical Apartheid: The Dark History of Medical Experimentation on Black Americans from Colonial Times to the Present.*[2]

The US Public Health Service's 40-year Tuskegee Experiment on syphilitic African American men provides the most well-known example of institutional racism in American medicine. The experimenters justified the practice of withholding cheap and available medication for syphilis based on the belief that the black race was too depraved to benefit from treatment. One doctor writing at the beginning of the 20th century expressed the view that the problem of syphilis and tuberculosis for the white race was also a solution that might ultimately facilitate "the end of the negro problem."[3]

In addition to Tuskegee, Washington also documents the genital mutilation of unanesthetized slave women, unanesthetized amputations, infecting or irradiating black prisoners, experimental contraceptive techniques, involuntary sterilizations, experimental smallpox inoculations, and the use of "stolen African American bodies for physician training." Even in the 1990s, experiments included the "jailing of poor black mothers who were unwitting research subjects in South Carolina" and the "infusion of poor black New York City boys with the cardiotoxic drug fenfluramine." More recently, the Office for Protection from Research Risks has

> ... suspended all research at such revered universities as Alabama, Pennsylvania, Duke, Yale, and even Johns Hopkins. Many studies enrolled only or principally African American, although some included a smattering of Hispanics. . . .

> These subjects were given experimental vaccines known to have unacceptably high lethality, were enrolled in experiments without their consent or knowledge, were subjected to surreptitious surgical and medical procedures while unconscious, injected with toxic substances, deliberately monitored rather than treated for deadly ailments, excluded from lifesaving treatments, or secretly farmed for sera or tissues that were used to perfect technologies such as infectious-disease tests.[4]

The government does not limit its prejudicial practices to blacks. Vera Hassner Sharav, MLS, contributed to the book *Vaccine Epidemic*, in which she documented several experiments conducted on non-US and disenfranchised populations. According to Sharav, the US Public Health Service and the National Institutes of Health conducted a vaccination experiment from 1946 to 1948 in Guatemala, where they infected nearly seven hundred institutionalized individuals with sexually transmitted diseases. In 1941, researchers from Longview State Hospital of the University of Cincinnati and from McLean Hospital of Harvard University exposed mentally ill patients to freezing temperatures for extended periods of time. In 1942, "US Army and Navy doctors infected four hundred prisoners in Chicago with malaria." From 1956 through 1972,

> . . . [d]octors deliberately infected "mentally retarded" children at the Willowbrook State School in New York with hepatitis in an experiment aimed at tracking the development of this viral infection, in pursuit of developing a hepatitis vaccine. Parents were coerced into agreeing to the experiment because participation in the study was a condition for admission to the institution.[5]

In addition to the hepatitis vaccine, Willowbrook Hospital also played a role in the development and eventual commercialization of the MMR vaccine. According to Dr. Andrew Wakefield, the children at Willowbrook had "major brain damage," cerebral palsy, and Down syndrome. ". . . [T]hey were easy to observe. They couldn't go anywhere. They lay in bed as vegetables. They were expendable. There was no informed consent whatsoever." Wakefield described these studies as "absolutely lamentable." He concluded,

> If you are going to extrapolate from putting a virus into people who are already brain damaged, and looking at the outcome for a virus that we know can cause encephalitis, inflammation of the brain and encephalopathy, and long term seizure disorders, then you are making a terrible mistake from the outset. How can you compare the outcome in those children who are already fundamentally brain damaged with those with a normal brain? It's just ridiculous.[6]

In 1965, members of the USPHS met at the Centers for Disease Control, where they discussed the public relations problems that might arise should the public become aware of the racist nature of the Tuskegee Study. Their strategy was recorded in the meeting minutes:

> Racial issue was mentioned briefly. Will not affect the study. Any questions can be handled by saying these people were at the point that therapy would no longer help them. They are getting better medical care than they would under any other circumstances.[7]

In 1969, physicians involved in the study met again where "one doctor argued that the study should be stopped and the men treated. . . ." He was overruled. Dr. James B. Lucas, the assistant chief of the Venereal Disease Branch, wrote in a memo: "Nothing learned will prevent, find, or cure a single case of infectious syphilis or bring us closer to our basic mission of controlling venereal disease in the United States." Lucas gave voice to the ongoing racist influence of the era when he concluded that the scientifically worthless study should continue "along its present lines."[8] And so it did until the story broke in the national press in 1972.

President Bill Clinton issued an official apology in 1997. He admitted that the USPHS betrayed "[m]en who were poor and African American, without resources and with few alternatives. . . ." He further stated,

> To our African American citizens, I am sorry that your federal government orchestrated a study so clearly racist. That can never be allowed to happen again. It is against everything our country stands for and what we must stand against is what it was.[9]

The CDC provides a brief summary of the Tuskegee atrocity on its website, noting that

> [t]he Tuskegee Health Benefit Program (THBP) is a congressionally mandated program that provides comprehensive lifetime medical and health benefits to the affected widows and offspring of study participants. There are 12 offspring currently receiving medical and health benefits.[10]

After the news of Tuskegee hit the airwaves, "the federal government took a closer look at research involving human subjects and made changes to prevent the moral breaches that occurred in Tuskegee from happening again."[11]

The CDC describes the changes in research practices that were initiated "to prevent a repeat of the mistakes made in Tuskegee," including the 1974 passage of the National Research Act, which created the National Commission for the Protection of Human Subjects of Biomedical and Behavioral Research.[12]

Informed consent is but one of many principles that was supposedly strengthened by the new law because, if it had been provided to the subjects and to the families of the Tuskegee Experiment, it would have never been conducted. Imagine what would happen to the vaccine program if the industry's insipid vaccine information sheets—which are often given to patients *after* vaccination—were scrapped and patients were instead informed of the following facts:

1. Congress has repeatedly produced scathing reports against the CDC and the FDA for their conflicts of interest with the vaccine industry.
2. Vaccines are tested against the safety profiles of other vaccines, not against an inert placebo.
3. Serious adverse events that occur in vaccine safety tests are routinely written off as not caused by the vaccine.
4. CDC officials committed felony crimes when they trashed documents that demonstrated a 236% increased rate of autism in African American boys and an 700% increased rate of "isolated autism"—meaning that no other medical issues were present—in children who received the MMR vaccine on schedule.
5. Merck whistleblowing scientists revealed that, under pressure from management to fake research efficacy in the mumps vaccine, they added rabbits' blood to research samples. The whistleblowers have filed suit in federal court against Merck for its part in orchestrating the fraud.
6. The oral polio vaccine is routinely given to immunocompromised people in developing countries including people with HIV and AIDS. This

practice results in the paralysis of tens of thousands of children every year and in the deaths of countless others.[13]

7. CDC scientists learned as early as 1999 that thimerosal dramatically increases the rates of several serious disorders including autism. The CDC continues to lie about the toxicity of thimerosal and aluminum to the present day.

8. The World Health Organization and the American Academy of Pediatrics support the use of thimerosal-containing vaccines—vaccines that have been banned in the USA—in developing countries.[14]

9. Pharmaceutical companies routinely test new products including vaccines on uninformed and sometimes unwilling subjects in developing countries.[15, 16]

10. The decision to deny compensation to over 5,000 US families of vaccine-injured autistic children was based on government-sponsored obstruction of justice.

11. The CDC refuses to study the health outcomes of vaccinated versus vaccine-free subjects.

12. Every new vaccine that is added to the schedule increases the risk of adverse events. The vaccine schedule has never been tested for safety.

13. The government is advancing a mandatory womb-to-tomb vaccination policy without religious or personal belief exemptions.

14. There are currently more than 250 vaccines in development, any number of which may be included on the mandatory childhood and/or adult schedules.

15. Vaccines represent the largest medical experiment and the largest medical fraud in the history of the world. Every person on the planet is either directly or indirectly affected.

The Tuskegee Syphilis Study was an affront to decency that never would have been conducted on white people. The horror of that experiment cannot be overstated, but the horror of the ongoing global vaccine experiment far exceeds it. When news of Tuskegee broke, elected officials stepped into action and brought the experiment to a close. However, after William Thompson blew the whistle in August 2014 on the racist nature of the CDC's felonious actions regarding the MMR vaccine, congressional bodies did nothing, that in spite of repeated pleas from Representative Bill Posey, as well as pleas from the public. The victims of Tuskegee numbered in the hundreds. The victims of the global vaccine experiment number in the billions. The surviving victims of Tuskegee received a presidential apology and lifelong compensation. The victims of vaccine injury most often receive hostility, scorn, and denial as to the cause of injury, as well as the denial of compensation.

Parents of vaccine-injured children surely sensed the irony in President Clinton's 1997 apology:

> Let us resolve to hold forever in our hearts and minds the memory of a time not long ago in Macon County, Alabama, so that we can always see how adrift we can become when the rights of any citizens are neglected, ignored and betrayed. And let us resolve here and now to move forward together.[17]

The government did indeed move forward, but with its systematic and strategic advancement of drug and vaccine testing based on substandard scientific principles, conflicts of interest, exploitation of vulnerable people, and fraud, demonstrating yet again "how adrift we can become when the rights of any citizens are neglected, ignored and betrayed."

In fact, even as President Clinton was delivering his speech at the nation's capital, government-funded scientists and doctors were testing toxic drugs and vaccines on orphaned children housed in the Incarnation Children's Center (ICC), a Catholic orphanage in New York City. *Source Watch* describes the circumstances as follows:

> The children ranged in ages from a couple years old to almost adult. Except for a few Hispanic kids, the children are African American, with a number of children in wheel chairs. The wheelchair-bound kids are being fed or drugged, or both, with a milky-white fluid dispensed through tubes coming out of hanging plastic packs. The tubes disappeared beneath their shirts. Inside, children in wheelchairs stared ahead, unable to focus. One wheelchair bound child was about 12. His head was oddly shaped and his eyes were widely space. His limbs and torso were slightly warped, shortened and weak-looking. He was an "AZT baby". Other children had similar faces, arms and legs. Amir, boy of about 6 sat at one of the tables. He had a stomach tube. He had also undergone multiple surgeries to remove "buffalo humps", what AIDS doctors call large, fatty growths from the necks and backs of people who take protease inhibitors. Five months later, he died in a hospital.[18]

The BBC exposed the story in a 2004 documentary titled *Guinea Pig Kids*. Merck, GlaxoSmithKline, Pfizer, Progenics Pharmaceuticals, Genentech, Chiron/Biocine, and others sponsored the drug trials, and New York City's Administration for Children's Services removed children from the homes of foster parents who refused to administer the toxic drugs. The BBC interviewed a 15-year-old boy who was forced to participate in the trials. He warned his peers to take the drugs or the doctors would insert a port into their stomachs to ensure compliance. Some of them didn't heed his advice.[19]

Liam Scheff, the investigative reporter and author who broke the story, corroborated the boy's testimony in his 2014 article titled "The House That AIDS Built." Scheff wrote,

> If the children refuse the drugs, they're held down and have them force fed. If the children continue to resist, they're taken to Columbia Presbyterian Hospital where a surgeon puts a plastic tube through their abdominal wall into their stomachs. From then on, the drugs are injected directly into their intestines.[20]

Amy Goodman with Democracy Now! interviewed Jamie Doran, the producer of *Guinea Pig Kids*. Doran said, "[W]e discovered they were carrying out tests which even under federal rules are certainly illegal. You have to be clear, to use foster children in experimentation, it's prohibited unless there is a direct benefit to those children."[21]

In 2004, The Alliance for Human Research Protection (AHRP) filed a complaint that led to investigations revealing that similar government-funded studies had been in operation in seven states, some since the late 1980s, involving nearly 14,000 children. Five to 10% of the subjects were foster children. AHRP declared, "The institutional culture of arrogance is demonstrably in evidence at both medical research centers and government agencies."[22]

The Simpsonwood meeting took place only three years after Clinton had apologized for the government's role in Tuskegee. Simpsonwood participants included representatives from the American Academy of Pediatrics, the American Academy of Family Physicians, the CDC, the FDA, the WHO, and others. They agreed that the risk associated with thimerosal was high enough that the neurotoxin should be removed from the American vaccine market, but not for vaccines used in developing countries.[23] According to William Thompson, a few years after Simpsonwood, a group of CDC scientists met together and threw away CDC research regarding their discovery that the MMR vaccine was injuring children, particularly African American boys.[24]

There is something deeply symbolic about throwing away damning evidence against the triple jab. By doing so, the scientists also trashed the lives of countless children and families. Robert F. Kennedy, Jr. estimates the number of African American boys who were harmed by receiving the MMR vaccine on schedule to be at least 100,000. Looking beyond the USA, the number of children who "could have been spared debilitating neurological injury if the CDC scientists had told the truth when Thompson and his team first discovered the increased risk in 2001" is truly staggering.[25]

Vaccine-informed black Americans are not surprised by racist governmental-sponsored research. The disregard shown to their children in AIDS research and the vaccine program are just more chapters in the saga of disregard shown to people of color for centuries around the world. In May 2016, Sheila Ealey, an African American mother of a severely vaccine-injured autistic son, addressed a full house in Compton, California, in a Q & A session that followed the mayor's complimentary screening of the movie *Vaxxed*. After recounting past examples of racist government-sanctioned experimentation, Ealey declared,

> Today, the American government, the CDC, has decided that my son's life and the lives of others like him are not worth it. They knew what they were doing when they sent that shot in the dark to cause this to happen to my son. But you see here's the difference: when you turn your face away from what's happening in one community, then the greed decides that it has no respect of person, race or nationality, and it trickles down to every other race of people. So now what we have is a holocaust. Our children are being maimed and they're being killed. And you've got a government sitting in Washington DC that doesn't think enough to subpoena Dr. Thompson who came out and said what they were doing.[26]

On another occasion, a group of African American women shared their thoughts after watching *Vaxxed*. One mother summed up the situation when she said, "The pharmaceutical companies are pimping the heck out of us."[27]

Yes, the pharmaceutical companies are indeed "pimping the heck out of" Americans and the rest of the world, and they're doing it in concert with governments and with the medical establishment. And economically disadvantaged Americans are experiencing the bulk of the "pimping" in the USA. Middle- and upper-class mothers, especially white mothers, are able to stand up to bullying doctors and say no to vaccinations. When poor mothers do the same, doctors and WIC nurses are more likely to report them to Child Protective Services, which sometimes leads to the removal of children from their mothers' care.[28] Cara Judea Alhadeff, PhD, visiting professor of Gender and Critical Pedagogy at UC Santa Cruz, explains the problem in greater detail:

> The poorest sectors of society (disproportionately black, single mothers) are severely punished if they do not conform. Consequences for those who attempt to exercise their health care freedom of choice through non-compliance include:
>
> • reduced or denied Women Infant Children (WIC) vouchers;
> • litigation;

- refused admittance to public school for even partially vaccinated (let alone fully unvaccinated) children; and
- now increasingly, court-ordered vaccination of children against parents' will.[29]

It's no wonder then that, in the words of parent educator Samsarah Morgan, "many will end up vaccinating their children, because they don't want to lose their housing, or they don't want their aid cut."[30]

Some people even believe that government-sponsored racist policy and practice is merely the tip of the iceberg designed to depopulate the world of poor people of color. They cite as evidence the government's development of "contraceptive vaccines." Vaccine believers dismiss such claims as just another tin-foil hat conspiracy theory posted on wacky websites. It's true, of course, that such people post that theory on their websites. What the vaccine believers seem to forget is that contraceptive vaccines are also discussed in what most people would consider to be reputable sources including US government records and the Rockefeller Foundation's Population Council. While population growth patterns are indeed a topic of crucial importance, it is not difficult to predict that entrusting population-related policy to known racists and eugenicists would result in racist and exploitive practices designed more for the benefit of the population architects than the benefit of The Herd. Established in 1952 by John D. Rockefeller III, the purpose of the Council from the beginning was the reduction of population growth, particularly among "undesirable" humans. Rockefeller appointed Frederick Osborn, a leader of the American Eugenics Society, as the Council's first president.[31] Among other organizations, the United Nations, World Bank, The Presidential Committee on Population and Family Planning, the Ford Foundation, and the American Assembly leant support to the Council.[32]

From that time forward, population control has been a central component of US foreign policy. In 1995, the *Journal of Policy History* published an article titled "World Population Growth, Family Planning, and American Foreign Policy" written by John Sharpless, associate professor in History and Demography at the University of Wisconsin. Sharpless wrote,

> The U.S. government position on world population growth as it emerged in the early 1960s was a fundamental departure in both content and commitment. We embraced the idea that one of the goals of American foreign policy should be the simultaneous reduction of both mortality and fertility across the Third World. It was not simply rhetoric. As the years passed, we committed a growing portion of our foreign aid to that end. The decision to link U.S. foreign-policy objectives with the subsidy

of family planning and population control was truly exceptional in that it explicitly aimed at altering the demographic structure of foreign countries through long-term intervention. No nation had ever set in motion a foreign-policy initiative of such magnitude. Its ultimate goal was no less than to alter the basic fertility behavior of the entire Third World![33]

The BBC produced a documentary in 1995 titled *The Human Laboratory* that provided an alternate perspective on the US government's "truly exceptional" aim "to alter the basic fertility behavior of the entire Third World." Professor Betsy Hartmann, author of *Reproductive Rights and Wrongs: The Global Politics of Population Control*, told the BBC,

> At the highest levels in Washington, population growth in the Third World has long been perceived as a national security threat. During the Cold War, of course, public fear and paranoia often focused on the nuclear bomb and in the post-Cold War period we're having the population bomb re-emerging as a threat. Now we're fearing these Third World peoples. Does this mean that you promote *Norplant* like a weapon in the war against population growth? Colleagues and I have looked through declassified documents and have found, much to our horror, that at the highest levels of government this has been an obsession. There is a national security memorandum, for example, which talked about the great need to control population growth in places like Brazil and the big countries and how this population was a definite national security threat.[34]

The first president of the Population Council, Frederick Osborn, and his colleagues were among the elites who promulgated the notion that third-world growth posed a threat to national security. Judging by its presence in more than 50 countries throughout Africa, Asia, Latin America, and the Middle East, it's safe to assume that its original premise remains in force. Naturally, the Council would hide its mission behind politically correct rhetoric including the following: "Our work allows couples to plan their families and chart their futures. We help people avoid HIV infection and access life-saving HIV services. And we empower girls to protect themselves and have a say in their own lives."[35]

No doubt, Wyeth used the same rhetoric in Bangladesh in 1981 to lure disadvantaged women to participate in the clinical trials of its contraceptive Norplant, which was licensed by the Population Council. No doubt, the women who suffered adverse effects from the implanted capsules did not feel empowered when the researchers "ignored [their] problems with the contraceptive and failed to remove the capsules even when asked repeatedly to do so."[36] According to the Population Research Institute, ". . . these results of the 'trials' were later represented as 'successful' and as an indication of how well women around the world had accepted Norplant."[37]

The Population Council sent Catherine Maternowska, a medical anthropologist, to Haiti on a Council fellowship to study Norplant's benefit to Haitian women. Rest assured her report will never grace the pages of the Council's website. No matter, the BBC aired her experience in the documentary *The Human Laboratory*, where Maternowska stated, "Side effects in the context of Haitian women's lives are horrible. With the *Norplant* users they were extremely severe. Bleeding could go on for 18 months. . . ." Maternowska also reported:

> One woman came in with an infection in her arm. She was a market woman, she carried heavy loads on her head and when she came in asking to get the insert out, the doctor complained and he complained and he looked at me and he was used to having me in the clinic and he said, "Oh Cathy, look at this woman, she's an animal, she wants her Norplant out, she's an animal. She has to be in the study and she wants it out now. What's her problem?"

> They proceeded to throw her literally onto the table, lie her down so that they could . . . take the Norplant insertion out. They threw her head to the [side like] this and they gave her the anaesthesia but before the anaesthesia had actually taken effect in her skin they started pulling the inserts out and making incisions and pulling the inserts out. Because [of] the infection in her arm it looked painful, it was red, it was swollen, and the muscle and sinew tissue had grown over the implants, they were pulling and she was wailing, she was crying why, why, and they continued calling her an animal.[38]

The disillusioned anthropologist concluded, "I think it's a sham, it's disgusting. . . . When someone's looking for . . . a solution to their poverty and what they find is something that just makes their poverty worse, it's a huge, huge sadness."[39]

Tuskegee and the experimentation on unwilling and unconsenting children as detailed above demonstrate that medical consent is of little concern to medical sociopaths. Contraceptive vaccines—if marketed as something else—would eliminate the bothersome need for consent. With or without eventual participant consent, the development of antifertility vaccines has been an international effort since the World Health Organization established the Task Force on Vaccines for Fertility Regulation in 1973. Clinical trials were well underway in the 1970s.[40]

The Netherlands-based organization Women's Global Network for Reproductive Rights (WGNRR) reports that the major players in "immunological contraceptive research" include

the World Bank, the UN Population Fund, USAID, Rockefeller Foundation, US and Canadian governments, and others. The major research teams include World Health Organization, National Institute of Immunology (India), The Population Council (USA), The Contraceptive Research and Development Program (USA), and the National Institute for Child Health and Development (USA).[41]

Rajesh K. Naz, professor of Obstetrics and Gynecology and director of the Division of Research at the Medical College of Ohio in Toledo, authored a 2005 paper in which he discussed the advancement in the efficacy of birth control vaccines. According to Naz, contraceptive vaccines (CVs)

. . . may provide viable and valuable alternatives [to other birth control methods] that can fulfill most, if not all, properties of an ideal contraceptive. Since both the developed and most of the developing nations have an infrastructure for mass immunisation, the development of vaccines for contraception is an exciting proposition.[42]

Researchers have focused their efforts on three different technologies to inhibit fertility: anti-sperm, anti-egg, and anti-fetus vaccines.[43] Dr. Naz wrote, "Vaccines targeting gamete outcome" were leading the way with the hCG vaccine tested in phase I and II clinical trials in humans.[44] Indian researcher GP Talwar explains that "Human chorionic gonadotropin (hCG) appears soon after fertilization of the egg and plays a critical role in implantation of the embryo leading to the beginning of pregnancy."[45] Talwar and nearly a dozen of his colleagues authored a 1993 paper in which they described how hCG vaccines stop the progression of pregnancy by inducing "antibodies against human chorionic gonadotrophin (hCG). This vaccine consists of a heterospecies dimer . . . linked to tetanus toxoid (TT) or diphtheria toxoid (DT) as carriers."[46]

In other words, the hCG vaccine causes the human immune system to attack hCG as a foreign invader, thus creating a novel autoimmune disorder in which the bodies of vaccine recipients respond to pregnancy as a disease. The difference between the autoimmune disorder resulting from the hCG vaccine and other well-documented vaccine-induced autoimmune disorders is that the former is intentional, not an unintended adverse event. Dr. Bonnie Dunbar, a more than 20-year veteran of contraceptive vaccine research, stated in a 2010 interview, "Our goal with our vaccine was to develop autoimmunity."[47][48]

Dunbar left the research to her colleagues after discovering that they had "completely destroyed the ovaries" in immunized research animals: "Unfortunately, we weren't just looking at preventing fertilization now; we generated a complete autoimmune disease, which is also known as premature ovarian failure."[49]

The Women's Global Network for Reproductive Rights took issue with the development of anti-fertility vaccines. It is important to note that WGNRR is not generally opposed to contraception or to abortion. To the contrary, the WGNRR supports the right of women "to realise the full sexual and reproductive health and rights of all people, with a particular focus on the most marginalised."[50]

As reported in a 2004 article written by Anita Hardon and published in the Dutch journal *Medische Antropologie*, the WGNRR launched the global *Call for a Stop of Research on Anti-Fertility Vaccines* in 1993.[51] The call was signed by 232 organizations from 18 countries. A portion of the document reads:

We, the undersigned, call for an immediate halt to the development of immunological contraceptives because of concerns about health risks, potential for abuse, unethical research, and the assumptions underlying this direction of contraceptive research.

. . . Immunological contraceptives will not give women greater control over their fertility, but rather less. Immunological contraceptives have a higher abuse potential than any existing method.

. . . Immunological contraceptives present no advantage for women over existing contraceptives.

. . . They interfere with complex immunological and reproductive processes. There are many potential risks: induction of autoimmune diseases and allergies, exacerbation of infectious disease and immune disturbances, and a high risk of fetal exposure to ongoing immune reactions.

. . . the concept of antifertility "vaccines" was conceived in a demographic-driven, science-led framework (WGNRR 1993).[52]

According to Hardon, "By May 1996, this call had been endorsed by 472 groups from 41 countries. Brazil (around 120 signatories), India (95 signatories) and Germany (around 60 signatories) account for more than half of the responses."[53] WGNRR even opposed the use of the word *vaccine* to label a product that "mimics an immunological disorder" rather than ". . . stimulating and increasing the body's ability to defend itself against a specific germ." The organization argued that using the word *vaccine* will prevent women from recognizing that the contraceptive induces rather than prevents disease.[54]

In 1991, global population architects met to discuss the impending "demographic crisis" due to unmanaged population growth. The ominous tone of the WHO's Human Reproduction Programme chairperson suggests that vaccine semantics were not high on their list of priorities:

> Foremost in my mind during these discussions was our difficulty in assessing the urgency of the demographic crisis. To the extent that the impact of that crisis increases, the need for more effective family planning methods must increase. At the very least, failure to develop something that might provide a more effective technology would be to take a grave and unnecessary risk.[55]

Knowing that population control has been a central tenet of US foreign policy for over half a century, that numerous governments and institutions have invested decades and millions of dollars into the development of contraceptive vaccines, and that medical ethics are sorely lacking in government-funded medical research, it would be naïve to think that contraceptive vaccines have not been tested on unsuspecting women in third-world countries. In fact, there's significant evidence that they have been tested.

The BBC's documentary *The Human Laboratory* exposed the odd occurrences in a "tetanus vaccine campaign" in the Philippines.[56] The vaccine was administered only to women of childbearing age and came in a three-shot series, unlike the usual one shot that—in theory, at least—provides protection against tetanus for 10 years. When health care workers noticed an increased rate of miscarriage, they considered the vaccines as the source of the problem. The Philippine Medical Association gathered some vials and sent them to the US FDA for testing. About 20% showed the presence of the hCG subunit. Nicaragua and Mexico later reported the same suspicious circumstances.[57]

The BBC interviewed Dr. Faye Schrater, a feminist immunologist who had written "a review article in which she supported the concern of women's health advocates about 'allergy, autoimmunity, irreversibility and teratology' and possible abuse and direct or indirect coercion by the state. . . ."[58] Schrater told the BBC,

> If there is a conspiracy to immunise the women of the Philippines with chorionic gonadotropin rather than tetanus, then it requires the knowledge of some member of a government, or two. It requires the participation of a manufacturer to link the chorionic gonadotropin physically to the tetanus toxoid—you can't just throw it in the vial and expect it to do its work. And it requires that it be mislabelled and that it be shipped

then to a centre who knows what's in it and who is going to distribute it in a guise of tetanus vaccine. Of course it's plausible and in fact it's probably not all that complicated. All it takes is money and desire and the willingness to lie. We have this long history, we, as women, of been either lied to or coerced in terms of contraception. We've been lied to in terms of either the dosage of hormones like in the pill, we've been lied to about the effects of *Norplant*, we have had *Norplant* coercively used and then refusal to remove it, women have been forced into sterilisation camps. There's a long history of medical science being used negatively on women's bodies and of women being lied to.[59]

In 2014, *Kenya Today*, an independent online news platform, posted a letter written by pro-vaccine Dr. Wahome Ngare, an obstetrician and gynecologist, representing the Kenya Catholic Doctors Association (KCDA). According to Ngare, in 1995 the Kenyan Catholic Bishops asked the Minister of Health to test the WHO's tetanus vaccine before releasing it to the public. "WHO opted to withdraw the vaccine instead of allowing it to be tested for HCG." WHO returned in 2014 and proceeded to vaccinate without prior testing for the presence of hCG. The Kenyan Catholic organizations questioned why "the WHO/ UNICEF sponsored tetanus immunization campaign . . . targeted . . . girls and women between the ages of 14 & 49 (child bearing age). . . ." In March 2014, KCDA secured samples of the suspect vaccine, and testing confirmed that it was ". . . laced with HCG. . . . Further, none of the girls and women given the vaccination were informed of its contraceptive effect." The Association concluded that the "WHO/UNICEF campaign is not about eradicating neonatal tetanus but is a well-coordinated, forceful, population control, mass sterilization exercise using a proven fertility regulating vaccine."[60]

In August 2015, *NPR News* reported that Kenya's

. . . Conference of Catholic Bishops declared a boycott of the World Health Organization's [polio] vaccination campaign, saying they needed to 'test' whether ingredients contain a derivative of estrogen. Dr. Wahome Ngare of the Kenyan Catholic Doctor's Association alleged that the presence of the female hormone could sterilize children.

NPR noted the "distrust [that] has been fueled by WHO's decision to blanket Kenya with polio vaccines, well over and above routine injections. . . ."[61]

In May 2016, Dr. Ngare and his colleague, Dr. Stephen Kimotho Karanja, also a gynecologist and obstetrician, were summoned to appear before the Medical Practitioners and Dentists Board "to respond to complaints . . . that you have given advice to the public on previous vaccination campaigns for Tetanus and Polio and the ongoing immunization. . . ."[62] On June 7th, Kimotho, a devout Catholic, posted the following statement (edited for spelling and grammar) on his Facebook wall:

> . . . I have been summoned by a cartel of medical mercenaries for a disciplinary hearing on why I have been informing the people the truth about the untested vaccines. I will still ask them why they refuse joint sampling and testing of the vaccines before they inject the people.
>
> I will also remind them that the Catholic Church tested the vaccines and found them tainted. . . .
>
> I do not fear them, for even if physical jailing was to result, I would happily submit for the sake of truth. Say a little prayer, fellow warrior, but know this is an excellent opportunity given by God for the rot in immunization to be exposed. . . . Peace.[63]

For those who struggle to even consider the existence of "medical mercenaries" who would use vaccines as a front to sterilize women in developing countries, consider the fact that the USA has a long history of forcibly sterilizing its own citizens for the greater good. California, one of only three states that has eliminated personal belief exemptions to vaccines, sterilized some 20,000 women with "undesirable traits . . . from the 1920s through 1976." Native Americans were targets of "[c]oerced sterilization and/or sterilization without consent . . . . Laws in many states for such sterilization remain on the books."[64]

In addition, the rate of infertility among American women has now reached epidemic levels with one in six couples diagnosed with infertility.[65] It would be irresponsible to suggest that vaccines are the sole cause of the problem. It would, however, be even more irresponsible to suggest that the ingredients in vaccines, some of which are known to reduce fertility, are not a potential source of the problem.[66]

Whether the evidence of intentional vaccine-induced sterility campaigns shakes the faith of devout vaccine believers is of little consequence. The fact remains that just as racism informed the policies of conquerors in former eras, it also informs the policies of modern profit-driven conquerors. Slavers once colonialized foreign soil, resources, and labor. Modern vaccine fascists colonialize the bodies of dark-skinned people with unethical medical experimentation and a smorgasbord of vaccines that are banned for use in wealthy countries. Modern medical colonialism is more insidious, however, because it's not delivered by sword-bearing crusaders, but by trusted institutions and professionals. Epic trauma will result from epic deception and exploitation, and it will eventually transform into hatred and violence against the perpetrators. Thus, the policies invoked by the grand eugenicists of the early- and mid-1900s and carried out by their modern successors will result in the very thing they sought to prevent: chaos, loss of control over resources, and destabilization of power.

Inasmuch as the transnational corporations and the governing bodies in wealthy countries are the same organizations that are advancing racist, violent, and misogynistic vaccine policy, changing that policy will only occur when the citizens of the world rise up and reclaim their bodies and their governments. On that note, another statement from Dr. Karanja is in order:

> I plead with you good people to stand up to these evil groups and refuse to be intimidated by them. We must faithfully serve our God and not Mammon. This is our Land, these are our children, we must fearlessly and courageously defend both.[67]

Chapter Twenty

INDOCTRINATING THE HERD

As previously discussed, herd immunity applies to natural immunity not to artificial vaccine-induced immunity, most people are vaccinated yet few are immunized, vaccines cause over 200 medical conditions including autism, the pharmaceutical industry regulates governmental regulatory agencies, and finally, fraud, corruption, and greed form the foundation of the Vaccine religion.

These facts and more beg the questions: Why do vaccine believers believe in the vaccine scam? Why do they entrust their children's bodies to the care of criminals? Why do they surrender their critical thinking skills to the myth, legend, and lore spoon-fed to them by the High Priests and Prophets of Vaccinology?

The answers are unflattering but simple: First, they need to believe. The thought that the sacred cow of public health is a sham is too much for many to bear. The implications run too deep. Second, emotions often play a larger role in human behavior than reason. This undeniable fact explains why teenagers smoke their first cigarettes, why addicts kill themselves with drugs, why smart people are attracted to abusive partners, why politicians support ill-conceived wars, why soldiers enlist to fight those wars, why obese people eat themselves to death, why anorexics starve themselves to death, and why workaholics work themselves to death.

Vaccine sociopaths in the Unholy Trinity control both the creation and the dissemination of the vaccine story. Humans respond to stories because stories evoke emotion, and those emotions play a larger role in human behavior than does reason. By and large, the industry manipulates The Herd via the pharma-funded mainstream media, and it manipulates the "healers" via pharma-financed medical education and pharma-funded medical journals. The story line and the plot may twist and turn depending on the target audience, but the goal is always the same: convince everyone—regulators, politicians, media, medical professionals, public health officials, parents, teens, and children—to vaccinate. The method is straightforward: appeal to emotion (primarily fear), not to reason. Appeal to myth, not to fact. Appeal to conformity, not to choice. Create the illusion that the story is built upon the rock of science, not the religion of Scientism.

Until fairly recently, traditional religion has provided the predominant paradigm that gives comfort in and purpose to pain, suffering, injustice, and death. Religion offered protection from bad weather, malignant spirits, vile people, and poor health. As the influence of religion decreased in modern society, the influence of the religion of Scientism took its place. Germs replaced evil spirits. Doctors replaced shamans. Pharmaceuticals replaced amulets and icons. And vaccines replaced prayers, ceremonies, and rites of passage.

It's interesting to note that one of the chief prophets of Vaccinology and self-avowed nonbeliever in traditional religion, Paul Offit, authored a book titled *Autism's False Prophets*. Offit went to great lengths—including outright fabrication—to assure his disciples that neither the MMR vaccine nor thimerosal has anything to do with autism. Beyond that, he claimed that biomedical treatments for autism don't work. *Generation Rescue's* cofounder, J.B. Handley, filed suit against Offit for inventing a conversation that never took place.[3] As a result, "Offit [corrected] the passage in his book," "Offit and Columbia University Press [each contributed] $5,000 to one of actress/activist Jenny McCarthy's favorite autism charities at UCLA," and "Offit [sent Handley] a personal letter expressing his regret for the lie he told."[4]

Offit is a paid storyteller. He peddles myths, legends, and lore as truth. Babies can safely receive 100,000 vaccines. Vaccines do not cause autism. Removing toxins injected into babies does not cure autism. He sells his story to believers who are desperate to shore up their fragile faith in the false religion of Vaccinology. His disciples subconsciously or consciously assume that the author of *False Prophets of Autism* must be the True Prophet, regardless of the fact that Offit doesn't treat patients with autism and that vaccines have turned Offit into a millionaire, making him not so much a prophet as profiteer.

Everyone has heard the claim that the media are crooked, corrupt, skewed, etc. In the USA, liberals despise Fox News, and conservatives despise just about every other media outlet. When it comes to vaccines, the industry recruits both major political ideologies to protect and increase its vaccine profits by filling the airwaves with its own story and silencing alternative accounts.

The media silence was deafening following Dr. William Thompson's August 2014 revelation of CDC fraud. It was equally deafening following Congressman Bill Posey's July 2015 explosive testimony in which he quoted Thompson saying that he and his CDC colleagues destroyed the evidence of the MMR's link to autism when they "reviewed and went through all the hardcopy documents that we had thought we should discard, and put them into a huge garbage can."[5]

Prior to the release of the movie *Vaxxed* in the spring of 2016, the media broke its code of silence with news outlets across the USA telling the public that the movie—a documentary that none of the critics had seen—was dangerous anti-vaccine propaganda. Del Bigtree spent nearly seven years as a producer for "The Doctors," a nationally syndicated daytime medical talk show. He walked away from his career to work with Dr. Wakefield in the production of *Vaxxed*, the story of the CDC "cover-up" and "catastrophe." Since *Vaxxed* began distribution in the theaters in the spring of 2016, Bigtree has routinely berated journalists and reporters for failing to cover what he describes as the biggest story of his career—a failure that extends far beyond the boundaries of journalism.

Much of the mainstream media has come out against the film without mentioning the unmentionable: the CDC committed research fraud. As Bigtree says, "If we cannot ask important questions about the safety of a vaccine then I fear for more than the health of our children, I fear for the health of our democracy."[6] Bigtree also said the media should

> . . . be held accountable for the weeks and weeks of covering a measles outbreak at Disneyland, terrifying people when only 644 people were affected. That's .000002% of the people in this country which effectively translates to zero, when one in 45 kids is now diagnosed with autism.[7]

Longtime critic of vaccine shenanigans, Levi Quackenboss, lashed out against the media nitwits who blasted *Vaxxed* without bothering to screen it first:

> Journalism is the reporting of events and facts to keep society informed. Jumping on the "anti-vax, dangerous, shut it down, fraudster, debunked" bandwagon and writing about a movie you've never even seen nowhere near qualifies as journalism.
>
> Emily Willingham at *Forbes*, I'm looking at you. *Los Angeles Times*, *New York Times*, and *Time Magazine*, I'm looking at you. I know damn well

that none of you saw an advanced copy of the movie before praising De Niro's decision under duress to pull it from the film festival, and you were all chomping to tell the masses why it's a dangerous movie. How do any of you call yourself journalists? [8]

Thompson and the *Vaxxed* team are not the first people to run up against the pharma-controlled media. Robert F. Kennedy, Jr. often writes and speaks about the cold shoulder he gets from traditional media as he did in a 2005 article titled "Tobacco Science and the Thimerosal Scandal." The attorney wrote, "I've met extraordinary resistance in my own efforts to publicize this [thimerosal in vaccines] debate. Newspapers have refused to carry an earlier editorial I wrote on this issue, regardless of the documentation I produced in hours-long meetings with editorial board members."[9] In 2015, Kennedy explained to TV host Jesse Ventura the reason the media refuses to take on the pharmaceutical industry, saying,

I ate breakfast last week with the president of a network news division and he told me that during non-election years, 70% of the advertising revenues for his news division come from pharmaceutical ads. And if you go on TV any night and watch the network news, you'll see they become just a vehicle for selling pharmaceuticals. He also told me that he would fire a host who brought onto his station a guest who lost him a pharmaceutical account.[10]

Investigative journalist Jon Rappoport sums up the state of the mainstream media as follows:

The press is a machine, a PR agency representing fear-mongering and vaccine-promoting organizations like the World Health Organization and the CDC. Logic and rationality aren't requirements for gainful employment as a reporter or editor.

I've spoken privately with many reporters over the years. They admit they know what lines they can cross and what lines they can't, what stories they can write and what stories they can't, if they want to keep their jobs. Forcefully contradicting what WHO or the CDC says about the cause of a disease is crossing the line.

Mainstream medical journalism is a walking corpse.[11]

Marcia Angell, MD, served for two decades as editor-in-chief at *The New England Journal of Medicine*. Her experience with the journal led to her 2004 book, *The Truth About the Drug Companies: How They Deceive Us and What to Do About It,* which provides a comprehensive analysis of the power Big Pharma holds over institutions including the media. It includes the following account:

> Morley Safer, of CBS's 60 Minutes, made hundreds of videos that resembled newscasts but were really promotional spots for drug companies. They were given to local public television stations to show between regular programs. Safer was hired by a marketing company called WJMK, on behalf of its pharmaceutical clients. The drug companies reportedly were allowed to edit and approve the videos, and Safer was paid six figures for one day in the studio. When he decided the "news breaks" (as WJMK called them) did not meet the standards of CBS News, the company decided to hire the retired CBS News anchor Walter Cronkite and CNN's Aaron Brown to replace him. Cronkite later pulled out of the deal and was sued by WJMK. His lawyer argued that he was defrauded into believing the advertising was journalism.[12]

With Pharma funding the news outlets and with HSS telling the media not to cover vaccine-informed people if they criticize the vaccine industry, reporters and journalists have two choices: 1. Walk away from their careers, as Del Bigtree did, or 2. Submit to their corporate overlords and turn tricks as "presstitutes." Most, of course, are no more inclined to abandon their careers than doctors are inclined to walk away from theirs.

An increasing number of people, however, recognize that mainstream media reporting in the US are propaganda and not news. As of 2009, the US ranked "49th out of 180 countries included in the [Reporters Without Borders] Press Freedom Index, joining the ranks of countries like Niger, Malta and Romania."[13]

Loss of confidence in the mainstream media is leading to the public's growing reliance on the Internet for news where independent sources abound. As would be expected, Big Business has done its best to seize control of the Internet by shutting down the neutrality of Internet search engines and through the proliferation of astroturf bloggers who pose as independent journalists, scientists, doctors, etc. Attkisson is one of the few journalists who has honestly reported on corruption, conflicts of interest, and other problems in the vaccine industry. In a 2015 TED Talk at the University of Nevada, Attkisson identified a few of the tactics astroturfers employ to obscure the truth:

> Sometimes astroturfers simply shove intentionally so much confusing and conflicting information into the mix that you're left to throw up your hands and disregard all of it including the truth. Drown out a

link between a medicine and a harmful side effect—say vaccines and autism—by throwing a bunch of conflicting paid-for studies, surveys, and experts into the mix confusing the truth beyond recognition.[14]

Attkisson shares additional insights on her blog:

The language of astroturfers and propagandists includes trademark inflammatory terms such as: anti, nutty, quack, crank, pseudo-science, debunking, conspiracy theory, deniers and junk science. Sometimes astroturfers claim to "debunk myths" that aren't myths at all. They declare debates over that aren't over. They claim that "everybody agrees" when everyone doesn't agree. They aim to make you think you're an outlier when you're not.

Astroturfers and propagandists tend to attack and controversialize the news organizations, personalities and people surrounding an issue rather than sticking to the facts. They try to censor and silence topics and speakers rather than engage them. And most of all, they reserve all their expressed skepticism for those who expose wrongdoing rather than the wrongdoers. In other words, instead of questioning authority, they question those who question authority.[15]

Authors Lou Conte and Wayne Rohde describe this disturbing trend:

America is being manipulated—"Astroturfed"—into believing that those who have made the connection between vaccine injury and autism are conspiracy nuts, into believing that doctors should be intimidated into suspending their own judgment and that parents have to be jailed for not giving their children a drug.

The authors further write, "People paid by the pharmaceutical industry should not be allowed to dictate public policy through fear, intimidation and Astroturf."[16] It's not surprising that they dub Paul Offit as "Vaccinology's 'Astroturfer in Chief.'"

An informal, nonscientific survey of Internet users coranked Professor Dorit Rubenstein Reiss and Paul Offit at number three on America's top 10 list of Astroturfers. (Moms Demand Action for Gun Sense in America and Everytown shared the number 1 position, while number 2 went to Media Matters for America.) Lower dishonors were awarded to "'Science' Blogs such as: *Skeptic.com*, *Skepchick.org*, *Scienceblogs.com* (Respectful Insolence), *Popsci.com* and *SkepticalRaptors.com*."[17]

It's important to note once again the power that the word "science" holds over the minds of adoring members of the religion of Scientism. When such members so much as hear the word *science*, their critical thinking skills vanish, which is, of course, the antithesis of science.

Dr. David Gorski, or "Orac" as he calls himself, is one of many bloggers responsible for turning the word "science" into an object of worship while burying real science under piles of disinformation. Orac denies his conflicts of interest with the pharmaceutical industry just as passionately as Offit denies that his vaccine-spawned wealth clouds his judgment. Gorski once hypocritically wrote that pharmaceutical industry shills should be outed, and then independent journalist Jake Crosby did just that by revealing Gorki's own Pharma connections through his employer, Wayne State University, to Sanofi-Aventis, one of the world's largest vaccine makers.[18]

Michael Belkin's healthy five-week-old daughter, Lyla Rose Belkin, died a few hours after getting the hep B vaccine. Belkin formed a band called *The Refusers*, named after the derogatory term used to describe parents—mostly parents of vaccine-injured children—who refuse to participate in further injury of their children with vaccines. He also blogs at *TheRefusers.com*. After Gorski the astroturfer slammed a song Belkin had written about the death of his daughter, Belkin's "First Do No Harm" video rose to the top 1% ranking in the Seattle Rock market. Belkin says the likes of Gorski can "take their immunization fanaticism to its ultimate pinnacle—and vaccinate themselves into oblivion . . . in a Jim Jones-style vaccine Kool Aid party. . . ."[19]

Sharyl Attkisson describes in her book *Stonewalled* how Wikipedia has been taken over by

> . . . powerful pharmaceutical interests that deftly use Wikipedia to distribute their propaganda and control the message. They maniacally troll specific Wikipedia pages to promulgate positive but sometimes-false information about medicines, vaccines, and their manufacturers; and delete negative but often-true information about the same topics . . . . This phenomenon is surely one factor contributing to shameful study results that compared several Wikipedia articles about medical conditions to peer-reviewed research papers, and found that Wikipedia contradicted medical research 90 percent of the time.[20]

Ninety percent! So much for Wikipedia's claim that it maintains a "neutral point of view."[21] Gorski contributes to the deluge of disinformation by anonymously editing Wikipedia, sometimes even quoting himself, the "surgical oncologist David Gorski."[22]

Mothers tend to have a powerful voice in the vaccine-informed movement. Their activism often arises from the guilt they feel from their own complicity with medical professionals in injuring their children. The industry's response to the authentic presence of vaccine-informed mothers is the contrived presence of "passionate influencers." In March 2016, Megan Media, a PR company, offered to pay mothers of young children to "raise awareness around childhood vaccination."[23] The writer who goes by the online name of "Professor" with Thinking Moms' Revolution wrote, "[I]t is a sure bet that none of the 'mommy blogs' produced in this astroturf campaign will be containing conflict-of-interest disclosures." The Professor said she wrote about Megan Media's ploy to turn mothers into industry cheerleaders "to show that what you see in the media is carefully crafted PR bullshit. The bullshit may change, but it is still bullshit designed to get people to shut down their critical thinking skills."[24]

The Megan Media story reveals how far vaccine sociopaths will go to control the vaccine story, but it doesn't reveal the identity of the sociopaths. Jeffry John Aufderheide, father of a vaccine-injured son and founder of *VacTruth.com*, dissected the relationships of multiple organizations supporting the website Voices for Vaccines (VFV), a well-known industry propaganda machine posing as a mommy blog. VFV claims to be a "parent-led organization."[25] It may be true that parents lead VFV, but they're not the parents VFV is referring to. The Task Force for Global Health owns VFV's website. According to Aufderheide, the Task Force is "the third largest charity in the United States," bringing in $1.66 billion a year.[26] Major funders include: Emory University, CDC, Bill & Melinda Gates foundation, Merck, Novartis, Johnson & Johnson, GlaxoSmithKline, Pfizer, and UNICEF. According to the Task Force's IRS Tax records:

> The Task Force for Global Health Inc. is an affiliate of Emory University, and as such, all Task Force employees are in fact Emory University employees. For both the President and Executive Vice President, Emory University includes these positions in its annual market review of compensated professionals in these categories. . . .[27]

Emory University owns 20% of the stock in a vaccine company called GeoVax, assists in developing vaccine technology, and receives milestone payments from its license and royalty agreements for an AIDS vaccine.

CDC employees also play a major role in VFV policy. It is no coincidence that the Task Force headquarters, Emory University, and the CDC are only about three miles apart, making for an easy commute. The Scientific Advisory board for Voices for Vaccines is also influenced by global vaccine architects from top to bottom.

If the board director, Alan Hinman, were to wear sponsorship pins on his suit lapel, he could model for the Bill & Melinda Gates Foundation, Novartis, Emory University, and the CDC. Hinman also sits on the Scientific Advisory board for Every Child by Two (ECBT) with his colleague Paul Offit. According to J.B. Handley, "ECBT is really just a Wyeth vaccine division marketing organization" or as he stated in 2008 with trademark brashness, "By nonprofit standards, ECBT is a rat-shit organization."[28]

Not surprisingly, the king of the rat-shit vaccine propaganda empire, Paul Offit, "Dr. 100,000 vaccines," also sits on VFV's scientific advisory board. That fact alone proves the ongoing prostitution of the word *science* in the service of one of the most corrupt industries on Earth.

Voices for Vaccines understands that its enmeshed web of relationships might raise concerns in the minds of mothers who are searching for nonbiased viewpoints on vaccination. Under the heading of "Independence," VFV responds to those concerns with the following statement: "To allay concerns about conflicts of interest, Voices for Vaccines does not accept donations from vaccine companies."

So few words, so much baloney.

Mothers are not the only demographic that's selectively targeted by industry propaganda. Political liberals are as well, and the source of the propaganda is none other than the American Legislative Exchange Council (ALEC), the Koch brothers-funded, corporate bill mill—the same organization progressives normally hate. Brandon Turbeville, the author of numerous books, shares the details of the hidden influence that the secretive conservative organization holds over the minds of liberals.[29] According to Turbeville, the same organization that writes legislation protecting the rights of gun owners plays a major role in the ongoing push to strip Americans of their right to abstain from mandatory vaccinations. Corporate interests, not ideology, are creating a country where its citizens can pack assault rifles while submitting to their mandatory shots.

The lies pumped out by vaccine sociopaths oddly resonate with progressives who profess a belief in equality and social justice. Yet there's no equality or social justice in ALEC-sponsored bills that withhold Temporary Assistance for Needy Families (TANF) assistance until economically vulnerable parents provide proof that their children are fully vaccinated.

ALEC capitalizes on liberal selective intolerance that would force everyone—regardless of a host of variables—to convert to their one-size-fits-all religion. Thus, liberals—the arch defenders of mothers, children, and minorities—unwittingly support their exploitation on behalf of maniacal corporate profiteers. Turbeville concludes his article by writing:

. . . [I]t is highly ironic that the political left should be the half of the paradigm that takes up the charge for mandatory vaccination laws. After all, it is the left (at the lower levels) who seems to live by the motto "If ALEC supports it, we oppose it." This time, all it took was some clever propaganda, trendy nudging, and social shaming and the left was marching right behind ALEC as militantly as if they were Republicans all along.[30]

Of course, the mainstream media aren't going to inform the public about the role ALEC plays in appealing to politically liberal sensibilities. Neither are they going to inform young mothers that the mothers in those mommy blogs are backed by billions of dollars from criminally run corporations. They won't expose the corporate roots of fake grassroots astroturfers, and the media definitely won't announce that they're pimping for Big Pharma, but they are. And pimping has never been more profitable.

The fact that the great majority of Americans and others around the globe continue to worship the golden calf of Vaccinology—while they remain ignorant of the sociopathic sculptors of the idol—is a testament to the power of the industry and the media to exploit human gullibility. The following chapter explores the fact that the industry not only exploits the gullibility of the vaccinated, it also exploits that of the vaccinators.

Chapter Twenty-One

INDOCTRINATING DOCTORS

Strange times are these in which we live when old and young are taught falsehoods in school. And the person that dares to tell the truth is called at once a lunatic and fool.

—Plato

You don't sell the drug, you sell the disease.[1]

—George Merck, founder of Merck

Big Pharma does not game the system;
Big Pharma owns the system.[2]

—Ben Swann

Americans tend to hold their medical professionals and healthcare system in high regard. And with good reason. Skilled practitioners perform life-extending medical interventions on a routine basis. But, as is evident by the information in the preceding chapters, the medical establishment is enmeshed in a rat's nest of corruption with government and industry, and of the three members of the Unholy Trinity—the pharmaceutical industry, the government, and the medical establishment—industry is the king rat. A brief examination of American history reveals that the original rats gained their wealth not through drugs, but through oil.

In the late 19th and early 20th centuries, John D. Rockefeller, Sr. and his brother William Rockefeller amassed the largest private fortune in history, primarily through Standard Oil. Their cutthroat business practices included "grand-scale collusion with the railroads, predatory pricing, industrial espionage, and wholesale bribery of political officials."[3]

While the Rockefellers were building their dynasty, the drug industry orchestrated the birth of the American Medical Association in 1847 to gain an advantage over nondrug therapies and to solidify the supply chain from manufacturer to consumer.[4] More than 50 years later, however, the drug-based AMA was still a weak organization compared to the influence held by chiropractic, homeopathic, and herbal-based medical practitioners.[5] That was due in part to the fact that the drugs of that era were no better and in some cases were worse than the products hawked by traveling snake oil salesmen.[6]

Since the AMA couldn't compete with the more effective medical practices of the day, it devised a plan in 1904 to delegitimize non-drug-based therapies through a medical ranking scheme conducted by its Council on Medical Education (CME). By 1910, it was evident that the plan had failed because the AMA was destitute, but the Rockefeller Foundation and the Carnegie Foundation stepped in to fund the CME, and over the following decades its tactics succeeded in making drug-based therapies, or allopathy, society's most accepted form of treatment.

The well-known talk show host, Robert Scott Bell, wrote,

> By 1925, over 10,000 herbalists were out of business. By 1940, over 1500 chiropractors would be prosecuted for practicing "quackery." The 22 homeopathic medical schools that flourished in 1900 dwindled to just 2 in 1923. By 1950, all schools teaching homeopathy were closed. In the end, if a physician did not graduate from [an] approved medical school with an M.D. degree, he couldn't find a job as a doctor.[7]

The driving impetus behind that shift was that the Rockefellers had expanded their business empire to include the pharmaceutical industry as well as the drug-intensive American medical establishment. Doctors were educated in Rockefeller-founded institutions with Rockefeller-supported curricula emphasizing the use of drugs manufactured by Rockefeller-owned pharmaceutical companies.[8]

E. Richard Brown, author of the 1979 book *Rockefeller Medicine Men: Medicine and Capitalism in America*, described the means by which "philanthropic capitalists" transformed social institutions,

> giving corporate philanthropy an historical role beyond the most visionary dreams of early philanthropic capitalists. This union of corporate philanthropy, the managerial-professional stratum, and the universities and science spawned the Rockefeller medicine men and their new system of medicine.[9]

It may have been a new system of medicine, but it was run on the same business principles that had turned the original oil robber barons into some of the most powerful men on Earth. In 1952, the *New York Times* described the power of the AMA on Capital Hill:

> Some rather expert observations of the art of lobbying as practiced in Washington assert that the A. M. A. is the only organization in the country that could marshal 140 votes in Congress between sundown Friday

night and noon on Monday. Performances of this sort have led some to describe the A. M. A. lobby as the most powerful in the country.[10]

The May 1954 edition of the *Yale Law Journal* reads:

As a consequence of its monopoly position, financial resources, and political strength, organized medicine is able to maintain a quasi-legal status in medical societies to appoint or recommend members of regulatory bodies. A.M.A. standards in medical education, training, and practice are usually adopted by law. In addition, A. M. A. inspection to determine whether its own standards have been satisfied is seldom subject to judicial review. Thus the political authority of the state itself has in effect been delegated to organized medicine.[11]

The medical establishment essentially claimed proprietary ownership of certain words such as "cure," "health," and "naturopath," and according to the naturopathic doctor T. W. Schippell, it used its power to put non-pharmaceutical-based practitioners who used those words out of business.[12] Dr. Richard Shulze, ND, MH, expanded on the establishment's control over language:

Medicine in our country has been on a crusade over the last 100 years to wipe out every other form of medicine. One of the things they did that was unique was they lobbied to make words legal only for them to use. Today in the US, only a medical doctor can diagnose a disease, prescribe something, and cure you. Nobody else can say "diagnose", "prescribe" and "cure". . . .

I can't as [an] herbalist, say that an herb will cure, even though a lot of prescription drugs are made from herbs.

. . . If I say that I go to jail. It isn't because the herbs don't work and the drugs are better, it's just because they have more money, they lobbied more and got the law passed in their favour.[13]

The assault on medical freedom was evident in the AMA's organized campaign to expose "mental health quackery"[14] as well as its decades-long battle to destroy the chiropractic profession. In 1987, a US judge ruled that the American College of Surgeons and the American College of Radiology had participated in a conspiracy with the AMA to prevent chiropractors from practicing in the United States. The *New York Times* reported:

The American Medical Association led an effort to destroy the chiropractic profession by depriving its practitioners of association with medical doctors and by calling them "unscientific cultists" or worse . . .

Judge Susan Getzendanner described the conspiracy as "systematic, long-term wrongdoing and the long-term intent to destroy a licensed profession" in a ruling late Thursday in an antitrust lawsuit filed in 1976.

The decision said the nation's largest physicians' group led a boycott by doctors intended "to contain and eliminate the chiropractic profession."[15]

The medical establishment was clearly out of control, in part because it derived its ethics from the out-of-control pharmaceutical industry, which derived its ethics from the out-of-control oil barons of the 1800s.

In 2015, Oprah Winfrey interviewed former US president Jimmy Carter, who essentially echoed the claim of Princeton University professor Martin Gilens and Northwestern University professor Benjamin I. Page that ". . . policymaking is dominated by powerful business organizations and a small number of affluent Americans . . ."[16] when he said, "We've become now an oligarchy instead of a democracy. And I think that's been the worst damage to the basic moral and ethical standards of the American political system that I've ever seen in my life."[17]

One need look no further than the lucrative pharmaceutical market to see the bitter fruit of amoral and unethical business practices in the American oligarchy. Following are a few of many examples published by the *New York Times*:

2007: " . . . Bristol-Myers Squibb and a subsidiary paid $515 million to settle federal and state investigations into marketing of its antipsychotic drug Abilify." (Bristol-Myers Squibb also manufactures vaccines.)

2009: "Pfizer paid $2.3 billion . . . , including $1.3 billion in the biggest criminal fine of any type in Unites States history, for off-label marketing of the painkiller Bextra and other drugs. Bextra was withdrawn from the market in 2005. The Pfizer fine included $301 million for off-label marketing of its antipsychotic drug Geodon." (Pfizer also manufactures vaccines.)

2009: "Eli Lilly paid $1.4 billion in January 2009 to settle investigations into illegal marketing of its antipsychotic drug Zyprexa. Lilly's settlement included a $515 million criminal fine, which, until the Pfizer case, was the largest such fine ever imposed on a corporation." (Eli Lilly manufactured thimerosal for vaccine use.)

2010: AstraZeneca was fined $520 million for marketing its blockbuster schizophrenia drug, Seroquel, for unapproved uses. The fine comes to just over 10% of its 2009 sales of $4.9 billion. The company signed a "corporate integrity agreement with the federal government over its marketing of Seroquel for unapproved uses" but did not face criminal charges, which raises the question Who are the real criminals? (AstraZeneca also manufactures vaccines.)[18]

In 2015, the *New York Times* published a scathing report on Johnson & Johnson's marketing of its blockbuster antipsychotic, Risperdal. Although not approved for use by children, J&J distributed "lollipops and small toys" in sample packages as part of its "back to school" marketing campaign. If truth in advertising were part of J&J's business ethics, it would have included bras for boys because insiders knew and hid the fact that Risperdal led 5.5 percent of boys to develop large breasts, 46DD in one case. The price of the bras could have come out of Alex Gorsky's $25 million salary. He was the crook in charge of marketing the drug to children and seniors. J&J paid out more than $2 billion in penalties and settlements. J&J punished Gorsky by promoting him to CEO.[19]

A sampling from US Department of Justice news releases reveals additional Big Pharma shenanigans:

2004: "Warner-Lambert to Pay $430 Million to Resolve Criminal & Civil Health Care Liability Relating to Off-label Promotion."[20]

2008: "Merck to Pay More than $650 Million to Resolve Claims of Fraudulent Price Reporting and Kickbacks."[21]

2010: "GlaxoSmithKline to Plead Guilty & Pay $750 Million to Resolve Criminal and Civil Liability Regarding Manufacturing Deficiencies at Puerto Rico Plant."[22]

2010: "Novartis Pharmaceuticals Corp. to Pay More Than $420 Million to Resolve Off-label Promotion and Kickback Allegations."[23]

2011: "U.S. Pharmaceutical Company Merck Sharp & Dohme to Pay Nearly One Billion Dollars Over Promotion of Vioxx®."[24]

2012: "Sanofi US Agrees to Pay $109 Million to Resolve False Claims Act Allegations of Free Product Kickbacks to Physicians."[25]

2012: "GlaxoSmithKline to Plead Guilty and Pay $3 Billion to Resolve Fraud Allegations and Failure to Report Safety Data."[26]

2013: "United States Sues Novartis Pharmaceuticals Corp. For Allegedly Paying Multi-Million Dollar Kickbacks To Doctors In Exchange For Prescribing Its Drugs."[27]

In 2013, Chinese officials exposed an elaborate criminal and prostitution operation that GlaxoSmithKline engineered to increase sales. Gao Fang, the head of the economic crimes investigation unit at the Chinese Ministry of Public Security, said GSK "has been investigated for bribery allegations in many countries. From our investigation, bribery is part of the strategy of this company." Several partners were involved in the operation, but Feng identified GSK as the main party responsible: "It is like a criminal organisation, there is always a boss. In this game, GSK is the godfather." It is interesting to note that Chinese authorities detained four Chinese nationals involved in the scheme, but Mark Reilly, the English head of GSK's China business, was allowed to leave the country.[28]

As if apologies from criminals engaged in elaborate, organized criminal activities mean anything, the *Daily Mail* reported that "the firm said it 'fully accepts' the facts of the investigation and the verdict and 'sincerely apologises' to patients and doctors."[29] Industry apologies might mean a bit more if the industry also stopped injuring and killing people for profit.

The consumer group Public Citizen reported in 2010 the unlikelihood of such an outcome since the pharmaceutical industry had overtaken the defense industry as "the biggest defrauder of the federal government." The Public Citizen report reads:

Of the 165 settlements comprising $19.8 billion in penalties . . . , 73 percent of the settlements (121) and 75 percent of the penalties ($14.8 billion) have occurred in just the past five years (2006-2010).

Four companies (GlaxoSmithKline, Pfizer, Eli Lilly, and Schering-Plough) accounted for more than half (53 percent or $10.5 billion) of all financial penalties imposed over the past two decades. These leading violators were among the world's largest pharmaceutical companies.[30]

It's important to remember that the US government is not only a victim of pharmaceutical organized crime, but it also profits from such crimes due to its much-heralded public-private partnership. One would think that it would be illegal for the government to do business with criminals, but, despite some past fines and settlements, the government rarely adequately prosecutes those corporations.

Using Merck's Vioxx scandal as an example, The Alliance for Natural Health USA (ANH-USA) explained in a 2011 article how the government's business relationship with industry prevents government officials from prosecuting drug companies for routinely injuring and killing people. After paying out billions of dollars to plaintiffs in Merck's Vioxx affair, the Department of Justice slapped the pharmaceutical giant with a $321 million criminal fine and one misdemeanor count of illegally introducing a drug into interstate commerce.

Additionally, Merck paid out $426 million to the federal government and $202 million to state Medicaid agencies to settle civil claims that its marketing caused doctors to prescribe and bill the government for Vioxx they otherwise would not have prescribed. ANH-USA explains both the reason and the implication for these nominal punishments:

> . . . [T]hese settlements are for rather minor infractions—not for delib-erately concealing the danger of a killing drug from patients, the medi-cal community, and their investors. Despite the serious consequences of Merck's actions, the government won't prosecute them for any serious charges—because, if they did and won, it would mean they would have to stop doing business with Merck in the future! Federal law makes it illegal for Medicare and Medicaid to do business with "an excluded or debarred entity resulting from serious criminal charges."[31]

Several books currently on the market describe the corrupting influence the pharmaceutical industry continues to hold over the medical establishment. One such book, *On the Take: How Medicine's Complicity with Big Business Can Endanger Your Health* by Jerome P. Kassirer MD, former editor-in-chief of the *New England Journal of Medicine*, details the perks—bribes—medical profes-sionals receive from industry in the form of anything-but-free "free" gifts, "free" meals, and "free" education.[32] *Publishers Weekly's* review of Kassirer's book sum-marizes the extent of these problems:

> "Some physicians become known as whores." This is strong language in Kassirer's mostly temperate but tough look at how big business is cor-rupting medicine—but according to Kassirer, one doctor's wife used the word "whore" to describe her husband's accepting high fees to promote medical products.[33]

In 2014, Amy Goodman, the host and executive producer of Democracy Now!, narrated a documentary titled *Big Bucks, Big Pharma* that:

> pulls back the curtain on the multi-billion dollar pharmaceutical indus-try to expose the insidious ways that illness is used, manipulated, and in some instances created, for capital gain. Focusing on the industry's mar-keting practices, media scholars and health professionals help viewers understand the ways in which direct-to-consumer (DTC) pharmaceuti-cal advertising glamorizes and normalizes the use of prescription medi-cation, and works in tandem with promotion to doctors. . . . Ultimately, *Big Bucks, Big Pharma* challenges us to ask important questions about the consequences of relying on a for-profit industry for our health and well-being.[34]

In 2016, six eminent British physicians answered the "important questions about the consequences of relying on a for-profit industry for our health and well-being." The *Daily Mail* covered the story in an article titled "How Big Pharma greed is killing tens of thousands around the world."[35]

Every company mentioned above also manufactures vaccines or vaccine ingredients that are less the fruit of science and more the products of a vaccine paradigm fostered by the industrial-medical-government complex. Its key players were trained to dole out drugs and vaccines to patients just as illicit drug pushers distribute pills and needles on street corners. And at least pushers aren't under the illusion that their products come to market through a science-based system of checks and balances.

Numerous sources report that Big Pharma and Big Medicine collude in creating and maintaining the illusion—from medical schools, to medical journals, and to medical conferences. Most, but not all, aspiring doctors bow their heads and submit to the indoctrination. In 2009, the *New York Times* ran a story about the influence of drug companies in Harvard's educational curriculum. Harvard medical students were not impressed when they learned that they are being trained to pimp for Big Pharma. One student said, "We are really being indoctrinated into a field of medicine that is becoming more and more commercialized." Another said, "Before coming here, I had no idea how much influence companies had on medical education. And it's something that's purposely meant to be under the table, providing information under the guise of education when that information is also presented for marketing purposes." According to Duff Wilson, the author of the article,

> The students say they worry that pharmaceutical industry scandals in recent years—including some criminal convictions, billions of dollars in fines, proof of bias in research and publishing and false marketing claims—have cast a bad light on the medical profession. And they criticize Harvard as being less vigilant than other leading medical schools in monitoring potential financial conflicts by faculty members.[36]

Marcia Angell is an outspoken critic of Pharma's influence over medical education and medical journals. As the editor-in-chief of the *New England Journal of Medicine* for over two decades, she witnessed the shenanigans first hand. Shortly before Angell stepped down from her position in 2000, she wrote an editorial titled "Is Academic Medicine for Sale?" The question was rhetorical. Angell's experience proved conclusively that such was the case.[37]

A reader made a pithy response in a later issue of the *Journal*: "Is academic medicine for sale? No. The current owner is very happy with it."[38] Happy indeed. Angell went on to document the happy relationship between industry and medicine in her 2004 book *The Truth About the Drug Companies: How They Deceive Us and What to Do About it.* According to Angell,

> No one should rely on a business for impartial evaluation of a product it sells. Yet the pharmaceutical industry contends it educates the medical profession and the public about its drugs and the conditions they treat, and many doctors and medical institutions—all recipients of the industry's largesse—pretend to believe it. So does the government. But "education" comes out of the drug companies' marketing budgets. That should tell you what is really going on. As in all other businesses, there is an inherent conflict of interest between selling products and assessing them.[39]

Angell also provided the mind-boggling figure "that the industry hosted over 300,000 pseudo-educational events in 2000, about a quarter of which offered continuing medical education credits."[40] The former editor asserts, "We need to end the fiction that big Pharma provides medical education. Drug companies are in business to sell drugs. Period. They are exactly the wrong people to evaluate the products they sell."[41]

Drug companies are also exactly the wrong people to control medical journals, but that doesn't stop them from doing so. Richard Smith was an editor for the *British Medical Journal* (BMJ) for 25 years. For the last 13 of those years, he was the editor and CEO of the BMJ Publishing Group. In 2005, the year after Smith stepped down from his position, he published a paper titled "Medical Journals Are an Extension of the Marketing Arm of Pharmaceutical Companies."[42]

In addition to quoting Marcia Angell and Jerry Kassirer, he also quoted Richard Horton, editor of *The Lancet.* They all came to the same conclusion: medical journals can't be trusted or believed. Smith confessed that it took him "almost a quarter of a century editing for the BMJ to wake up to what was happening." Smith pointed out that journals could go under financially if they were to adhere to journalistic and scientific integrity:

> Many owners—including academic societies—depend on profits from their journals. An editor may thus face a frighteningly stark conflict of interest: publish a trial that will bring US$100,000 of profit or meet the end-of-year budget by firing an editor.[43]

Smith also laid to rest the myth that the peer review process safeguards against error because the process is subject "to bias and abuse."[44] Beyond bias and abuse, the BMJ demonstrated that the process doesn't work when it sent 300 reviewers a short paper that included eight deliberate errors. Smith told *The Times Higher*

Education in 2015, "No-one found more than five, the median was two, and 20 per cent didn't spot any. If peer review was a drug it would never get on the market because we have lots of evidence of its adverse effects and don't have evidence of its benefit." Referring to peer review, Smith concluded, "It's time to slaughter the sacred cow."[45]

There is rich irony in the fact that Richard Horton, the editor of *The Lancet* in 2004, made the statement that "[j]ournals have devolved into information laundering operations for the pharmaceutical industry."[46] Horton would know because he's the editor who announced in a 2010 press conference that the Andrew Wakefield et al. paper was "fatally flawed," not because the information presented in the case series was incorrect, but because "the claims in the original paper that children were 'consecutively referred' and that investigations were 'approved' by the local ethics committee have been proven to be false."[47] Wakefield described in his book *Callous Disregard* the role Horton played in the retraction of the paper and Wakefield's eventual delicensure.[48]

The Wakefield et al. paper was retracted for the same reason that the CDC's fraudulent 2004 DeStefano et al. paper was not retracted: industry profit. In addition, Dr. Brian Hooker's 2014 paper, a paper that criticized the CDC's 2004 paper, was retracted for the same reason.[49]

Last, if scientific integrity really were more than just a slogan, any and all papers concocted to hide the thimerosal-autism link and connected in any way to felon and wanted fugitive Poul Thorsen would have long since been retracted. Sadly, all of these cases are proof that the bond between medicine and Rockefeller money is good for business and bad for medicine, consumer health, and freedom. American citizens now have a medical system that is ranked as the USA's third leading cause of death due in large part to the number of people who die taking medications even as prescribed.[50]

Inasmuch as healthy diets and lifestyles don't fit into the drug-based American healthcare system, the medical establishment can also take partial credit for the part it plays in the two leading causes of American death—heart disease and cancer. In their defense, many doctors fail to provide sound nutritional advice because they haven't been trained to recognize any remedy unless it comes in a pill or a syringe. The curriculum in most medical schools includes little more about nutrition than it includes about the substantiated risks of vaccines.[51]

Emeritus Professor of Biochemistry at Cornell T. Colin Campbell, coauthor of the best-selling book *The China Study*, expounds upon this appalling situation:

> You should not assume that your doctor has any more knowledge about food and its relation to health than your neighbors and coworkers. It's a situation in which nutritionally untrained doctors prescribe milk and sugar-based meal-replacement shakes for overweight diabetics, high-meat,

high-fat diets for patients who ask how to lose weight and extra milk for patients who have osteoporosis. *The health damage that results from doctors' ignorance of nutrition is astounding* [emphasis in original].[52]

David Ayoub, MD, discussed in a 2010 presentation how hard it was for him when he realized that

> ... everything that you may have learned in medical school about health care potentially now is inaccurate and it was a lie to promote nothing more than the drug companies that really control healthcare education, and much of the healthcare system here in the United States.[53]

The disillusioned physician learned that institutional ignorance was "more the rule than the exception in healthcare." Said Ayoub,

> Where there's a profit to be made by the drug industry you can bet that the research on causation has been suppressed, has been converted to mostly genetic research which there is no therapy for, and it maintains enormous profit for the industry that is selling drugs to treat these conditions.[54]

It comes as no surprise, then, that many of the same people who believe that health comes in pills and potions also believe that a healthy immune system comes through a needle . . . with or without patient consent. In 2015, The AMA updated its policy on vaccination proclaiming that the people it purports to serve have no right to vaccine-related religious, philosophical, or medical self-determination: "Under new policy, the AMA will seek more stringent state immunization requirements to allow exemptions only for medical reasons."[55] Is it really a good idea to have the AMA—a key player in America's third leading cause of death—advocating for vaccine policy that strips Americans of their right to decline AMA-mandated vaccines?

Not all medical trade groups share the AMA's fascist relationship with the government-pharmaceutical complex, but the power of the AMA cannot be overstated. More than 150 years of history demonstrate that AMA policies and practices are designed to control government, contain and eliminate non-drug-related therapies while expanding the market for the pharmaceutical industry, and training medical professionals to hawk its patented products.

As a result, Americans now bear the burden of having the world's most expensive healthcare system coupled with some of the worst health outcomes among developed and developing nations. Under such circumstances it's growing ever more difficult to function as a vaccine-informed medical provider. That dilemma will be explored in greater detail in the following chapter.

Chapter Twenty-Two

GODS, PAWNS, AND
PERPETRATORS

Power is in tearing human minds to pieces and putting them together again in new shapes of your own choosing.

—George Orwell

I know that most men, including those at ease with problems of the greatest complexity, can seldom accept even the simplest and most obvious truth if it be such as would oblige them to admit the falsity of conclusions which they have delighted in explaining to colleagues, which they have proudly taught to others, and which they have woven, thread by thread, into the fabric of their lives.[1]

—Leo Tolstoy

Most doctors tend to have explicit trust in the scientific pronouncements of high-ranking authority figures. It's rare to find physicians who challenge established thinking and professionally very risky to do so.[2]

—Alan Cantwell, MD

Every day vaccine reactions happen, yet doctors won't report them and deny they exist. The very people who should speak the truth stay silent to protect their wallets, reputations, and practices. Their dishonesty betrays those they are supposed to protect. Vaccine damaged families are treated so badly and exemptions are under threat because policy matters more than honesty.[3]

—Suzanne Humphries, MD

The relationship between physicians and patients has the potential to be respectful, nurturing, and healing. But just like any human interaction, especially those that have an unequal balance of power, the doctor-patient relationship can also be abusive and traumatizing. Unfortunately, the system that trains new entrants in the medical profession is, by and large, itself abusive. The tactics to which medical students are exposed and that some medical professionals use on their patients bear striking similarities to those that abusers utilize to maintain control over others.

Once victims of domestic violence have escaped from the control of their abusers, they frequently compare their experiences with other escapees and discover that abusers tend to wield similar weapons to subjugate their victims. Those typically used in domestic abuse include: power games, mind games, isolation, clinginess, guilt, jealousy, harsh language, restricted access to support systems, using support systems to sanction abuse, degradation, denial, minimizing, blaming, threats, intimidation, economic abuse, etc. Another favorite among abusers is the threat of taking, hurting, or killing their victims' children. Similar tactics appear in other abusive relationships in which a power differential is present: teacher-student, police officer-citizen, captor-prisoner, employer-employee, and yes, even doctor-patient.

The power differential between physicians and patients is among the greatest in modern society. The Unholy Trinity—Pharma, the medical establishment, and the government—exploits the power differential with its brain-numbing repetition of phrases such as "Ask your doctor" or "Only your doctor knows if (insert name of blockbuster drug) is right for you." Not that asking one's doctor is inherently bad, but being told, "Only your doctor knows," *is* inherently unhealthy. Such advice keeps adults locked in a perpetual state of dependence on physicians, who are, after all, only human beings themselves. Patients who submit to such authority are like small children before a parent, or as adults might relate to God. More troubling still is that the system tends to train physicians to act as if they *are* God. Russell Blaylock, MD, addressed the phenomenon in a 2008 presentation:

> We're seeing an arrogance that exceeds all arrogance that we've seen in medicine before . . . they're teaching medical students that you are the brightest people on Earth. Medicine is so far advanced, you know things that no one else could know, and therefore you don't have to listen to your patients because you know what's best. And so you no longer interact with your patients in deciding on procedures and treatments; you tell them what to do. And if they don't do it, you tell them to get out of your office.[4]

In the Western medical model, the "God complex" from which many doctors suffer is not a problem to be corrected; it's a position to be celebrated. Those who suffer are the patients, and authoritarian physicians are often rewarded—not fired—for chronic misuse of power over patients. This situation might be more justifiable if the treatment doctors prescribed resulted in recovery from chronic illnesses, but that is seldom the case. Modern, drug-based, treatment protocols mask symptoms far more often than they heal disease. And the "side effects"—unwanted direct effects—often result in yet another prescription, and then another, etc. In such a system it is no wonder that medical treatment is ranked as the third leading cause of death in the USA. Doctors can and do get away with murder.

The modern medical establishment casts physicians in the roles of both victim and perpetrator. For many students of medicine, the initial desire to heal is destroyed in a highly competitive and soul-sapping system that includes endless shifts, sleep deprivation, poor nutrition, constant indoctrination by pharma-funded propaganda, exploitation and objectification of patients, crushing debt, and abusive advisers. Suicide is the most common cause of death among medical students. Alcohol and other forms of substance abuse are common. Of those who survive the hazing process, most take up careers in which many of the same abusive dynamics operate. No wonder medical professionals take their own lives at a higher rate than any other profession.[5]

Nowhere is the abuse of power in the medical system more evident than it is with vaccine policy and administration. Medical schools fail to provide upcoming doctors with rudimentary training in the science of vaccines. They're "given extensive training on how to talk to 'hesitant' parents—how to frighten them by vastly inflating the risks during natural infection," says Suzanne Humphries, MD. "They are trained on the necessity of twisting parents' arms to conform, or fire them from their practices. Doctors are trained that NOTHING bad should be said about any vaccine, period"[emphasis in original].[6]

The author of *The Vaccine Book: Making the Right Decision for Your Child*, Bob Sears, MD, said it this way:

> Doctors, myself included, learn a lot about diseases in medical school, but we learn very little about vaccines, other than the fact that the FDA and pharmaceutical companies do extensive research on vaccines to make sure they are safe and effective. We don't review the research ourselves. We never learn what goes into making vaccines or how their safety is studied. We trust and take it for granted that the proper researchers are doing their job. So, when patients want a little more information about shots, all we can really say as doctors is that the diseases are bad and the shots are good.[7]

TV's *The Doctors* cohost Rachael Ross, MD, summed up this appalling situation when she told an audience following the screening of the movie *Vaxxed* in May 2016:

> They don't teach us about the ingredients; they don't teach us about the studies behind it. . . . what they teach us is that they've always been given and that they cure diseases and that you just do it. And honestly from the

outside looking in now and in saying this to all you people, I almost feel like an ass. . . . I am just blindly following like a robot following through with this with no real data, no real information, didn't know what was in them . . . that's part of what makes us all feel real bad, and it's part of why physicians are very resistant to this information . . . You have to sit at home and re-digest everything that you've learned and come to terms with the damage that you've potentially caused over the years.[8]

OB/GYN Kathryn A. Hale published a blog titled "I saw *VAXXED* and I was shattered!" in which she described her transition from vaccine believer to vaccine informed. She had declined the flu shot for the first time the previous year and had already stopped addressing the issue of vaccines unless asked directly by a patient. Watching *Vaxxed* led her to agree with the CDC whistleblower, Dr. William Thompson. In Hale's words, "There is a definite link between the MMR vaccine and autism. Children are being damaged and something needs to be done." Echoing Humphries and Ross, Hale said,

There is much that I have learned recently that I was not taught in medical school and is not part of my Continuing Medical Education. Don't be afraid to ask questions. Don't settle until you have an answer. Don't presume that physicians know everything there is to know about vaccine safety. The MMR vaccine is a case where we only knew what we had been told and that was a lie.[9]

As long as medical professionals remain ignorant of numerous vaccine safety issues as well as endemic industry corruption, they remain unable to provide informed consent. According to the CDC, lack of informed consent is not a problem because "There is no Federal requirement for informed consent relating to immunization."[10] Of course there isn't. Informed consent would require informed doctors who would then provide accurate information to their patients. The result would be a physician-led mutiny against an abusive medical system as well as decreased rates of vaccine uptake. The faith of even the most zealous believer would be shattered.

However, in the age of the Internet, an increasing number of medical providers—many following their patients' lead—are learning the truth about vaccines. Theirs is an unenviable position because truth and current vaccine policy are incompatible companions. Del Bigtree, producer of *Vaxxed*, described the situation in an interview with ABC:

The real sad thing is the [number] of doctors I've spoken to that say, "Del, I know that vaccines are causing autism, but I won't say it on camera because the pharmaceutical industry will destroy my career just like they did to Andy Wakefield." And that's where we find ourselves: being bullied by an industry that doesn't really care about our children.[11]

The fear of receiving the same wrath visited upon Wakefield is so common that his name has morphed into a frightening verb as expressed in a statement by Mollie Schreffler, editorial assistant for the *Autism File Magazine*:

One other thing I find disturbing is the number of doctors I'm hearing from who tell me that they know that vaccines are linked to autism but that coming forward with the truth will destroy their careers. They literally say, "I don't want to get Wakefielded."[12]

In 2016, Dr. Nick Delgado made the astounding statement that he had spoken to some 500 doctors in the previous three years. He asked them privately if they would be willing to share their views on vaccinations. They told him, "No, I can't talk about it." Their response to his "Why not?" was "Because my license is at risk and if I do talk about it, I can't defend my colleagues if they're in court."[13]

The experience of integrative cardiologist Dr. Jack Wolfson demonstrates that doctors' fear of losing their licenses is entirely reasonable. Wolfson spoke out against the damage caused by vaccines in a 2014 NBC news interview in Phoenix, Arizona, and a 2015 CNN interview.[14, 15] He also posted an article he described as a ". . . scathing condemnation of parents who blindly follow their doctor's advice, loading up their children with vaccines."[16] His efforts resulted in 38 complaints to the medical board with many medical doctors calling for his license to be revoked. The Arizona Osteopathic Medical Board reviewed his case and decided that he has the First Amendment right to make such statements. After his name was cleared, Wolfson addressed his colleagues in a blog, writing,

Do people really want to live in a country where doctors cannot have opinions outside of those promoted by pharmaceutical companies and the doctors on their payroll? Should doctors like me shut up about pharmaceutical dangers and useless procedures? . . .

I am free to speak my mind and speak the truth, as a doctor, a father, and an American. I urge you and urge all doctors to come out of the shadows and from under the rock where they hide. Open your eyes and open your mouth.

There are hundreds of us out there on the front line defending the sanctity of children. Join us.[17]

Like Wolfson, Daniel Neides, MD, the medical director and chief operating officer of the Cleveland Clinic Wellness Institute, believed that he was free to criticize the sociopathic vaccine industry and other sources of environmental toxins. He did so in a scathing 2017 online article, writing

> I am tired of all the nonsense we as American citizens are being fed while big business—and the government—continue to ignore the health and well-being of the fine people in this country. Why am I all fired up, you ask?
>
> I, like everyone else, took the advice of the Centers for Disease Control (CDC)—the government—and received a flu shot. I chose to receive the preservative free vaccine, thinking I did not want any thimerasol [*sic*] (i.e., mercury) that the "regular" flu vaccine contains.
>
> Makes sense, right? Why would any of us want to be injected with mercury if it can potentially cause harm? However, what I did not realize is that the preservative-free vaccine contains formaldehyde.
>
> WHAT? How can you call it preservative-free, yet still put a preservative in it? And worse yet, formaldehyde is a known carcinogen. Yet, here we are, being lined up like cattle and injected with an unsafe product. Within 12 hours of receiving the vaccine, I was in bed feeling miserable and missed two days of work with a terrible cough and body aches. . . .
>
> For those who want to dive in further, help me understand why we vaccinate newborns for hepatitis B—a sexually transmitted disease. Any exposure to this virus is unlikely to happen before our second decade of life, but we expose our precious newborns to toxic aluminum (an adjuvant in the vaccine) at one day of life.[18]

The Cleveland Clinic pledged its allegiance to the Vaccine religion by firing Neides for promoting "harmful myths and untruths about vaccinations," thus demonstrating that the fear vaccine-informed medical professionals feel is well founded.[19]

The original Wakefielded physician, Andrew Wakefield, said that doctors tell him all the time that they'd like to speak up but are afraid of what it would do to their careers. Wakefield says he has little patience or tolerance for such people anymore. They took an oath to "First Do No Harm," and in remaining silent, they violate that oath and what it means to be a doctor.

On a surface level, it might appear that vaccine-informed physicians and victims of domestic violence are in the same boat: both are afraid to speak their minds for fear of what their abusers might do to them. But victims of domestic violence do not earn millions of dollars over their careers in exchange for their silence. Pediatricians often earn from 50% to 80% of their income from administering vaccines,[20] and many receive year-end bonuses for reaching vaccine target levels.[21] A pediatrician told a Minnesota audience in 2016 that he loses $700,000 a year because he doesn't push vaccines according to the US vaccine schedule.[22] The trade journal *Family Practice Management* published an article in 2015 titled "Immunizations: How to Protect Patients and the Bottom Line," in which the author, a medical doctor, boasted of his skills at buying cheap vaccines to maximize profits. One of the commenters, also a medical doctor, crunched the numbers and concluded, "If a practice just did 4 [pediatric patients] per hour," it would take in "$48,000/40 hr week, $2,400,000/50 weeks (allowing 2 wks for holiday closure)."[23]

In 2016, Blue Cross Blue Shield of Michigan published a Provider Incentive Program booklet. According to the booklet, doctors who meet a 63% vaccination compliance rate in their pediatric practice receive a $400 payout for each eligible member. To get the payout, children must receive the following vaccines on or before their second birthday:

- (4) DTaP* vaccinations
- (3) IPV* vaccinations
- (1) MMR vaccination
- (1) VZV vaccination
- (3) HiB* vaccinations
- (3) Hepatitis B vaccinations
- (4) PCV* vaccinations
- (1) HepA vaccination
- (2 or 3) RV* vaccinations
- (2) Influenza** vaccinations

*Vaccinations administered prior to 42 days after birth are not counted as a numerator hit.

**Vaccinations administered prior to 180 days after birth are not counted as a numerator hit.

The only acceptable exclusionary criteria are "[c]hildren who are documented with an anaphylactic reaction to the vaccine or its components."[24]

Such incentive programs teach doctors that "anaphylactic reaction" is the only one that matters. Every other reaction is money in the bank. Documented encephalopathy? Seizures? Respiratory arrest? No problem. Like Pavlov's dogs, physicians are conditioned to salivate at the sight of unvaccinated babies. Vaccination incentive programs have demonstrated to vaccine-informed parents that jabbing children has far more to do with their doctors' financial health than with their kids' "preventive health." Dr. Suzanne Humphries wrote:

> Can we trust any doctor with any intervention if they are getting kick-backs for using it? No. Can we trust doctors who get kickbacks and then abuse and humiliate and intimidate and coerce you to take their interventions that make them rich? Heck no.[25]

It's no wonder that unscrupulous pediatricians sometimes refuse to treat the children of vaccine-informed parents, a practice that, until August 2016, violated AAP policy.[26, 27, 28] Over a century ago, William Osler, MD, chastised his colleagues:

> You are in this business as a calling, not as a business; as a calling which exacts from you at every turn self-sacrifice, devotion, love and tender-ness to your fellow men. Once you get down to a purely business level, your influence is gone and the true light of your life is dimmed. You must work in the missionary spirit, with a breadth of charity that raises you above the dead level of a business.[29]

In the climate established by vaccine sociopaths, compliant pediatricians view their policies as justifiable means to protect the public, but their actions turn the trust-based, doctor-patient rapport into a power-and-control-based, perpetrator-victim relationship. Jeffrey Benabio, a doctor employed by Kaiser Permanente, published an article in *Dermatology News* in 2017 in which he referred to the power differential between patient and doctor as "asymmetric" or "light paternalism" and said, "It's game on," when patients refuse a flu shot "for flawed reasons." He advised doctors to use their "authority approach" to over-come objections. Benabio failed to see the irony in his words when he stated, "There's a reason why tobacco companies once used doctors in white coats to sell cigarettes—we can be quite persuasive."[30] Yes, modern-day vaccine poison peddlers have replaced tobacco poison peddlers from the past. Parents would be well advised to flee from such physicians and seek care from providers who respect patients' medical autonomy. In the words of vaccine researcher Neil Z. Miller, "You should be thankful that this dysfunctional relationship with your health practitioner has been terminated."[31]

By kicking patients out of their practice, doctors not only protect their fiscal health, they also shield their belief in the vaccine paradigm. Vaccine-informed parents know things that vaccine-believing doctors don't or can't bring them-selves to know. The information such parents share with pediatricians not only threatens their income, it also threatens their careers and indeed their identities.

The psychological energy needed for vaccinators to sustain their faith in vaccines is a stunning testament to the power of even the brightest minds to believe in fairy tales written to protect the profit of sociopaths.

Upton Sinclair was probably referring to meatpackers when he said, "It is difficult to get a man to understand something when his salary depends upon his not understanding it." If the writer had made a similar observation about physicians, it may have read like this: "It is difficult to get a doctor to understand something when his investment in time, energy, education, his career, prestige, salary, bonuses, incentives, retirement accounts, stock options, gifts, memberships, affiliations, privileges, and influence depend upon his not knowing it." With so much to lose, one might more reasonably expect the Pope to convert to Judaism.

But stranger things have happened. The Association of American Physicians and Surgeons (AAPS) is a medical trade organization that has somehow managed to maintain its ethics in a cesspool of medical corruption. AAPS members aren't afraid to rub shoulders with Andrew Wakefield, so in 2011—only one year after the GMC had stripped the scapegoat of his license—Wakefield was invited to speak at the AAPS's 68th annual meeting, where he stated that pediatricians are bribed with incentives for meeting vaccination targets, turning them into "middlemen," something he described as a "tragedy."[32]

Why would the AAPS ask Wakefield to deliver the keynote address if he was a charlatan? Jane Orient, MD, provides an indirect answer to that question in an 18-page letter submitted to the US House of Representatives' Committee on Government Reform 11 years before the United Kingdom's General Medical Council struck off Wakefield from the medical register:

> AAPS revenue is derived almost exclusively from membership dues. We receive no government funding, foundation grants, or revenue from vaccine manufacturers. No members of our governing body [the Board of Directors] have a conflict of interest because of a position with an agency making vaccine policy or any entity deriving profits from mandatory vaccines.[33]

Free of conflicts of interest, the AAPS is also free to speak the words that thousands of vaccine informed doctors are afraid to speak. Among other things, the AAPS told the Committee on Government Reform,

> An intelligent and conscientious physician might well recommend AGAINST hepatitis B vaccine, especially in newborns, unless a baby is at unusual risk because of an infected mother or household contact or membership in a population in which disease is common [emphasis in original].[34]

The implication is clear: only unintelligent and unconscientious physicians would recommend the hepatitis B vaccine to low-risk babies. Such physicians are responsible for damaging an entire generation of children—especially boys— as noted in a 2018 paper published in the *International Journal of Environmental Research and Public Health*. Researchers analyzed the data from 1990 to 2005 and found that boys who received three doses of the thimerosal-containing Hepatitis B vaccine were more than nine times more likely to receive special education services than boys who did not receive the vaccines.[35] The World Mercury Project commented on the paper as follows:

> Extrapolating to the US population as a whole, this means that almost 1.3 million US boys born from 1994-2000 received special education services directly attributable to receiving three doses of thimerosal-containing HepB vaccine—costing taxpayers over $180 billion.[36]

Replacing one neurotoxin for another, unintelligent and unconscientious physicians continue to harm children with the Hepatitis B vaccine to this day. Paul Thomas, MD, lamented that fact in a 2017 interview:

> So it's TOXINS, TOXINS, TOXINS, and then your baby's born, and the first thing they do is give your baby a hepatitis B vaccine with a huge dose, 250 mcg. of aluminum, TEN TIMES THE MAXIMUM TOXIC DOSE, according to the FDA. [The FDA] has had an active policy up since 2000 stating not to exceed 5 micrograms/Kg/day of parenteral aluminum[37] [emphasis in original].

Of course, vaccine-informed nurses find themselves in the same situation as vaccine-informed doctors. But some of them recognize that silence is complicity, and they refuse to be complicit in the abusive vaccine culture. These brave professionals have organized two online groups: Nurses Against Mandatory Vaccines and Nurses Against All Vaccines. As of 2015, more than 22,000 American nurses had refused to surrender their medical autonomy by submitting to mandatory jabs. Some have been fired as a result.[38] A mother of a vaccine-injured child described her encounter with a nurse who bravely broke the code of vaccine silence:

> My daughter had an adverse reaction and the doctor said it was normal and that I was overreacting. The nurse pulled me aside and told me I wasn't overreacting and that some kids do have adverse reactions to vaccine. She said not to tell anyone she told me. Then I started researching

and was appalled at what they hid from me. I tried confronting the doctor to ask why he didn't have me sign a consent form or tell me any of the vaccine risks but he would never take my calls.[39]

Another mother fared even worse because no one warned her of the risk of vaccines to her infant. The midwife who cared for the woman felt a great burden for the part she had played in the senseless death of her client's baby, and, as the editor of the *Midwifery Today* magazine, she later wrote,

> Vaccines are my pet peeve in life. The only "SIDS" case I have had in my practise (20 yrs, 800 births) was a little boy named Sam. His Mom had him in hospital with no meds and no intervention. She was someone I judged to be "too conservative" for me to mention the risks of vaccines.

> Her baby had thrush at six weeks, so she took him to the doctor and he received an antifungal treatment for the thrush, then she drove to the public health clinic and he was given oral Polio and DPT shot. He never woke up for his 3:00 am feed. . . . I'll never forget getting the news he was dead. I told his Mom about my judgement of her and my cowardice to tell her about vaccine risks, and she slammed her fist into the kitchen wall. I promised her I would do everything I could to stop this health holocaust and to never let another client vaccinate without information about the risks.[40]

Similar tragedies play out every day across the USA and around the world.

Perhaps the most encouraging stories that emerge from the abusive vaccine culture are professionals who—sometimes in spite of their best efforts—abandon the faith of their colleagues and join the ranks of the vaccine informed. Patti White, a nurse, testified before a congressional subcommittee in 1999. She described the encounters she and her colleagues were having with parents who were "calling and asking how [to] exempt their children from the hepatitis B vaccination." The nurses spent six months "studying documents, books and research articles published by internationally respected doctors and scientists. . . ." White told the subcommittee,

> You must understand that we began this study to reassure our parents and show them the truth about how safe vaccines are. Unfortunately, our sincere, honest, dedicated study has caused a complete reversal of our once strongly held beliefs. Instead of being able to reassure the parents, we have found ourselves being drawn deeper and deeper into this

unbelievable controversy over vaccines that is raging among physicians, scientists, researchers, parents, and the government.[41]

After expressing her guilt for dismissing parental concerns over the vaccine, White concluded,

> We are all now faced with a moral dilemma: will we protect the "sacred cow of conventional vaccine philosophy" or will we stand up and speak out for the "health and well being of innocent children"? We choose children. We wonder, which will our government choose?[42]

Nearly two decades have passed since that courageous nurse posed the question, and the answer grows more clear with every addition to the vaccine schedule: the government has consistently chosen the interests of Big Pharma over the interests of American citizens.

One of the more inspiring stories to emerge in recent years comes from the state of Washington from a physician by the name of Sam Eggertsen, a family practitioner who faithfully pushed vaccines while slamming Andrew Wakefield. One mother stood up to the doctor, saying he was wrong about vaccines and Wakefield. Unlike most doctors, Eggertsen decided he'd better find out what his patient was talking about. Not only did the practitioner have the humility to learn from his patient, he also had the courage to document and share his findings on his YouTube channel in a lengthy presentation packed with exactly the same information vaccine sociopaths keep from the public when they can.

Eggertsen begins his video by acknowledging his initial contempt for Wakefield and finishes with words of praise, saying, "Looking at the evidence, I must now agree with my patient that Andrew Wakefield is not a fraud, and if I ever meet Dr. Wakefield, I will give him my apology for having said so." Eggertsen's transition from vaccine believer to vaccine informed represents the embodiment of professional integrity and medical ethics. And in the context of the current abusive and coercive treatment of doctors by the medical institution, Big Pharma, and the government, his public alignment with Wakefield is boldly heretical. His is a rare gift to the medical community and to humanity. When asked about his concern over possibly losing his job for questioning vaccine orthodoxy, Eggertsen replied, "I have worried about this but feel that the issue is too important not to say something. I am deeply troubled about mandatory vaccination."[43]

Mandatory vaccination is the biggest threat to patient health and freedom. It is the means by which vaccine-informed medical professionals are eliminated from the medical system when they refuse to submit to mandatory vaccinations or refuse to force patients and parents to submit.

Various websites are dedicated to telling the stories of countless patients who have experienced classic abuse from indoctrinated medical professionals. Perhaps the most well-known site is the National Vaccine Information Center's Cry for Vaccine Freedom Wall, which contains hundreds of accounts of abusive public health officials and medical providers.[44]

It's a horrible irony that some of the same professionals who ask patients if they're experiencing domestic violence employ many of the same tactics that batterers use to force patients and parents to submit to unwanted vaccinations, and they're evident in the victims' stories on the NVIC Cry for Vaccine Freedom Wall and on numerous other websites.

Typical accounts of abuse include: putting parents down for choosing not to vaccinate their children, making them feel guilty by telling them the children will suffer calamity by withholding vaccines, limiting their access to vaccine-related information including vaccine package inserts, withholding information about vaccine exemptions, vaccinating children against parental will when they are not present, dismissing or denying vaccine injury and not taking parental concerns about it seriously, refusing to report vaccine injury to the Vaccine Adverse Event Reporting System (VAERS), threatening not to treat sick children until they are fully vaccinated or until a parent has signed a "vaccination contract" giving the clinic complete control over vaccination choices, threatening to kick parents out of a medical practice for not vaccinating, threatening to report to child protective service agencies for choosing not to vaccinate, requiring non-vaccinating parents to sign a document stating that they are endangering their children, or commanding and expecting compliance.

It would be untrue to suggest that all medical providers abuse patients and parents regarding vaccinations. It is true, however, that the misuse of power permeates the entire vaccine system, and medical providers are both victims and abusers in that system.

This is not a new phenomenon. British physician Walter Hadwen's medical career spanned the late 19th and early 20th centuries. The outspoken critic of both the theory and the practice of vaccination was arrested nine times for refusing to vaccinate his own children. Later, he was charged with manslaughter because he refused to participate in the fashionable practice of killing people with toxic smallpox and diphtheria vaccines. Hadwen had no respect for his colleagues who refused to stand up to the tyrannical vaccine culture of the time. The eloquent public speaker stated in 1925,

It is the great commercial manufacturing firms who are providing the brains for the medical man of to-day. [Applause and laughter.] We are deluged with circulars of ready-made medicines for every ailment under the sun. There never was a day when a medical man had less need for the use of his brains than he has at the present time. The commercial firms do all the thinking for him. [Hear, hear.] With a pocket syringe and a case of concentrated tabloids he can go forth a veritable medical Don Quixote to do battle with every imaginary foe. [Laughter.][45]

The US has its own history of jailing vaccine informed medical professionals including naturopathic doctor and chiropractor, Herbert M. Shelton, in the 1940s.[46] Shelton's victimization by an abusive system led him to conclude, "Medical science is a form of delusional madness from which few medical men ever recover. Backed by commercialism, this madness runs roughshod over the life and health of the people."[47]

Medical journalist Larry Husten writes of the problem of "eminence-based medicine" and "the culture of medicine, which rewards the hubris of eminence and actively punishes or offers subtle disincentives to anyone who question[s] this process." According to Husten,

> Medical training is disturbingly similar to military training, where immediate and unreflecting obedience is the goal. Both basic training and residency are designed to break down the mindset and instincts of a young person in order to mold them to the needs of the profession. In both, the submission to authority is a central tenet.[48]

The need to submit is so extreme that numerous healthcare professionals have been known to guard the secret of senior colleagues who commit medical atrocities including the routine performance of unnecessary and dangerous surgeries and sexual abuse of patients.[49] If the culture of medicine sanctions acts such as these, one must ask the question: who is more sick, doctors or their patients?

Dr. Suzanne Humphries, coauthor of *Dissolving Illusions* and authority on the vaccine-related false historical narrative, echoes Husten's concerns, stating that the medical culture has turned most doctors into "little more than blind slave-technicians who follow the dogma they were taught and were rewarded for repeating, even as the truth unfolds in front of them dictating otherwise."[50] Humphries describes the abusive nature of the medical establishment, beginning with her struggle against the dangerous practice of routine vaccination of kidney-impaired patients, in her 2016 autobiography, *Rising From the Dead*.[51] Like many other vaccine-informed professionals, she eventually found peace and healing outside the confines of the medical establishment.

Dr. Russell Blaylock, a harsh critic of self-identified vaccinologists, stated,

> In this modern age, we are witnessing the absolute regimentation of man, where people are given instructions and expected to follow them

without question. Physicians are more regimented than at any time in history, which is ironic because they were always considered the most independent thinking of the professionals. Today they do what they are told without question.[52]

James Meehan, MD, lashed out against pediatricians in a 2017 Facebook post, writing,

I have ZERO RESPECT for vaccine profiteers that are so financially biased, confirmation biased, indoctrinated, and willfully ignorant of the evidence that clearly shows vaccines cause injury, disease and REGRESSIVE AUTISM, that they aggressively lobby lawmakers to make vaccines mandatory, and deny parents the essential knowledge about the risks of toxic ingredients injected into their babies. . . .

They are complicit accomplices in the murder-by-vaccine crimes that have made American infants THE MOST VACCINATED and THE MOST LIKELY TO DIE in the first year of life. . . .

Every pediatrician, family practitioner, or vaccine profiteer that isn't rising up against the corruption of the science of vaccines perpetrated by the CDC is betraying their oath to "first, do no harm." They are on the wrong side of history. . . .

The blood of every vaccine injured or killed child is on the hands of every pediatrician that parroted lies like "vaccines do not cause autism" and "the science is settled". . . .

The vaccine industry will soon face the backlash as doctors, scientists, and parents across America become aware of your crimes, rise up to oppose your lies, and hold you accountable for the vaccine injury holocaust you've caused[53] [emphasis in original].

Tyrannical paradigms give birth to and nurture tyrants, and few are more tyrannical than the global vaccine paradigm. Almost everyone has been victimized by both its dogma and its application. For every account of abusive medical providers found in books, documentaries, and on the Internet, countless more go unshared. The victims of those encounters may be too traumatized, too scared, too hurt, too angry, too isolated, too overwhelmed, or too busy taking care of their vaccine-injured children to express themselves in print or on video.

For the sake of brevity, only two comments from abusive doctors will be provided here, the first from a family practitioner and the second from an elite member of the Vaccine religion. After a mother wrote about her son's vaccine injury in a Facebook post, a physician responded with the following:

Ms. [last name], what "massive" reactions? Forgive me, but I hear overly-dramatized stories of anecdotal medical incidents so often that I must ask. Was there:

-death?

-permanent damage?

-intubation and a mechanical ventilator followed by admission to the ICU?

-hospitalization (beyond the common "overnight observation to calm Mom down" variety)?

Or was it more like the very common fever, rash, irritability, and/or "acting funny" (per Mom)?

Madam, "your concerns" are a matter for your diary, not the Medical Record. For Christ's Sake, I cannot count the number of times that an ACCURATE diagnosis would have been "Child Fine, Mother Neurotic" [emphasis in original].[54]

In 2018, Peter Hotez, dean of the National School of Tropical Medicine at the Baylor College of Medicine, gave a lecture at Duke University in which he made the outrageous claim that members of the vaccine-informed community are members of a "hate group." According to Hotez, "[Anti-vaccine organizations] camouflage themselves as a political group, but I call them for what they really are: a hate group. They are a hate group that hates [our] family and hates [our] children."[55]

Unfortunately, the attitude of both physicians quoted above is not a rare occurrence. It reflects the all-too-common patronizing and misogynistic attitude fostered in medical school and rewarded in medical practice. Tens of thousands of parents attest to the fact that "professionals" of their ilk infest medical clinics like the cancers that infest an increasing numbers of children's bodies. Appointments with such individuals result in emotional and, far too often, physical injury.

Dr. Marty Makary, a Johns Hopkins University researcher and author of the book *Unaccountable*, states that

. . . the patients that get the best care . . . are those that are highly informed, get second opinions, ask about treatment alternatives, and come in with a loved one or family member either in their doctor's visit or in their hospital room to be a safety net to make sure everything is going smoothly and is well coordinated.[56]

Needless to say, infants, toddlers, and children are more at risk of being harmed and are more in need of protection from dangerous doctors than any other group of people. Parents would do well to remember Makary's advice and act as bodyguards for their children when avoiding medical professionals is not an option.

It's more than evident that the system is broken and a growing number of parents are angry. A member of the Thinking Moms' Revolution expressed herself on the organization's website:

> I'm upset that it's 2016 and Western medicine has their heads still firmly planted up their rear-ends when it comes to nutrition and health. I'm bitter about the fact that now, more than ever, moms are being ostracized for daring to challenge their doctors and tell them there is a better way. There are more and more cases of parents [who] are being threatened with CPS [Child Protective Services] action if they disagree with a diagnosis from a doctor. I might feel completely differently if I didn't see it every day. But it's simply not the case. Western medicine has been an utter failure in helping chronically ill people get better. An utter disappointing and abysmal failure.[57]

Thinking Moms' Revolution also published an article written by Alicia Davis Boone, mother of a daughter injured by the Gardasil vaccine. Boone's interactions with medical professionals following her daughter's injury demonstrate how the vaccine paradigm turns intelligent and empathic caregivers into abusers:

> There is never compassion, empathy, words of encouragement, or any sort of softness in the voices of the medical community. It is just a surreal experience from start to finish, and as parents it leaves us angry, frustrated, desperate, and scared. The people we are taught to go to for help when we are sick are dismissive and cold. No concerned looks, no sense of urgency. Our society has encouraged and enabled an environment for these victims and their families that is confrontational, combative, and the victims are bullied and called crazy. . . .

> We are told to report allergic and adverse reactions be they serious or not, but when we do we are shut down. We are told no way, no how could it be, because it is "rare." What sense does that even make? It is rare, so no, that symptom is not caused by Gardasil or any other vaccine. . . . Every single day doctors are dismissing vaccine injury, and it is placing our children in deadly situations.[58]

J.B. Handley, father of a vaccine-injured child and cofounder of *Generation Rescue*, took well-known astroturfer Dr. David Gorski to task in a 2012 blog dedicated to unmasking "Orac," one of several names Gorski uses online. Handley directed his words at Gorski, but they apply equally to thousands of other doctors:

> A real doctor would care deeply about these real reports from tens of thousands of real parents with real babies. A real doctor would be asking real questions. A real doctor wouldn't be satisfied with the paltry science that's actually been done. A real doctor would realize that studying only one vaccine and one excipient doesn't come close to understanding what is actually being done to our babies in the real world. A real doctor wouldn't play word games with "autism" and "autism like-symptoms." A real doctor wouldn't assert that vaccines don't cause autism when only one vaccine has been analyzed.[59]

Rather than jail doctors for refusing to vaccinate their patients, as has been done in the past, Handley advocates for the jailing of doctors who—for whatever reason—repeatedly jab sick children. In a blog titled "Vaccines Don't Cause Autism, Pediatricians Do," Handley wrote,

> If a doctor sticks six vaccines into a child while the child is taking antibiotics for an ear infection and Tylenol for a cold, he's not a doctor, he's a criminal, and should be hauled into jail on the spot for assault and battery. If the child also happens to have eczema, long-term diarrhea, and has missed a milestone or two, perhaps the charge should be attempted murder.[60]

Way back in 1958, the American Academy of Pediatrics specifically listed eczema as a contraindication for vaccination saying,

> Eczema vaccinatum is frequently iatrogenic and uniformly preventable.

> The following steps are recommended for prophylaxis: 1) No child with atopic eczema or other skin disorder should be vaccinated. 2) No child should be vaccinated if any member of his family has eczema or other skin disorder. 3) Parents of children with eczema should be notified at the onset of the disease of the danger from vaccination contact. 4) If a sibling of a child with atopic eczema is vaccinated, he must be completely separated from that child for at least 21 days.[61]

How many millions of children have medical professionals injured since then because they've forgotten what was well known to their predecessors some 60 years ago?

But it gets worse. Many doctors are so indoctrinated with the lie that vaccines are safe that they're blind to vaccine injury even when it happens right in front of them and at their own hands. In 2005, Marie Hansen's one-year-old son, Dylan, had just received the MMR vaccine when he had a seizure and repeatedly stopped breathing. Fifteen minutes later, the pediatrician administered the varicella vaccine, disregarding the manufacturer's warning in the package insert: "M-M-R II should be given one month before or after administration of other live viral vaccines."[62, 63]

Such behavior is unconscionable, and the system that protects and rewards such doctors is beyond unconscionable. If young Dylan had seized following the administration of *any* other drug—yes, vaccines *are* drugs—it would have been clearly noted in his medical record and have been a contraindication for further use of that drug for the rest of his life. But Dylan will never be able to warn doctors of his reaction to vaccines because the injury he experienced left him severely autistic and mute. How many more children will be injured before the AAP publishes the following statement: "The condition known as Autism Vaccinosis is frequently iatrogenic and uniformly preventable"?

Parents are not the only people outraged at the contemptible vaccine culture developed in the US and exported around the world. After the hepatitis B vaccine was added to the US schedule, Thomas Stone, MD, wrote a scathing "Open Letter to Pediatricians on the Flu Vaccine." He went to great lengths to describe the malfeasance and corruption that brought the swine flu vaccine to market in 1976. He reminded pediatricians that the same system that created "the greatest public-health fiasco in the history of the United States thus far" was the system that licensed, approved, and commercialized the hep B vaccine. Then he stated,

> These new vaccines have been RAMRODDED through these SAME kind of "EXPERT" panels, with the SAME "RUBBER STAMP" mentality, with the SAME total disregard for the safety, health and well-being of those innocents who were and are subjected to these SAME fraudulent assurances of effectiveness and safety. ONLY THIS TIME IT WILL BE INFANTS AND CHILDREN who, unlike those adults who chose to trust the CDC and their "experts," they WILL NOT have a CHOICE, or as it seems, even a CHANCE.

> These are the SAME people who will manage the forced/coerced vaccination of our babies and children with 20 or more injections most of which are for mild or non-fatal illnesses, and NONE of which are to be studied for safety or effectiveness. With their tiny IMMUNOLOGIC functions OVERWHELMED and/or OVER-COMMITTED to these

useless vaccines, their synthetic immune system will be unable to counter an organism of even low virulence.

And these are the SAME people who have gone into the medical business to solve the "health-care crisis"—which they created.

Are you going to use this SAME degree of CAUTION with your tiny patients [emphasis in original]?[64]

Camille Hayes, a nurse, described in a YouTube video her transformation from ardent vaccine believer to self-identified anti-vaxxer. In addition to being angry with believers who refuse to see the facts about vaccines, she's angry with medical providers who prescribe endless combinations of drugs rather than prescribe a healthy diet and lifestyle. Hayes asks, "Why are there so many diseases that are idiopathic? Because we're a bunch of idiots, that's why!"[65]

The evidence is incontrovertible: vaccine believers within the medical profession are both victims and abusers in an abusive system that has injected their minds with equal portions of ignorance and arrogance. Their million-dollar conflicts of interest multiply with every addition to the vaccine schedule. Their prejudice against and hostility toward vaccine-informed parents and patients is understandable but inexcusable. Their opinions on the subject of vaccines—whether offered in their medical offices, the courtroom, or in legislative halls—are worse than worthless; they're dangerous. And such professionals who advance the cause of medical tyranny through mandatory vaccinations are sworn enemies of their patients, of public health, and of democracy.

Battered women are most at risk when they leave their abusers, because at that moment abusers elevate their violence in a last-ditch effort to control their victims. Similarly, the government-medical-industrial complex is gearing up in a last ditch effort to prevent vaccine-informed parents and patients from leaving The Church of Vaccinology.

It's long past time for the growing body of vaccine-informed medical professionals to end their silent complicity with their mercenary colleagues. It's time for them to end their silent complicity with a tyrannical and violent medical system. As the younger generation would say, it's time for them to grow a pair. Or, as Del Bigtree stated emphatically on July 1, 2016, the day medical tyranny was officially instituted in California, it's time for doctors to "be brave."[66] If they fail to do so, they further sully their profession. Only those who've stood up and spoken out against the corruption of the medical profession are worthy to be called healthcare professionals. Suzanne Humphries is one such doctor. The nephrologist/researcher/author finished her classic work, *Dissolving Illusions*, with both a final slam against her "blind slave-technician" colleagues and a final warning to parents:

Until the minds of pediatricians are emancipated, parents will remain the best line of defense for their children. The reality . . . is that vaccinology, as portrayed to the public today, amounts to writing religion on the back of ignorance.[67]

The ignorance Humphries speaks of is planned and purposeful, an ignorance built upon a religious foundation of unimaginable depravity. The depth and breadth of that depravity is the subject of the following chapter.

Chapter Twenty-Three

THOU SHALT HAVE NO OTHER GOD BEFORE THE GODS OF VACCINOLOGY

For we wrestle not against flesh and blood, but against principalities, against powers, against the rulers of the darkness of this world, against spiritual wickedness in high places.

—Ephesians 6:12

To someone whose god is science, vaccination makes sense. But to someone whose god is God, it is appalling.[1]

—Isaac Golden, PhD

Vaccination is a barbarous practice, and it is one of the most fatal of all the delusions current in our time, not to be found even among the so-called savage races of the world.[2]

—Mahatma Gandhi

Many ancient civilizations performed the ritual of human sacrifice for the benefit of their communities, or in other words, for the Greater Good. In most cases, those who were sacrificed were selected because of their virtue or bravery. The honored recipients were fully informed of their coming demise and felt assured that their bloodshed and deaths would benefit the living. The ritual was practiced in the most holy edifices and on display for all to see. There was no deception, deceit, denigration, or denial.

Human sacrifice did not end with ancient civilizations. Indeed, literal human sacrifice is one of the primary legacies of the modern Vaccine religion. In the early 1900s, scientists forcibly aborted—murdered, that is—fetuses from "feeble minded women" for vaccine research.[3] In more recent years, hundreds of babies have been delivered live, then dissected, and harvested. When "successful," their tissue is rendered artificially semi-immortal, giving scientists tons of human tissue upon which to culture disease antigens. When "successful," the tissue from the sacrificed human beings and disease antigens are mixed with a host of other toxicants and injected back into other human beings, ostensibly in the service of the Greater Good, the utilitarian ethic of modern practitioners of Public Health effectively trashing the Hippocratic Oath to First, Do No Harm.[4]

Beyond the practice of using aborted human fetal tissue, practitioners routinely sacrifice the health of all vaccine victims to one degree or another by means of original antigenic sin,[5] chronic inflammation and pain, hosts of diseases and conditions including neurological destruction, as well as the unnumbered and unrecognized dead.

And finally, the High Priests of Vaccinology have succeeded in sacrificing the human race itself by bastardizing human DNA through the unintentional process of insertional mutagenesis as well as the planned and purposeful transformation—destruction, that is—of the human genome (more in Chapter 24).[6, 7, 8] It is no wonder then that Vaccine Sociopaths keep these and numerous other facts hidden from vaccine believers by means of deception, deceit, denigration, and denial. Murder, the intentional poisoning of infants, toddlers, pregnant women, and the elderly, and the corruption of the human race tend to leave a bad taste in the mouths of most people.

The Public Health profession has a long history of notable accomplishments that has resulted in improved health. Advocating for the removal of environmental toxins including raw sewage, unsanitary water, and lead paint are a few examples of success. Limiting access to tobacco and junk food has also yielded positive results. But the public health profession went horribly wrong when it shifted its focus from the removal of environmental toxins to the control and prevention of infectious diseases. By doing so, professionals became the primary source of environmental toxins injected directly into the bodies of virtually all human beings on the planet via toxic vaccines and the unwitting tools of the profit-driven pharmaceutical industry. As the years have passed their love affair with poisoning people has only increased.

Where vaccine injury, vaccine failure, vaccine contamination, and vaccine-induced death should have resulted in the termination of the barbaric practice of vaccination, it has resulted instead in calls for mandatory vaccination of virtually all people and for an assortment of punishments against those who refuse to comply. Just as religious crusaders of yesteryear were willing to go to any length—including murder—to convert "heathens" to their faith, modern vaccine crusaders are willing to go to any length—including the violation of constitutionally protected religious rights—to convert everyone to the Vaccine religion. And the number of casualties from the ancient crusades pales in comparison to the casualties in the ongoing, global, vaccine-induced, womb-to-tomb holocaust.

In their frenzied state of mind, the crusaders are blind to the fact that their surrogate markers for health—ever-increasing numbers of toxic vaccinations inflicted upon ever-increasing numbers of vulnerable people, increased antibody titers, and even the decreased incidence of disease—have resulted in the sickest generation in American history, where the most vaccinated individuals are the most unhealthy and indeed the most susceptible to a large number of diseases and conditions including even the diseases for which they were vaccinated. Thus, Public Health has become the number one enemy to individual health. And when individual health is destroyed, public health is destroyed, as well.

Jane M. Orient, MD, eloquently addressed the warped ethics of the public health profession in a critique published in the *Journal of American Physicians and Surgeons*:

> In Hippocratic medicine, the physician is working for the good of the individual patient, and the voluntary nature of the patient-physician relationship is axiomatic. The New Ethics, however, is attempting to replace the Hippocratic model with a public health model. The empha-sis is on prevention and on optimizing "population health," not individ-ual outcomes. A "right to healthcare" is proclaimed, and few notice that the right to refuse healthcare is being overridden by a duty to accept it in the name of public health. An expert committee replaces the individual patient as the decision maker. Mandatory vaccination is the leading edge of the new ethic. The policy to require annual influenza vaccination as a condition of working in a medical facility illustrates the dogmatism of the public health model and how it trumps individual autonomy, the Hippocratic ethic, and also evidence-based medicine.[9]

Fortunately, the US Constitution protects religious freedom and thus inoculates the vaccine informed against vaccine zealots far more safely and effec-tively than any vaccine ever protected against a disease. In addition to having an abundance of scientific-based arguments against vaccination, people of faith can cite an impressive list of religious-based reasons to exempt themselves from the filthy ritual of vaccination. Following are a few of the challenges in the vac-cines themselves as well as in vaccine policy, the vaccine program and paradigm, and the vaccine industry as perceived by the majority of religious individuals, especially those who consider respecting natural processes and upholding social justice as sacred obligations:

- Human beings are created in God's image. Babies are born exactly as the Creator designed, with immune systems functioning exactly as they are meant to function. God did not make a mistake. Babies are not born vaccine deficient.
- Vaccines injure and kill people.
- Mandatory vaccination violates God-given agency.

- Virtually every ingredient in vaccines defiles the sanctity of human bodies, including cells from aborted human fetuses, human albumin, neurotoxins and heavy metals such as aluminum and mercury, bacteria, cells from monkey and dog kidneys, cells from the brains of mice, chicken embryos, serum derived from calf fetus blood, beef extract, cells from cabbage moth and armyworms, genetically modified (unnatural) organisms, live or attenuated viruses (including sexually transmitted viruses), retroviruses, cleansers, adjuvants, stabilizers, preservatives, and known and unknown contaminants. It is well documented that viruses and retroviruses injected into the body via vaccines embed themselves in human DNA and are passed from generation to generation.
- Early vaccine research used fetal tissue obtained by forced abortions performed on "feeble minded" women.[10]
- The workings of the human body—from individual cells to the trillions of nonhuman microbes found on and within human bodies—are miraculous and beyond understanding. It is nothing more than human arrogance to think that the production of vaccine-induced antibodies does not also result in a cascade of known and not-yet-known human processes that adversely affect cells, tissues, organs, systems, persons, families, communities, ecosystems, and future generations.
- Vaccines currently under development are designed to permanently alter DNA, the consequences of which scientists cannot possibly predict or understand.[11, 12]
- Most vaccines enter the body through injection, an unnatural, dangerous, and destructive process.
- Vaccine-induced immunity is artificial, temporary, incomplete, dysfunctional, and it interferes with natural immunity.
- Vaccines work against the body's natural systems, especially the systems of newborns and young children.
- The developing life within a mother's womb is sacred. To vaccinate a pregnant woman with a host of known neurotoxicants is sacrilege and is equivalent to if not worse than drinking alcohol during pregnancy.
- Breast milk is a natural form of immunization—a precious gift from mother to child. Vaccinations are an unnatural form of immunization.
- Breast milk inhibits (fights against) the immune response of vaccines, demonstrating the body's resistance to the unnatural process of vaccine-induced immunity.
- Natural immunity confers many health benefits extending to the next generation in utero and through breast milk. Preventing girls from contracting diseases through vaccination also prevents them from being able to protect their future offspring as God or nature intended.

- Vaccine research routinely exploits people of color, the undereducated, and the poor.
- People in developing countries are vaccinated with ingredients banned in wealthy nations. They are also over-vaccinated in ways that would never be tolerated in developed countries.
- Anti-fertility vaccines are used without consent on people in developing countries.
- Hepatitis B is a disease common to prostitutes and IV drug users. Babies are at virtually no risk of contracting hepatitis B in developed countries. This is a moral affront to children.
- A one-size-fits-all vaccine policy discriminates against the genetically vulnerable and others in individual circumstances.
- The vaccine program is founded upon greed, lies, fraud, shoddy science, and corruption. To participate in the program is to collude with criminals.
- Government bureaucrats are now assigned the task of judging the sincerity and authenticity of people claiming religious-based vaccine exemptions that sometimes results in secular zealots grilling people of faith and telling them what they're supposed to believe.[13]
- Granting religious exemptions based on church membership rather than individual belief is unconstitutional religious discrimination.
- Mandatory vaccinations violate the protected right of freedom of religion.
- "Thou shalt have no other Gods before me" (Exodus 20:3). The vaccine program is a secular religion filled with false prophets offering false salvation from evil (germs) with its false and dangerous religious sacrament of vaccination.

Speaking of false prophets, Paul Offit, the Prophet of vaccine profit, authored a book in 2015 titled *Bad Faith: When Religious Belief Undermines Modern Medicine*.

Offit, a nonbeliever, used his book to mock people of faith while perched atop his own house of cards—the citadel of pseudoscientific certainty. Mark Oppenheimer wrote a review of Offit's book in the *New York Times*. Oppenheimer, a vaccine believer, was not impressed with Offit's treatment of ". . . the false conflict that some perceive between medicine and religious faith. . . ." Offit condescendingly believes that if people of faith properly understood their own religion, they'd be among the first to partake in the holy sacrament of vaccinations. But Oppenheimer bought neither Offit's arguments nor his tone, writing,

. . . Dr. Offit's book is more a fervent attack job than an earnest attempt to understand people with different, if misguided views. His book is thinly sourced and poorly researched, seeming at times as if he began with a conclusion and then went in search of evidence. . . .

But when Dr. Offit tries to give context to religious people's choices, his anger blinds him.[14]

Obviously, the purpose of Offit's book is not to entreat the members of the faith-based community to give up their silly beliefs about religious freedom, God, and other such nonsense. Rather, its purpose is to incite anger among the rank-and-file soldiers of the vaccine-believing army and convince them that if religious people are too deluded to enter the Vaccine church on their own, the "scientifically minded" have no choice but to cancel religious freedom, take away babies if necessary, and vaccinate the hell out of them . . . for the good of The Herd, of course.

Offit displayed his blindness and anger in a 2017 article ironically titled "MISSISSIPPI MIRACLE: The Unhealthiest State in America Has the Best Vaccination Rate." Puzzled, Offit asked, "How did a state with the worst overall health in the nation score the best vaccination rates?" To the vaccine informed, the answer is hiding in plain sight in the question. Offit concluded otherwise, writing,

> Today, 47 states have religious exemptions to vaccination. Using religion as an excuse to perform a profoundly unreligious act, parents in these states have the right to allow their children to catch and transmit potentially fatal infections. Our country would do well to follow the state that stood up for its children in 1979.[15]

Marjorie Ordene, MD, disagrees with Offit, from both scientific and religious perspectives. Ordene's return to her Jewish faith aligned with her adoption of holistic medical practices. As a physician, she had witnessed devastating vaccine injury in her practice that led her on a search for more truth. She eventually took a stand against her husband, family, and various colleagues and decided that no one would vaccinate her son. Years later, Ordene wrote,

> My problem was I knew too much. I knew that the mercury levels far exceeded safe doses, even for adults, but that in the interests of public health, the EPA had ignored its own standards. I also knew of the connection between measles virus and autoimmune disease, such as MS, a development that doesn't manifest until years later, and therefore is difficult to ascribe to vaccination. On the other hand, I also knew that autism is a complex condition with no single cause, and that, as

with any disease, it likely requires a genetic predisposition. So, in other words, Avi was probably safe. Yet, knowing what I knew, I couldn't bring myself to take the chance, not when childhood diseases were no longer a threat. It just didn't seem necessary.[16]

Scientific reasoning and spiritual values also inform the medical practice of Dr. Richard Moskowitz, MD. The Jewish physician and author wrote in his article titled "The Case Against Immunization":

> For the past ten years or so, I have felt a deep and growing compunction against giving routine vaccinations to children. It began with the fundamental belief that people have the right to make that choice for themselves.

> But eventually the day came when I could no longer bring myself to give the shots, even when the parents wished me to. I have always believed that the attempt to eradicate entire microbial species from the biosphere must inevitably upset the balance of Nature in fundamental ways that we can as yet scarcely imagine. Such concerns loom ever larger as new vaccines continue to be developed, seemingly for no better reason than that we have the technical capacity to make them, and thereby to demonstrate our right and power as a civilization to manipulate the evolutionary process itself.

> Purely from the viewpoint of our own species, even if we could be sure that the vaccines were harmless, the fact remains that they are compulsory, that all children are required to undergo them, without sensitivity or proper regard for basic differences in individual susceptibility, to say nothing of the values and wishes of the parents and the children themselves.[17]

Moskowitz concludes with both a denouncement of the state-sponsored pharmaceutical sacrament of vaccination and a testimony of his religious beliefs:

> I cannot have faith in the miracles or accept the sacraments of Merck, Sharp, and Dohme and the Centers for Disease Control. I prefer to stay with the miracle of life itself, which has given us illness and disease, to be sure, but also the arts of medicine and healing, through which we can acknowledge and experience our pain and vulnerability, and sometimes, with the grace of God and the help of our friends and neighbors, an awareness of health and well-being that knows no boundaries. *That* is my religion; and while I would willingly share it, I would not force it on anyone [emphasis in original].[18]

Unlike Offit, people such as Ordene and Moskowitz—and there are many— have little if any influence over CDC policy. No doubt, many aspiring CDC bureaucrats are so taken in by the millionaire's sophistries that they endorse his self-appointed position as Pharaoh over enslaved religious Americans. But the strategy presented in the 2016 version of the Division of Health and Human Services' National Adult Immunization Plan is subtler. HHS plans to proselytize "trusted leaders" within "faith-based and community organizations," in order "to promote the importance of adult immunization," and to turn such leaders into "adult immunization champions." The government—ever sensitive to the concerns of its diverse citizenry—claims its targeting community and faith-based organizations because they ". . . play an especially important role in reducing racial and ethnic disparities in adult immunization, as they can deliver education that is culturally sensitive, linguistically appropriate, and tailored to specific subpopulations."[19] As the conspirators in the CDC's fraudulent 2004 MMR study disposed of the evidence of the disproportionate vaccine-induced harm to African American boys, were they focused on delivering "education that is culturally sensitive, linguistically appropriate, and tailored to specific subpopulations," or were they perhaps focused on protecting their own self-interests?

Trusted leaders in the African American community view influential blacks who pimp for the CDC and Big Pharma as sellouts. Of course, the real leaders are, to use a religious phrase, filled with righteous indignation. Nation of Islam Western Regional Minister Tony Muhammad summed up the situation when he addressed a full house in Compton, California, following a screening of the movie *Vaxxed*:

> What we are finding out is that the pharmaceutical industry is one of the richest lobbying groups in the world and they are now financing many pastors. . . . And they need to be brought up on charges of treason for what's going on with our boys. . . .[20]

Muhammad has been chastising religious leaders for their complicity with government fraudsters ever since Robert F. Kennedy, Jr. informed him about the CDC fraud. In 2015, he repeatedly spoke out against California's proposed mandatory vaccination bill, SB 277, likening it to the government's infamous Tuskegee experiment. In addition, he supported a protest held at CDC's Atlanta headquarters in the fall of 2015. Citing CDC fraud that resulted in preventable injury to African American boys, he told members of the California Legislative Black Caucus that supporting SB 277 was "a traitorous act," warning them that they would not be welcome in the black community if they voted for the coercive bill.[21]

Sheila Ealey, an African American Baptist, was featured in *Vaxxed* with her severely vaccine-injured son. Following the screening in Compton, Ealey delivered a sermon reminiscent of the finest Baptist preachers. She told the audience that she never could have imagined sharing the stage with a Muslim preacher, but their common goal of saving their children from the conspiring forces of evil had brought them together.[22]

Del Bigtree, producer of *Vaxxed*, also addressed the predominately black and Latino Compton audience. Frustrated that the great majority of religious leaders stood by while the lying pediatrician, Richard Pan, and others of his ilk stripped the faith-based community of their medical freedoms, Bigtree asked, "Where are our religious leaders? . . . Where are our ministers? Where are our priests fighting for religious exemptions? Our entire country—the First Amendment—was founded on freedom of religion, freedom of belief."[23] Then he addressed the fact that the misplaced faith in fascist pseudomedicine was trampling the rights of religious people:

> So we're left with faith, with the theory put out by the pharmaceutical industry and our doctors. We're left with faith that the pharmaceutical industry that makes billions of dollars is actually looking out for our health, not for their stockholders and their bottom dollar. We're left with faith that our doctors are actually looking into these studies done by the pharmaceutical industries themselves, done by the CDC and people that walk off and get better jobs at the pharmaceutical industry when they're done. . . . And I'd say with faith like that we have to call medicine for what it is: it's a religion. And I should be able to deny that religion like you can deny mine. But we have a freedom of religion in this country, and we should be able to stand in our religion, wherever that takes us: fully vaxxed, semi-vaxxed, not vaxxed, . . . it doesn't matter, it's your choice.[24]

Reverend Lisa Sykes has been a staunch activist for vaccine safety for many years. In 2008, her influence contributed to a resolution issued by the United Methodist Church to "ban the presence of any mercury compound in pharmaceutical products or vaccines, prescribed or over-the-counter." In addition, the Church issued a call for

> . . . the Global Alliance for Vaccines and Immunizations, United Nations Children's Fund (UNICEF), Rotary International, the Bill and Melinda Gates Foundation, as well as any other organization from which vaccines are purchased, [to] join The United Methodist Church in the educating the public about and advocating for mercury-free drugs and vaccines.[25]

The American Academy of Physicians and Surgeons posted a "template exemption" on its website to help its member physicians exercise their religious right to abstain from mandatory vaccinations. The template includes several references from the New Testament but can easily be adapted for other religions as needed.[26]

Examples of other religious-based exemption letters are also easily found online. It's important to note that some officials have ruled against religious exemptions when they cite scientific and/or medical arguments against vaccination. Yes, that's a nonsensical stance, but be aware. Exemptions are more likely to be approved if exemption letters steer clear of the numerous scientific problems with vaccines.

One the simpler examples of a religious-based exemption letter is posted online. The letter, which was approved by Idaho officials, reads as follows:

> We, [parents' names], as the parents of the child [child's name], hereby assert that the immunization of this student would be contrary to the religious beliefs of this child. Therefore, this child shall be exempt from all suggested and/or required immunizations to attend public school in Idaho and shall be permitted to attend school except in the case of a vaccine preventable disease outbreak in the school.[27]

Simpler still, an Alaskan father was provided with a religious-based vaccine exemption form that asked him to identify the name of the church he belonged to that did not support vaccinations. In the space provided, he wrote, "None of your damn business." The school approved the exemption.[28]

Megan Heimer, an online Christian blogger, published a sassy entry in 2014 titled "God Does Not Support Vaccines" in which she referenced several scriptures to back up her claim. In response to people who say Christians should thank God for vaccines, Heimer wrote,

> The same people thanking God for vaccines are the same ones who downplay and disregard the thousands of references in His word to how we should eat, live, and take care of our bodies. The Bible does not reference vaccines specifically, but it does reference pharmaceutical medication . . . to which vaccines belong. You know what the Bible calls this? Sorcery (Gal 5:20, Rev 9:21, 18:23, 21:8, and 22:15). Actually the Greek word for sorcery is "pharmakeia." Pretty ironic don't ya think?[29]

Abundant arguments against the theory and the practice of vaccination are found in both scientific and religious literature, and both are essential. The sociopaths running the vaccine paradigm have created a false religion to lure people of faith into believing that vaccines are consistent with human morals, ethics, and values. Attorney William Wagner addresses this concept from a legal perspective in the highly recommended book, *Vaccine Epidemic*:

The government . . . increasingly substitutes itself for God, as the source of our liberty. The paradigm shifts under this evolving legal philosophy. To evaluate state action that has an impact on parental decisions, the state replaces self-evident, unalienable standards with its own morally relative, utilitarian assessments. Thus the freedom of conscience and the sanctity behind parents directing the upbringing of their children no longer serve as moral benchmarks against which to measure whether government vaccination laws are right or wrong, good or bad, just or unjust. Instead, parents are told that questions regarding vaccination laws are public policy matters for the government to decide. Moreover, parents should not bother asking to participate in the debate if our view of the world is informed by religious principles since we are told we must only adopt public policy informed by secular dogma—without regard to any sacred, conscientious, or moral considerations.

Beware. When the government eliminates a self-evident moral element from the law, it removes any moral reference point with which to measure whether laws are right or wrong, good or bad, just or unjust.[30]

While some religious people dutifully roll up their sleeves for every shot on the vaccine schedule, the architects of the vaccine program are maneuvering behind the scenes to remove religious and philosophical exemptions from the rest. For decades, Barbara Loe Fisher has been one of the strongest voices against vaccine tyranny. As a cofounder and president of the National Vaccine Information Center, Fisher put out a video in January 2016 titled "Knowledge is the Antidote for Vaccine Orthodoxy" in which she said, "Those embracing vaccine orthodoxy have a right to their beliefs, but they should not be given the legal right to persecute and punish fellow citizens refusing to convert. Tyranny by any other name is still tyranny."[31]

Religious communities that generally avoid the tyranny of vaccinations have lower rates of a host of medical problems including autism, asthma, allergies, and ADHD. UPI reporter Dan Olmsted made such an observation in 2005 when he interviewed several people in American Amish communities and found lower rates of vaccination accompanied by a vastly lower rate of autism. Dr. Heng Wang, medical director, physician, and researcher at the DDC Clinic for Special Needs Children, created specifically to treat the Amish in northeastern Ohio, told Olmsted that he was only aware of one autistic child among a population of 15,000 Amish who lived in the area.[32]

Mayer Eisenstein, MD, made similar observations from his decades spent serving the Amish community in Lancaster County, Pennsylvania. Eisenstein gave a presentation at the annual AutismOne conference in 2012, saying,

Since 1973, my medical practice, Homefirst Health Services, has cared for more than 40,000 children who were minimally vaccinated or not vaccinated at all. We also have virtually no autism, asthma, allergies, respiratory illness, or diabetes in our unvaccinated children, a telltale revelation when compared to national rates.[33]

Dr. Frank Noonon also worked with the Amish in Lancaster County for over 25 years. He offered yet another testimony regarding an absence of autistic kids in his practice: "You'll find all the other stuff, but we don't find the autism. We're right in the heart of Amish country and seeing none, and that's just the way it is."[34]

Others dispute the doctors' claim, but the fact remains that the Amish experience far less autism than people from more highly vaccinated communities. A 2012 letter to the editor in the *Journal of Allergy and Clinical Immunology* reported that the Amish also suffer from far lower rates of "allergic sensitization" compared to other agrarian communities.[35]

By contrast, the members of The Church of Jesus Christ of Latter-day Saints, commonly known as the Mormons or LDS, headquartered in Salt Lake City, Utah, reportedly vaccinate at one of the highest rates in America. The LDS Church has a long history of funding vaccination programs in developing countries, and church leaders have repeatedly issued public statements advising members to vaccinate, suggesting that those who fail to do so are acting out of "ignorance and apathy."[36, 37]

It is important to note that many members interpret such pronouncements as the word of God and believe God to be pro-vaccine. Eschewing drugs, alcohol, tobacco, coffee, and tea while also injecting repeated doses of toxic chemicals into the bodies of their babies is oddly consistent with the values of the majority of LDS members. This phenomenon likely explains why, according to a 2008 CDC study, predominately Mormon Utah boasted the highest rate of autism in the country.[38] Of course, the CDC isn't pinning Utah's record-breaking rate of autism on the Beehive State's love affair with pediatric jabs. In fact, based on a lawsuit filed in January 2016 by Judith Pinborough-Zimmerman against her employer, the University of Utah, it appears that the CDC is doing everything it can to erase the damning statistics from the study. Zimmerman alleges that the University of Utah published data that contained uncorrected errors amounting to significant research misconduct.[39]

As the author of the 2016 book *Master Manipulator: The Explosive True Story of Fraud, Embezzlement, and Government Betrayal at the CDC*, James Ottar Grundvig is an expert on CDC fraud. Grundvig refers to Zimmerman as the Utah whistleblower. He speaks emphatically about the purpose of the research misconduct, saying, "What they are continuing to work on is a giant lie, a cover up for a failed CDC health program and for HHS having wasted years and millions of dollars in not mitigating the autism epidemic."[40]

More than 100 years ago, several groups left the larger Mormon Church to continue the practice of polygamy. One of the more infamous breakaway groups eventually made its way to Texas, where the members lived in a compound generally isolated from their fellow Texans. After authorities raided the compound in 2008 and removed 416 vaccine-free children, they found them to be "healthy and robust,"[41, 42] demonstrating once again the obvious fact that nonpoisoned children are healthier than poisoned children.

Religious organizations that use tyranny and coercion to force people to join and that refuse to allow members to leave are known as cults. Most cults manage to pull off their treachery for a limited time on a limited number of people before they crumble. The Vaccine religion—cult, that is—is uniquely successful as a cult, having drawn in and enriched many of the most powerful, wealthy, and evil people and organizations on Earth and having deceived the vast majority of the world's inhabitants into blind submission to the apparently endless orgy of poisoning by vaccination.

People of modern sensibilities are quick to describe the ancient practitioners of human sacrifice as savages. If such is the case, then they were rank amateurs compared to the savages who administer and profit from the modern day ritual of harming to one degree or another 100% of vaccine victims. Murdering human fetuses, harvesting and growing diseases on their tissue, and mixing the putrid mess with a hellish concoction of animal DNA, heavy metals, retroviruses, carcinogens, mutagens, etc., and then pronouncing it clean before injecting the filth back into pregnant women, infants, toddlers, and the aged is pure savagery. Lying to the public about xenotropic murine leukemia virus-related virus (XMRV), SV40, dozens of others viruses, the link between thimerosal and autism, the link between the MMR vaccine and autism, the supposed dangers of benign and beneficial childhood illnesses, and the benefit, efficacy, and necessity of worthless and dangerous vaccines is savagery. Mandating toxic vaccines while denying their toxicity and refusing to compensate for the countless injured and dead vaccine victims is savagery. Denying the constitutionally protected right of a free and public education to the healthy children of the growing number of vaccine informed parents is savagery. And, of course, one of most savage acts of all is the planned and purposeful bastardization of the human genome and human race through DNA vaccines.

Clearly, the Vaccine cult is one of the most oppressive, tyrannical, dangerous, and savage of all cults in the history of the world. If humanity is to survive, the vaccine-informed public must shut it down and bring the High Priests of profit and savagery to justice for their ongoing and unfathomable crimes against humanity.

Chapter Twenty-Four

STICKING IT TO
YOUR FUTURE

If you want a picture of the future,
imagine a boot stamping on a human face—forever.
— George Orwell

As discussed previously, the vaccine program was out of control by the latter half of the 1800s, and compulsory vaccination was enforced with fines and jail sentences. But if the vaccine-believing doctors and lawmakers of that era were to observe today's vaccine program, even they would be flabbergasted at both its power and its absurdity.

Compulsory vaccination in the past meant the public had to submit to one vaccine for one disease. Compulsory vaccination laws were passed based on the correct understanding that smallpox is a communicable disease coupled with the incorrect belief that pus from sick cows protected against the spread of smallpox. The laws were passed, in all likelihood, by well-meaning leaders attempting to protect their families and communities. Based on the information they had at the time, the greater good argument made at least some sense. In addition to the practice of vaccination, sick and infected people were isolated from the greater population to limit disease transmission, a practice that also makes sense, and quarantine continues to be used effectively today in developing countries to limit the spread of polio and other infectious diseases.

By contrast, the only sense to be made of modern mandatory vaccination laws is business sense. From a public health perspective, the laws are absurd from beginning to end. Consider a few of many farcical points resulting from the passage of California's SB 277:

1. The theory of vaccine-induced herd immunity is based on the belief that an approximate vaccination rate of 95% will prevent disease outbreaks. It's well known that the efficacy of vaccines diminishes over time, thus the need for boosters or yearly revaccination in the case of the flu vaccine. Therefore, most adults are no more immune to the diseases

targeted by vaccines than are vaccine-free children. Vaccinating school-aged children has little effect on reaching the fabled population-wide 95% vaccination rate.

2. The premise for banning nonvaccinated children from their constitutionally protected public education is that they endanger the health status of vaccinated children, who are, in theory, protected from "vaccine preventable diseases." If the vaccinations don't protect against the non-vaccinated, then why take the risk of getting them in the first place?

3. According to immunologist Tetyana Obukhanych, PhD, author of *Vaccine Illusion*,

    > . . . due to the properties of modern vaccines, non-vaccinated individuals pose no greater risk of transmission of polio, diphtheria, pertussis, and numerous non-type b H. influenzae strains than vaccinated individuals do, non-vaccinated individuals pose virtually no danger of transmission of hepatitis B in a school setting, and tetanus is not transmissible at all . . . .[1]

    Therefore, banning children from school who have not received these vaccines is nothing more than state-sponsored discrimination, which would be less glaring if children recently vaccinated with live virus vaccines were also banned from school for a month or so following vaccination and if the carriers of hepatitis B, HIV, and HPV-related STDs were also banned from school, but such is not the case.

4. The idea that separating vaccine-free children from vaccinated children in the public school setting for 6 out of 24 hours five days a week somehow protects vaccinated children is beyond illogical. If a public health official living in Leicester, England, in the 1860s had suggested that healthy non-vaccinated individuals should be quarantined from their peers in like manner, that individual would have been tarred and feathered, consigned to the mad house, or both. If there is to be any logical use of banning children from school, it must be based on health status rather than vaccination status. If such a policy were implemented, sick, diseased, and recently vaccinated children would be the ones banned from school, not healthy vaccine-free children. In 1999, the Association of American Physicians and Surgeons addressed this issue in testimony before the US House of Representatives' Committee on Government Reform:

Federal policy of mandating vaccines marks a profound change in the concept of public health. Traditionally, public health authorities restricted the liberties of individuals only in case of a clear and present danger to public health. For example, individuals infected with a transmissible disease were quarantined. Today, a child may be prevented from attending school or associating with others simply because of being unimmunized. If there is not an outbreak of disease and if the child is uninfected, his or her unimmunized state is not a threat to anyone. An abridgement of civil rights in such cases cannot be justified.[2]

George Fatheree, a Harvard-educated attorney and father of a severely vaccine-injured son, testified before the California Assembly Committee on Health on June 9, 2015, where he articulated the practical implications of attempting to implement SB 277. Among other points, Fatheree informed the committee that the bill unfairly discriminated against California's most vulnerable students, including the economically disadvantaged, children with non-English-speaking parents, the homeless, and special needs children with IEPs who call for socialization with their nondisabled peers. In regard to the latter point, Fatheree stated, "So . . . SB 277 is in direct conflict with Federal education law and will be preempted." He further argued that

there's no compelling state interest to eliminate a personal belief exemption, especially given that it's used by such a small percentage of the population. . . . The bill is also not tailored which is a requirement for it to be held constitutional. It applies to every kid, it applies to every disease whether the disease is communicable or not. It applies to diseases that have been eradicated from US shores for decades like diphtheria. So [there are] serious constitutional problems.[3]

If legislators had listened to Fatheree, SB 277 would have suffered an ignominious death on that very day. But they didn't listen; nor did they listen to numerous others who opposed the repressive legislation. Barbara Loe Fisher, representing the National Vaccine Information Center, testified before the committee with her usual clarity:

This bill is not about measles or pertussis. It is about taking power away from mothers and fathers to make medical risk decisions for their minor children and handing it over to doctors to implement a one-size-fits-all policy with no personal accountability for the children who become casualties of that policy. Many parents refuse to violate their deeply held religious, spiritual and conscientious beliefs that compel them to protect their children. . . . The prospect of non-complying parents being charged with truancy and fined or potentially sent to jail if they cannot homeschool will foster mistrust and fear of health officials and the medical profession.[4]

Yes, the purpose of SB 277 is about stripping parents of their right to make medical risk decisions for their minor children, but as Fisher alludes to in her statement, the stripping only applies to the poor and working-class citizens of California. Those who possess sufficient gold in the Golden State have the means to exclude their children from vaccine mandates by educating their children in home-based private schools.

The architects of mandatory vaccination legislation hold hostage the protected right of free public education from those who can't afford other options. The ransom required to regain what was illegally stolen—free access to public education—is free access to the bodies of their children.

How do California citizens feel about SB 277? Nearly 800 citizens made statements before the Senate Education Committee in April 2015. Of that number 743 opposed SB 277, while only 53 supported it.[5]

Prior to the passage of SB 277, Senator Richard Pan, cosponsor Ben Allen, and several other supporters of the bill repeatedly stated that doctors would be free to exercise full clinical judgment with medical exemptions and that the government would not interfere with that process. Barbara Loe Fisher disagreed, warning that 99.99% of children would not qualify for medical exemptions. George Fatheree testified that he couldn't get a medical exemption for his daughter based her older brother's severe vaccine injury.[6] California Governor Edmund G. "Jerry" Brown, Jr. added his voice to the mix in a letter dated June 30, 2015, addressed to the Members of the California State Senate. After he stated his intent to sign the bill, Brown wrote,

> The Legislature, after considerable debate, specifically amended SB 277, to exempt a child from immunizations whenever the child's physician concludes that there are "circumstances, including but not limited to, family medical history, for which the physician does not recommend immunization . . ."
>
> Thus, SB 277, while requiring that school children be vaccinated, explicitly provides an exception when a physician believes that circumstances—in the judgement and sound discretion of the physician—so warrant.[7]

In June of 2016, the Public Health Department in Santa Barbara issued a letter that proved that the assurances from Governor Brown, Pan, and his colleagues were just more lies in a string of lies that duped legislators into passing the repressive bill.[8] Whether most were party to or victim of the lie is unknown. The letter was addressed to school superintendents, principals, and child care center directors, and in the words of independent journalist Jefferey Jaxen, it

. . . demands all permanent and temporary medical exemptions on file for the 2016-2017 California school year be faxed to the Immunization Program citing the authority of a newly formed Medical Exemption Pilot Program. From there, "Immunization Staff" will determine if the once-promised medical exemptions will be allowed.[9]

Repressive laws around the world similar to California's SB 277 prevent The Herd in developed countries from leaving the Vaccine religion. Such laws add another tier to the global two-tiered vaccine program with the elite remaining free to abstain from vaccinations as always, but with the poor and working-class citizens coerced into receiving every vaccine according to the vaccination schedules in their respective countries. The poor and working classes in developing countries are forced—sometimes at gunpoint—to receive vaccines that are banned in developed countries such as the oral polio vaccine, DTP, and thimerosal-containing vaccines. Repressive regimes build walls and prisons to corral The Herd, control behavior, and punish dissent. Mandatory vaccination accomplishes the same purpose.

California is only one of dozens of states caught up in the wave of coercive vaccine-related legislation following the 2015 Disneyland measles hysteria. Virginia defeated a bill (HB 1312) described as "[t]he most oppressive forced vaccination bill introduced in any state. . . ." Had it passed, it would have eliminated the religious belief exemption, and, according to vaccine safety advocate Cathy Jameson, it would have also prohibited

. . . state licensed doctors and nurse practitioners from exercising professional judgment and delaying administration of or granting a child a medical exemption that does not conform with narrow federal vaccine contraindication guidelines.[10]

The truth of the matter is that vaccines have absolutely nothing to do with public education. Vaccination legislation is tied to it for one reason and one reason only: the majority of parents would reject some or all vaccines for their children if the government did not force them into submission: "No jabs, no school." And the majority of school administrators would reject the role of vaccine cop if the government didn't tie vaccination rates to school funding.

The Northern Utah Immunization Coalition (NUIC) described the process in a PDF document under a section appropriately titled "What is the Method to This Madness?":

• Schools are required to file a report in November and June of each school year.

- In November, the schools must submit an immunization report to the Utah State Health Dept identifying children who are conditional admissions or out of compliance with the Utah School Rule.
- If a student is out of compliance on the June report, the Utah Immunization Program will collect the information and submit it to the Utah State Office of Education (USOE) to determine weighted pupil unit funds for each public school district in accordance with USOE policies and Utah Statutory Code (Section 53A-11-301).
- This means decreased funding for schools. Without money, schools don't function.[11]

But don't believe for a second that vaccine sociopaths are satisfied only with free access to the bodies of children. They already have a coercive adult vaccination plan in the works and their syringes lined up and ready to stick it to adults. In recent years, the National Vaccine Program Office published its latest version of the National Adult Immunization Plan (NAIP). The 67-page document is a masterpiece of propaganda and Orwellian doublespeak. According to the Plan, "the benefits of vaccination are not realized equally across the U.S. population. Adult vaccination rates remain low in the United States, and significant racial and ethnic disparities also exist."[12] The full vision of the Plan is revealed in the following paragraph:

> The U.S. Department of Health and Human Services National Vaccine Plan (NVP), released in 2010, is a road map for vaccines and immunization programs for the decade 2010–2020. While the NVP provides a vision for improving protection from vaccine-preventable diseases across the lifespan, vaccination coverage levels among adults are not on track to meet Healthy People 2020 targets. The National Vaccine Advisory Committee and numerous stakeholder groups have emphasized the need for focused attention on *adult vaccines and vaccination*. . . . The National Adult Immunization Plan (NAIP) outlined here results from the recognition that progress has been slow and that there is a need for a national adult immunization strategic plan [emphasis in original].[13]

Vaccine architects propose to solve the unfortunate disparity in racial, ethnic, and age-related vaccination rates by employing the same strategies they use to get parents to submit to vaccinating their children: deception, coercion, and extortion.

Aiding "federal and nonfederal partners" and stakeholders, the NAIP "aims to leverage the unique opportunity presented by the implementation of the Affordable Care Act." The CDC further explains on its website:

Under the Affordable Care Act, non-grandfathered, private health plans will cover a range of recommended preventive services with no cost-sharing (such as copays and deductibles) by the beneficiary, including vaccinations recommended by the CDC's Advisory Committee on Immunization Practices (ACIP).[14]

These anything-but-free "free" services cover pediatric vaccines as well as the following vaccines for adults: Hepatitis A, Hepatitis B, Herpes Zoster, Quadrivalent Human Papillomavirus vaccine for females, Influenza, MMR, Meningococcal, Pneumococcal, DTP, and Varicella.[15]

The Affordable Care Act also plays a role in the coercive practice of mandated flu shots for healthcare workers. A member of the Colorado Health Care Workers Against Forced Vaccination organization described how Centers for Medicare and Medicaid Services (CMS) reduces payment amounts to hospitals based on "summary data on influenza vaccination of healthcare personnel."[16] The Advisory Board, a health care advisory organization, crunched the numbers in a 2013 article to show how the CMS plan spanks the bottom line of healthcare organizations:

> For the first time this year, hospitals are being asked to report influenza vaccination rates among health care personnel under Medicare's quality-reporting program, or pay a fine. The American Hospital Association (AHA) estimates that a 100-bed hospital that fails to comply could forfeit $320,000. . . .

> After implementing a mandatory vaccine or mask program in 2009, Nashville-based HCA—with 162 hospitals and 204,000 employees—increased its vaccination rate above 90% for the past three consecutive flu seasons. Before that, coverage at HCA facilities ranged between 20% and 74%.[17]

"Vaccine or mask" is only part of the strategy that the plan employs to "[i]mprove community demand for adult immunizations." The CMS trains health care organizations in the art of "Influenza Vaccination Strategies." The strategies are necessary because "National health care worker vaccination rates are hovering around 40%. . . ."[18]

The tactics of the Vaccine Big Brother range from innocuous to outright malevolent:

- Implement declination forms (i.e., all health care workers will receive the vaccination unless they sign a form declining the administration of the vaccine). Declination forms can improve their employee vaccination rates substantially from one year to the next.

- Provide small financial or nonfinancial incentives, such as gift cards to local coffee shops, or introducing competition among departments within the organization.
- If employee has contraindications for the influenza vaccination, require that he/she wear a mask throughout the flu season.
- Provide education materials or lunch and learn type sessions for staff and make use of internal staff newsletters.
- Make the vaccinations mandatory for employees. Consequences of non-vaccination may result in termination or suspension of employment.[19]

As discussed previously, if the mask requirement were based on hard science, flu vaccine recipients would be forced to wear them, not those who abstain from the vaccine. And as also discussed, the mandatory flu vaccine requirement is a fiscal-based policy masquerading behind the thin façade of public health seen most starkly in the firing of a pregnant nurse for refusing the jab.[20] And why not? According to the Plan, pregnant women are an "adult population."[21]

Other examples of coercive and punitive vaccine legislation targeting adults abound. Shortly after California legislators betrayed the majority of their constituents with the passage of SB 277, Governor Brown signed into law SB 792, requiring parents who volunteer at public and private daycare and preschools to submit to the MMR, TDaP, and yearly flu shots. Those who refuse are now barred from volunteering in the classroom.[22]

The University of California system jumped on the Disneyland hysteria bandwagon by requiring students to submit to vaccinations for "measles, mumps, rubella, chickenpox, meningococcus, tetanus, and whooping cough, under a plan set to take effect in 2017."[23] Del Bigtree, producer of *Vaxxed*, blasted the university's regents in a public meeting in June 2016, telling them that vaccines are neither safe nor effective, that the CDC is a cesspool of corruption, and that mandatory vaccinations violate the religious and philosophical beliefs of some UC students.[24]

Not only do mandatory vaccinations violate religious and philosophical beliefs, they violate common sense, logic, and basic math skills, traits that are apparently lacking among UC administrators. Robert F. Kennedy, Jr. made a few computations on meningitis vaccine mandates and found them to make sense only for those who profit from the mandates:

My opposition to new meningitis mandates for every New York State seventh and twelfth grader has nothing to do with autism and everything to do with arithmetic. . . . Meningitis is a rare disease that [affected] only 390 people nationally last year. FDA and industry testing show the meningitis vaccine to be unusually low efficacy and high risk. The manufacturers' inserts predict that 1% to 1.3% of inoculated children will suffer "serious adverse effects." CDC's Pink Book forecasts that 0.3% of these will die from the vaccine. Of the 400,000 New York school children inoculated annually, some 4,000 will become ill and nine will die in order to prevent around four people from contracting the disease. At between $84 and $117 per shot, and with the requirement for a two-shot series, the law is an $80 million annual windfall for vaccine manufacturers at taxpayer expense. This math makes sense only to the pharmaceutical companies and the Albany politicians who have taken their money.[25]

The trend is clear: access to employment, public education, public space, public services, public transportation, health insurance, etc., will increasingly be tied to vaccination status. Welcome to the world of the future, where wealthy people and their fellow elites will be the only ones free from the scourge of compulsory vaccinations.

To gain a better view of the dystopian vaccine culture of the future, one need look no further than America's current armed forces. Whether young people join the military to be all that they can be, to defend their country, to fight the war on terrorism, or just to keep themselves off the streets and out of jail, few if any have any idea that when they commit to give their all for their country, their "all" includes the unconditional use of their bodies to test vaccines and other pharmaceutical products.

According to Heather Fraser, author of *The Peanut Allergy Epidemic*, this is not a new development. Fraser wrote, "The tradition of compulsory injections for US soldiers began in World War I (1914-1918) with vaccines for typhoid, cholera, tetanus, smallpox, and other diseases."[26]

The *New York Times* reported in 1918 that "Elmer N. Olson of Goodrich, Minn. . . . refused to submit to vaccination. He was tried by general court-martial and sentenced to fifteen years in the disciplinary barracks at Fort Leavenworth."[27] Dr. William Osler explained in his book *Influence of Vaccination Upon Other Diseases* why military personnel such as Olson would risk court-martial and imprisonment over vaccination:

> Our recent "vaccination" wars have presented a dismal picture of paralysis among the soldiers with large hospital wards filled with paraplegics (paralysis of both sides) and hemiplegics (paralysis of one side.) Thus we see that the doctors know and the government knows what vaccination is doing to our service men and civilians. Why have they turned their "blind side" to it and allowed it to continue?[28]

Osler's use of the phrase "vaccination wars" is thought-provoking. War profiteers teach soldiers that they war against tyranny and terrorists in the same way that vaccine profiteers teach The Herd that vaccines war against the terror of germs. Both classes of profiteers are the real terrorists, and both profit from the exploitation of the bodies of American military personnel.

If doctors and the government were blind to the racket of vaccination wars a century ago, their blindness has only increased. Following is the US military vaccination schedule as of 2003, a schedule that makes the vaccinations of the First World War look bland by comparison:

Anthrax	6 doses + annual
Hep A	3 + boosters
Influenza A & B	1 Annual
Jap Enceph	3 + biannual
MMR (Live)	1
Meningococcal MGC	1 every 3 years
Pneumococcal 123; PPV-23	1
Polio Inactivated IPV	1 booster dose
Rabies	3 doses
Smallpox (Live)	1 every 10 years
Td; TT	1 every 10 years
Typhoid Injectable	1 every 2 years
Varicella (Live)	2 doses if needed
Yellow Fever (Live)	1 every 10 years.[29]

Representative Dan Burton's committee totaled the amount of mercury US soldiers of the 1990s could potentially be exposed to from thimerosal-containing vaccines. By the EPA's standards, the maximum safe limit for a 180-pound person is 8.16 micrograms per day, yet soldiers were receiving from 110.5 micrograms to 135.5 micrograms in one day. As documented in the committee's Mercury in Medicine Report, the following account demonstrates that the US military is not only guilty of poisoning its soldiers, it's also guilty of failing to acknowledge the poisoning and failing to initiate effective medical protocols to treat and recover vaccine-wounded soldiers:

The Committee received documentation from one Air Force pilot who suffered from serious symptoms of Gulf War Syndrome. After failing to have his medical issues resolved through the military or the Veterans Administration (VA) medical system, Captain Frank Schmuck, a pilot, became so ill that he was no longer able to fly. He sought medical treatment outside the military medical system and was tested for heavy metals, and was found to have toxic levels of mercury in his system. After chelation therapy, he returned to good health and has resumed flying. Gulf War Syndrome victims are not routinely tested for heavy metal toxicity or treated with chelation therapy by the military or the VA.

Given the lack of progress in finding other successes with recovery from this condition, this is an issue that both the Department of Defense (DOD) and the VA should be aggressively evaluating on behalf of Gulf War veterans.[30]

Mercury is only one component of the military's toxic and abusive vaccine program, and Captain Schmuck is one of the more fortunate victims of that program. Most lack the resources or knowledge to seek out and obtain medical treatment provided by vaccine-informed medical professionals outside the military system. Several veterans have shared their stories in documentaries, on the Internet, and in congressional hearings. The 2003 documentary *Direct Order* reveals the widespread and common injuries that American soldiers suffered at the hands of their own government that forced troops to submit to its experimental and unapproved anthrax vaccine.[31] Tech Sgt Jeff Moore, one of the soldiers interviewed in the film, stated,

> The crew was pulled aside and told to march into this tent. They were told they were going to be given a shot, it was classified. And it had to do with livestock and they were not to talk about it and there were to be no side effects from it and that the shot would not be annotated into their shot records.[32]

Of course, "There would be no side effects" is an edict, a policy statement, or in military parlance, a direct order. Lieutenant Doug Rokke backed up Moore's statement in an interview included in the documentary *Beyond Treason: Depleted Uranium & Anthrax*. Rokke said,

> Our team was tasked to put together the anthrax vaccine program, but we were also ordered to not record lots, batches, doses, who got them, what their reactions were, when they got them, or how many they got. Direct orders.[33]

Lieutenant Rich Rovet testified before the House Committee on Government Reform in July 1999, saying that soldiers who violated orders by suffering vaccine injuries were accused of being "malingerers, liars, and hypochondriacs." Their symptoms included dizziness, ringing in their ears, joint pain, muscle pain, memory impairment, constant fatigue, numbness and tingling in various parts of their bodies, photosensitivity, miscarriage, swollen and painful testicles, cardiac problems, chills and fever greater than 48 hours post-vaccination, rash, swelling, and medically confirmed hyperthyroidism. The lieutenant further stated,

> All through the squadrons on base, people are afraid to come forward for they are going to lose their flying status and lose their career if they come forward. For every one individual that comes forward, there are three individuals that will not.[34]

OGR Committee member, Representative Benjamin A. Gilman, affirmed Rovet's statement at the same hearing when he offered the following:

> It appears that this vaccination program was initiated in a hasty manner, before a proper amount of research on the effectiveness and safety of the vaccine was completed.

> Even more distressing has been the reports of deliberate downplaying of adverse reactions among our military personnel who have received the shots to date. These reports, of course, are all too familiar for those of us who investigated the Gulf War Syndrome issue.

> Then as now, there was the all-too-frequent case of commanders who are more interested with following the official public relations message rather than being concerned with the welfare of the personnel under their command.[35]

Col. Felix Grieder refused to sacrifice the welfare of the personnel under his command. In 1999, Grieder shut down the vaccination program at Dover Air Force Base after he learned that his soldiers were being used as guinea pigs to test both the anthrax vaccine and the adjuvant squalene. The move ended Grieder's military career.[36]

The *Delaware News Journal* reported that it had "uncovered documents and videos that reveal that Pentagon officials lied; that US troops were given an experimental concoction of anthrax vaccine laced with squalene." According to the *Journal*, squalene is

> a fat-like substance that occurs naturally in the body. Squalene boosts a vaccine's effect, but some scientists say injecting even trace amounts of it into the body can cause serious illness. Many soldiers have suffered permanent harm as a result.[37]

The *Journal* wrapped up its article with this statement: "Dozens of Web sites and support groups are dedicated to linking autoimmune disorders to the shot. The vaccine has been the subject of several scientific studies that conclude it could be a factor in making soldiers sick."[38] Gary Matsumoto makes the same case in his book *Vaccine A: The Covert Government Experiment That's Killing Our Soldiers—and Why GI's Are Only the First Victims.*[39]

Congressman Gilman's final statement in the Anthrax Vaccine Adverse Reactions hearing put the Pentagon on notice: Congress was not going to ignore the ethical and medical issues surrounding the military's experimental use of the anthrax vaccine. "Mr. Chairman," said Gilman, "these hearings are important, as they help keep the Department of Defense focused on an uncomfortable issue and remind both officials at the Pentagon and the members of the public of Congress' determination to fully address this subject."[40]

Just over two months later, President Bill Clinton signed Executive Order 13139 euphemistically titled Improving Health Protection of Military Personnel Participating in Particular Military Operations.[41] The Order authorizes the use of unapproved and experimental products on members of the armed forces without informed consent or in some cases without any consent at all.[42]

The president may not have been aware of the fact that the protection he offered military personnel with his Executive Order was unconstitutional and it also destroyed the protection embodied in the Nuremberg Code, which was written to protect individuals against inhumane experimentation like that carried out by the Nazis on prisoners. The first tenet of the code reads, "The voluntary consent of the human subject is absolutely essential."

The following year, Clinton approved mandatory vaccinations for the entire US military. A company named Bioport "was given a single source contract to supply and manufacture anthrax vaccine to the entire 2.5 million military members." Bioport was coowned by former Joint Chiefs of Staff Admiral William J. Crowe. Crowe was the first military commander to endorse Clinton for presidency in 1992.[43] Apparently, World War II didn't bring an end to fascism.

When *Direct Order* came out in 2003, it included a brief summary of the military's use of the anthrax vaccine including the following:

Since 1998, when the vaccinations began, nearly 500 active-duty service-members have refused the vaccine, and more than 100 have been court-martialed. According to government figures, approximately 500 to 1,000 pilots and flight crew members have quit, resigned or transferred from the Air National Guard or reserves rather than take the vaccine.[44]

Sheila Ealey's family was not only impacted by severe childhood vaccine injury, her husband, a career military man, was given a choice: get the anthrax vaccines or get out. Ealey described the experience with power and indignation in the Q & A session following the screening of the movie *Vaxxed* in Compton, California:

> My husband served 26 years in the military and he wanted to make one more promotion and stay 30 years, but he was going to be forced to take five injections of anthrax. Five injections of anthrax! Let me tell you, he got out. . . . We were in the military when this happened to my son. And what I can tell you is the military has the highest rate of [autism compared to] any other population and you are not allowed to bring any charges against anything medically related against the military if you're active duty or retired.

> This is a new form of slavery.

> Democracy in this country is deteriorating as I speak. You're under fascism and medical tyranny. And the only way to take it back . . . is to stand up and rise up. You have to stand for something. You have to be willing to put your life on the line for this cause, because if not, your children are not going to make it and you're not going to make it. The pharmaceutical industry has developed a client from the womb to the grave and it breaks you. Autism breaks you. It's the most expensive disability of all disabilities.[45]

Ealey was not the first to label the practice of mandatory vaccination as slavery. In 1902, John W. Hodge, MD, published a book titled *The Vaccine Superstition* in which he wrote, ". . . compulsory vaccination ranks with human slavery and religious persecution, as one of the most flagrant outrages upon the rights of the human race." The doctor made a total of 22 equally powerful statements arising from

> . . . a careful consideration of the history of vaccination gleaned from an impartial and comprehensive study of vital statistics, and pertinent data from every reliable source and after an experience derived from having vaccinated 3,000 subjects. . . .[46]

The National Vaccine Information Center provides a timeline of important vaccine-related events. One such event occurred in October 2004, when

> US District Court Judge Emmet Sullivan issued an injunction blocking DOD from ordering US soldiers [to] receive anthrax vaccine without their informed consent, citing the reactive anthrax vaccine's "experimental" status because the FDA had never licensed it as effective for use against weaponized inhalation anthrax. [DOD would subsequently

get around the injunction by requesting the Secretary of Health and Human Services utilize recently acquired Project Bioshield powers and issue an "Emergency Use" authorization.][47]

Project Bioshield is essentially the civilian equivalent of Clinton's 1999 Executive Order. The Associated Press shared more on the subject on July 21, 2004:

President Bush on Wednesday signed legislation to develop and stockpile vaccines and other antidotes to chemical and germ attacks, saying the measure will "rally the great promise of American science and innovation to confront the greatest danger of our time."

The legislation, called Project BioShield, provides the drug industry with incentives to research and develop bioterrorism countermeasures. It speeds up the approval process of antidotes and, in an emergency, allows the government to distribute certain treatments before the Food and Drug Administration has approved them. . . .

U.S. officials are hoping that Project BioShield will yield enough new-generation anthrax vaccine to dose 25 million people. Federal health officials also hope that the $5.6 billion program will provide antidotes for botulism and anthrax, a safer smallpox vaccine and a long-awaited children's version of an anti-radiation pill.[48]

George Orwell once said, "Every war when it comes, or before it comes, is represented not as a war but as an act of self-defense against a homicidal maniac." George W. Bush sounded just like an Orwellian character when he made the following statement in the Rose Garden as he signed Project BioShield into law:

Every American can be certain that their government will continue doing everything in our power to prevent a terrorist attack and if the terrorists do strike we will be better prepared to defend our people because of the good law I sign today.[49]

Project BioShield authorized the government to spend "$5.6 billion in funding over 10 years. . . ."[50] Part of those funds were used to turn existing pathogens into life forms that were even more pathogenic. Richard Ebright, a professor of biochemistry at Rutgers University and director of the Waksman Institute of Microbiology, didn't think Bush's "good law" was all that great in 2004, but he grew even more dismayed to see President Obama breathe new life into the Project in 2013 with a five-year extension and another $2.8 billion. Ebright said in an interview with *The Verge* in 2013, "It's hard to imagine that someone thought creating new pandemic pathogens would be a good strategy for defending against pandemic pathogens. It reflects the clear lack of anyone in charge."[51] The biochemist may be right, but it may also reflect clear evidence that the *wrong people* are in charge, since they are some of the same people who've been orchestrating vaccine policy for decades.

Carl Franzen, the author of *The Verge* article, wrote that the most disconcerting fact among several disconcerting facts is that

> the very same parent agency in charge of funding drugs for the national stockpile, HHS, is also the one that is separately funding research into new diseases that could result in a bioterror or accidental infection, which would in turn demand a response from the national stockpile.[52]

In Ebright's words, "The activities of Project Bioshield are directly undermined by HHS funding the development of potential bioweapons agents. These are clear cross purposes. Would any sane government do that? Absolutely not."[53]

Would a government that is run by sociopaths "do that"? Absolutely. It would, it has, it is, and unless stopped, it will continue to do so.

Vaccine terrorists have capitalized on the alleged threat of bioterrorism to turn the stockpiling of vaccines into a third vaccine market. Unlike the pediatric and adult vaccine markets, the vast majority of stockpiled vaccines will most likely never be used. They will remain in warehouses until they expire, are disposed of, and then replaced with more vaccines. Every step in the cycle will transfer billions of dollars from taxpayers into the pockets of profiteers and politicians for products that the public will likely neither see nor use. Idle vaccines sitting in a stockpile also don't bear the costs associated with vaccine injury, death, and litigation. This scam will grow like cancer until sane minds bring it to an end.

An analysis of vaccine-injured military personnel could lead to the conclusion that vaccine injuries are the largest case of "friendly fire" in the history of the US military. But such is not the case. "Friendly fire" is defined as the inadvertent or accidental killing of fellow soldiers. There is substantial evidence to suggest, a fraction of which is presented in this chapter, that at least some of the vaccine-induced injury to military personnel, as well as the denial of and the failure to treat such injury, is not friendly. It's government-sanctioned experimentation in violation of ethical codes and decency, providing yet another example of the misuse of power over powerless people.

The full extent of the government's misuse of power is seen in the US military's plan to develop human biofactories through genetic modification attempting to use "living, breathing humans as their own antibody factors."[54]

It is, or at least it should be, a self-evident fact that individuals, corporate entities, and governments do not have the right to alter human DNA. Neither do they have the ability to contain their laboratory creations. The fact that the US military—the world's greatest purveyor of violence and greatest source of environmental pollution—is supporting such research should be a cause of great concern. The combined hubris, ignorance, and quest for power in such an endeavor holds the potential to unleash myriad known and yet unknown consequences, including the destruction of the human race.

There's great irony in the fact that those who believe they're fighting for freedom from tyranny don't have the freedom to control what their own government tyrants inject into their bodies. It's also a great irony that the majority of American civilians are all too willing to allow vaccine sociopaths to protect them in the same way military personnel are protected: by allowing their medical and religious freedoms to be trampled.

Orwell was right: "Freedom is slavery."

Sane voices are far too few, but they give cause for hope. In 1999, one month before military personnel described their vaccine injuries to the Oversight & Government Reform committee, the Association of American Physicians and Surgeons testified before the OGR's Subcommittee on Criminal Justice, Drug Policy, and Human Resources. Their statement is more relevant today than ever before:

> Public policy regarding vaccines is fundamentally flawed. It is permeated by conflicts of interest. It is based on poor scientific methodology (including studies that are too small, too short, and too limited in populations represented), which is, moreover, insulated from independent criticism. The evidence is far too poor to warrant overriding the independent judgments of patients, parents, and attending physicians, even if this were ethically or legally acceptable.
>
> AAPS opposes federal mandates for vaccines, on principle, on the grounds that they are:
>
> - An unconstitutional expansion of the power of the federal government.
> - An unconstitutional delegation of power to a public-private partnership.
> - An unconstitutional and destructive intrusion into the patient-physician and parent-child relationships.
> - A violation of the Nuremberg Code in that they force individuals to have medical treatment against their will, or to participate in the functional equivalent of a vast experiment without fully informed consent.
> - A violation of rights to free speech and to the practice of one's religion (which may require one to keep oaths).[55]

US Representative Ron Paul, a medical doctor, gave a speech in 2011 titled "Government Vaccines — Bad Policy, Bad Medicine" as the keynote speaker at the International Medical Council on Vaccination. He said,

> No single person, including the President of the United States, should ever be given the power to make a medical decision for potentially millions of Americans. Freedom over one's physical person is the most basic freedom of all, and people in a free society should be sovereign over their own bodies. When we give government the power to make medical decisions for us, we in essence accept that the state owns our bodies.[56]

Ten months prior to making this statement, the U.S. Supreme Court ruled that drug companies would no longer be liable for vaccine injuries even when the companies were aware of design defects and could have made a safer vaccine. In the words of Barbara Loe Fisher:

> From now on, drug companies selling vaccines in America will not be held accountable by a jury of our peers in a court of law if those vaccines brain damage us but could have been made less toxic. . . .
>
> If you get paralyzed by a flu shot or your child has a serious reaction to a vaccine required for school and becomes learning disabled, epileptic, autistic, asthmatic, diabetic or mentally retarded, you are on your own. . . .
>
> This is not public health. This is exploitation of a captive people by a pharmaceutical industry seeking unlimited profits and by doctors in positions of authority, who have never seen a vaccine they did not want to mandate.
>
> It is a drug company stockholder's dream, a health care consumer's worst nightmare and a prescription for tyranny. [57]

Supreme Court Justice Sonia Sotomayor penned a brilliant dissenting opinion to the Supreme Court's ruling with Justice Ruth Bader Ginsburg joining her:

> The majority's decision today disturbs that careful balance based on a bare policy preference that it is better "to leave complex epidemiological judgments about vaccine design to the FDA and the National Vaccine Program rather than juries." . . . To be sure, reasonable minds can disagree about the wisdom of having juries weigh the relative costs and benefits of a particular vaccine design. But whatever the merits of the majority's policy preference, the decision to bar all design defect claims

against vaccine manufacturers is one that Congress must make, not this Court. . . . By construing §22(b)(1) to pre-empt all design defect claims against vaccine manufacturers for covered vaccines, the majority's decision leaves a regulatory vacuum in which no one—neither the FDA nor any other federal agency, nor state and federal juries—ensures that vaccine manufacturers adequately take account of scientific and technological advancements. This concern is especially acute with respect to vaccines that have already been released and marketed to the public. Manufacturers, given the lack of robust competition in the vaccine market, will often have little or no incentive to improve the designs of vaccines that are already generating significant profit margins. Nothing in the text, structure, or legislative history remotely suggests that Congress intended that result. I respectfully dissent.[58]

According to Sotomayor, by ruling in favor of the industry, the Supreme Court usurped the authority of Congress. In August 2016, the US Department of Health and Human Services/CDC issued a Notice of Proposed Rulemaking (NPRM) that, if implemented, would not only usurp the authority of Congress, but also trample the US Constitution and the Bill of Rights. By doing so, it would solve, once and for all, industry's growing problem of how to control the vaccine-informed public. Titled "Control of Communicable Disease," the proposal purports to "provide additional clarity to various safeguards to prevent the importation and spread of communicable diseases affecting human health into the United States and interstate."[59]

What the HHS/CDC really intends to do is give itself the power to detain healthy people en masse without appeal. Restricting public travel appears to be one of the main hammers the government will use to pound the public into submission, including submission to mandatory vaccination.

Less than three months later, President Obama signed an Executive Order titled "Advancing the Global Health Security Agenda to Achieve a World Safe and Secure from Infectious Disease Threats."[60] The presidential order appears to be nothing more than the global version of the CDC's "Control of Communicable Disease" agenda, essentially calling on the entire world to march in lockstep with the USA's Global Health Security Agenda. It is highly unlikely that the timing of the two documents is coincidental. Inasmuch as the CDC's financially driven mission to control and prevent disease has resulted in billions in profit and millions of dysfunctional, damaged, and diseased people, and inasmuch as controlling and preventing population growth is a cornerstone of US foreign policy, the people behind this agenda likely represent a far greater threat to the human race than the world's infectious diseases combined.

George Orwell's prophesied future is within sight. With the government's boot pressing ever harder on the face of humanity, well-meaning but misguided medical professionals may soon be free to forcibly inject virtually every human being with every toxic vaccine manufactured by one of the most corrupt if not the most corrupt institutions in the world: the pharmaceutical industry. Perhaps the most frightening aspect of this scenario is the fact that millions of individuals appear more than happy to surrender their right to life, liberty, and the pursuit of happiness in exchange for their own destruction. Shawn Siegel, a noted modern-day anti-vaccinationist, shares his admiration for those individuals who have thus far pulled off one of the greatest crimes in the history of the world:

I simply have to admire the hubris, the gall, of the global cartel who many decades ago commandeered the vaccination paradigm, morphing it into a most surreal program—an Auschwitz Lite; an Auschwitz with gates flung wide open, into which people flock willingly; eagerly. Should they all hang by the neck 'til dead, as they deserve, my admiration will endure.[61]

Who will be left hanging in the end remains yet to be seen.

Chapter Twenty-Five

WILLIAM THOMPSON, *VAXXED,* AND THE GREAT AWAKENING

———◄┼———————┼►———

For there is nothing covered, that shall not be revealed; neither hid, that shall not be known. Therefore whatsoever ye have spoken in darkness shall be heard in the light; and that which ye have spoken in the ear in closets shall be proclaimed upon the housetops.

—Luke 12:2-3

There comes an hour when protest no longer suffices. After philosophy there must be action. The hand finishes what the idea has sketched.

—Victor Hugo

Knowledge will forever govern ignorance; and a people who mean to be their own governors must arm themselves with the power which knowledge gives.

—James Madison

Until they became conscious they will never rebel, and until after they have rebelled they cannot become conscious.

—George Orwell

Health literacy is a growing problem.[1]

—Glen Nowak, CDC

On August 27, 2014, William Thompson publically confessed that he and a number of his CDC colleagues had committed scientific fraud when they attempted to bury the association between the MMR vaccine and autism. A portion of his press release follows:

> My name is William Thompson. I am a Senior Scientist with the Centers for Disease Control and Prevention, where I have worked since 1998.

I regret that my coauthors and I omitted statistically significant information in our 2004 article published in the journal *Pediatrics*. The omitted data suggested that African American males who received the MMR vaccine before age 36 months were at increased risk for autism. Decisions were made regarding which findings to report after the data were collected, and I believe that the final study protocol was not followed. . . .

I am providing information to Congressman William Posey, and of course will continue to cooperate with Congress.[2]

By and large, the Unholy Trinity responded to Thompson's confession with silence, as did the mainstream media presstitutes.

Andrew Wakefield was not surprised by the confession. He and Brian Hooker—the scientist who had recorded four of numerous telephone conversations with Thompson—had been strategizing for months. They knew that the best way to protect Thompson from harm and even from death was to go public with the story.

One week before Thompson would become known as the CDC whistleblower, he exchanged texts with Wakefield's wife, Carmel, saying, "I do believe your husbands [*sic*] career was unjustly damaged and this study would have supported his scientific opinion. Hopefully I can help repair it."[3] On the day of the press release, text messages shared between Wakefield and the CDC scientist reveal something of the history between the two men as well as something of the character of the vaccine industry's most reviled enemy:

Wakefield: Is the press conference real?

Thompson: Yes!

Wakefield: Thank you. This was the right and honorable thing to do, Andy.

Thompson: I agree. I apologize again for the price you paid for my dishonesty.

Wakefield: I forgive you completely and without any bitterness.

Thompson: I know you mean it, and I am grateful to know you more personally.[4]

Since having his license unjustly revoked, Wakefield had moved to Texas, where he and a few of his many supporters had established the Autism Media Channel. By doing so, Wakefield and his team became the media. Whether due to serendipity, karma, or, as many believe, the will of God, Wakefield was uniquely positioned to tell Thompson's story with authority unmatched by anyone on Earth.

Del Bigtree, former producer of the daytime TV show "The Doctors," recognized the CDC whistleblower's story as the biggest of his career and stated that he had no choice but to walk away from his job and offer his expertise in the production of a documentary about the affair.

When *Vaxxed* came out, the media could no longer remain silent, so they blasted the film, many doing so even before they'd seen it. When the public finally got its chance to view the documentary, most agreed that the evidence was indisputable: the agency in charge of protecting the health of America's children had sacrificed those children upon the bloody altar of the Vaccine religion.

Vaxxed changed and is changing the public dialogue. Although the film is anything but anti-vaccine, it is antitreachery. Which means, of course, that it is anti-vaccine because the vaccine scam is treacherous. Wakefield himself, a strong supporter of safe or at least safer vaccines, has told numerous audiences, "I do not believe that any vaccines currently on the market meet the criteria for safety and efficacy."[5]

Thompson's admitted fraud makes the stench of industry propaganda all the more foul. After viewing *Vaxxed*, even lifelong defenders of the vaccine program realize that to be pro-vaccine is to be pro-hogwash.

Perhaps the most disturbing part of the CDC whistleblower's saga is the reaction of the medical establishment in general and, more particularly, the response from the American Academy of Pediatrics. If the AAP were truly "Dedicated to the health of all children," the organization would have stormed the CDC the day after Thompson went public. The guild leaders would have demanded transparency and answers. They would have retracted the fictional 2004 paper authored by Thompson and his fellow perpetrators of fraud. Most important, they would have instructed pediatricians to stop using the MMR vaccine until Congress had investigated Thompson's claims and the matter had been resolved. Rather than do any of those things, they ignored Thompson altogether, just as the media had done.

The AAP remained silent until September 2015, when US presidential candidates, including Ben Carson, MD, agreed during a nationally televised debate that too many jabs administered too soon were injuring too many American children.[6] Less than 24 hours later, Karen Remley, MD, the AAP's executive director, issued a formal response on behalf of the AAP "to correct false statements made during the Republican presidential debate last night regarding vaccines." Every sentence reeks of lies and Orwellian doublespeak, the official language of The Church of Vaccinology:

Claims that vaccines are linked to autism, or are unsafe when adminis-tered according to the recommended schedule, have been disproven by a robust body of medical literature. It is dangerous to public health to suggest otherwise.

There is no "alternative" immunization schedule. Delaying vaccines only leaves a child at risk of disease for a longer period of time; it does not make vaccinating safer.

Vaccines work, plain and simple. Vaccines are one of the safest, most effec-tive and most important medical innovations of our time. Pediatricians partner with parents to provide what is best for their child, and what is best is for children to be fully vaccinated.[7]

Armed with the shield of vaccine risk denialism, it's no surprise that when *Vaxxed* hit the big screen the following spring, pediatricians, who don't "part-ner" with parents in the least, were among its most outspoken critics, many denouncing it even though they had no intentions of viewing it. One Arizona pediatrician said she had no time for "hocus pocus movies" while Colorado's Pediatrician of the Year called *Vaxxed* "a work of fiction."[8, 9]

A small allowance might be made for ignorant pediatricians whose trust was betrayed by the CDC and the AAP. But when anyone chooses to remain in a self-imposed state of ignorance, they become coconspirators with fraudsters. Such physicians are pimps to industry and slaves to the anti-science Vaccine religion.

The words of Carl Sagan apply to the unfortunate souls who model one of the saddest lessons of history:

If we've been bamboozled long enough, we tend to reject any evidence of the bamboozle. We're no longer interested in finding out the truth. The bamboozle has captured us. It's simply too painful to acknowledge, even to ourselves, that we've been taken. Once you give a charlatan power over you, you almost never get it back.[10]

The President of the Utah Chapter of the American Academy of Pediatrics, William E. Cosgrove, MD, FAAP, proved Sagan's point when he wrote a let-ter to key state officials including the speaker of the house, the governor, the executive director of the Utah Department of Health, and members of the state senate.[11]

Without ever referring to Thompson, Cosgrove categorically denounced *Vaxxed* and then set out to "delineate fact from fiction." His attempt to do so proved that he himself is both a victim of Thompson's fraud and a perpetra-tor of harm against vaccine-injured children and their families. In the church in which Cosgrove worships, vaccines are safe and effective. He and his fellow white-robed High Priests look down on The Herd from their exalted position and proclaim that "it is certainly easier to blame an immunization, or the doctor, or the government, than to blame their own genetics; to blame themselves."

Harris L. Coulter, the author of *Vaccination, Social Violence, and Criminality: The Medical Assault on the American Brain*, provided the perfect response to Cosgrove more than twenty years before the pediatrician had penned his patronizing point of view:

> The physician is irresistibly impelled to characterize the "new morbidity" as "emotional," or perhaps "congenital," because these disabilities can then be blamed on the child or the parents. In fact, the responsibility should be placed squarely at the physician's own door. The vaccination program is intrinsically dangerous, which was never recognized or admitted, and has been implemented across the board in a careless way—without due concern for contraindications.[12]

Cosgrove concluded his epistle as follows:

> While it is easy for you to empathize with the troubled parents in your districts, and to hurt with them, please recognize that decisions about vaccines, especially public policy decisions, must be based on science, data re-confirmed in careful replication studies, and cool cognition, not the heat of emotion, nor the blindness of fear.[13]

In a church and paradigm based on fear and filled with irony, one of the greatest ironies is the cool detachment of pediatricians who've long since lost the ability "to empathize with troubled parents"—pediatricians whose unquestioning faith in corrupted science and corrupted institutions renders them blind to the role they play in destroying the health and vitality of unborn children, preterm infants, newborns, and toddlers.

Anti-vaccine activist Shawn Siegel defines the system and the mental process "professionals" such as Cosgrove use to blame the faulty genetics of patients rather than blame themselves and their toxic vaccines:

> Plausible deniability: The ability of pediatricians and other MDs, through a stream of corrupt information disseminated to the medical establishment and the general public by the CDC and other public health entities, to deny any connection between severe adverse reactions and the vaccinations given only minutes or hours before; or, acknowledging the connection, to misrepresent them as normal.[14]

The AAP provided more corrupt information to the public in August 2016, just two weeks after the HHS/CDC had posted its tyrannical proposal to detain citizens without cause, clamp down on public travel, and enforce mandatory vaccinations, and only a few days after Judge Dana Sabraw had denied the preliminary injunction against the implementation of SB 277.[15] After ensuring the public that pediatricians are "the best source of answers" for "vaccine hesitant parents," AAP President Benard P. Dreyer, MD, FAAP, stated in a press release, "Non-medical exemptions to immunizations should be eliminated."[16] Why? Because unimmunized children acquired measles in the 2015 Disneyland epidemic. Of course. Unimmunized kids got measles, so every kid should be forced to get every jab of every vaccine. That makes perfect sense if you head up a cartel whose members make a significant portion of their income from vaccines.[17] But for parents of vaccine-injured or dead children, Dreyer's pronouncement chills the soul.

The AAP insults vaccine-informed parents and dishonors the injured and deceased with the following statement: "Parents are expected to consider the best interest of their child in medical decision-making, focusing on their child's medical, emotional, and social needs, rather than their own social or emotional interests."[18] The AAP also used the occasion to reverse its previous policy regarding the treatment of unvaccinated children, authorizing pediatricians to kick them out of their practices.[19]

Twenty years ago when AAP leaders and pediatricians had less access to the truth, the hubris and self-inflicted ignorance of doctors like Dreyer and Cosgrove were more forgivable and the humility of men like Wakefield was more remarkable. But to deny today the obvious role of vaccines in the epidemic of ADHD, asthma, allergies, autoimmune disorders, autism, etc., is criminal.

Several scientific bodies have declared that man-made environmental toxicants play a large role in the global epidemic of neurodevelopmental disorders in children. The government journal *Environmental Health Perspectives*, a monthly peer-reviewed journal of research and news published with support from the National Institute of Environmental Health Sciences (NIEHS), National Institutes of Health, and the U.S. Department of Health and Human Services, published "The TENDR [Targeting Environmental Neuro-Developmental Risks] Consensus Statement" in its July 2016 issue. The 47 signers of the statement, all government scientists, declared:

Children in America today are at an unacceptably high risk of developing neurodevelopmental disorders that affect the brain and nervous system including autism, attention deficit hyperactivity disorder, intellectual disabilities, and other learning and behavioral disabilities. These are complex disorders with multiple causes—genetic, social, and environmental. The contribution of toxic chemicals to these disorders can be prevented.

The scientists further assert:

> . . . [T]he current system in the United States for evaluating scientific evidence and making health-based decisions about environmental chemicals is fundamentally broken. To help reduce the unacceptably high prevalence of neurodevelopmental disorders in our children, we must eliminate or significantly reduce exposures to chemicals that contribute to these conditions. We must adopt a new framework for assessing chemicals that have the potential to disrupt brain development and prevent the use of those that may pose a risk.[20]

Yes, the government's system "for evaluating scientific evidence and making health-based decisions about environmental chemicals is fundamentally broken." And the government's misnamed "Control of Communicable Diseases" proposal, Judge Sabraw's refusal to protect constitutionally guaranteed personal belief exemptions, and the AAP's goal to forcibly vaccinate virtually every American infant and child clearly illustrate that nowhere is the government more broken than in its own vaccine program.

The Thompson saga is but a microcosm of corruption in a system based on fraud, and the stories of the vaccine injured depicted in *Vaxxed* and in hundreds of other documentaries, books, articles, blogs, and online videos recount but a fraction of the pain, grief, and anger experienced by billions of people who have been betrayed by the Unholy Trinity and The Church of Vaccinology.

Falsus in uno, falsus in omnibus—"false in one, false in all"—is a concept referred to in legal matters. If the Unholy Trinity—Big Pharma, Big Medicine, and Big Government—were brought up on charges for perpetrating some of the largest crimes against humanity through its global vaccination program, the principle of *falsus in uno, falsus in omnibus* would entitle jurors to doubt all of the Trinity's many claims knowing that it has been lying in part—a *very* big part.

Vaccine believers and sociopaths are fond of saying that the success of the vaccine program is its biggest problem. They're right, but not in the way they mean it. People are not abandoning vaccinations out of ignorance, apathy, or because they no longer fear infectious diseases. They're not vaccinating because they're afraid of the sociopaths who've been sticking it to the public with increasing numbers of unnecessary and scientifically unjustifiable vaccines. In other words, they fear those who create, manipulate, and profit from public fear, and, for many, that fear has transformed into anger that increases with every jab added to the already bloated vaccination schedules. Each new stick multiplies the synergistic toxicity and results in more injuries and deaths.

As has been shown, the Unholy Trinity is making a last-ditch effort to prevent The Herd from leaving the fold. It's the biblical equivalent of the desperate attempts of Pharaoh to prevent Moses and the Children of Israel from leaving bondage and tyranny. Pharaoh needed slaves to produce bricks. Modern pharaohs and workers of magic need slaves to ingest, imbibe, and inject a wide range of patented, bioengineered products including vaccines made from an ungodly mix of heavy metals, viruses, retroviruses, bacteria, oncogenic cell lines, glyphosate, aborted fetal tissue, contaminated cells from cows, primates, insects, and who knows what else. The description of the plagues visited upon ancient Egypt pales in comparison to the plagues that have resulted and will yet result from the mandatory poisoning of fetuses, infants, toddlers, children, pregnant women, and the elderly.

With over 700 synthetic chemicals now detectable in humans, the children of today and tomorrow are cursed from conception onward.[21] It's no wonder that MIT professor Stephanie Seneff predicts that up to half of America's children and 80% of its boys will suffer from autism and related disorders within the next 20 years.[22]

Vaccine-related informed consent, parental rights, and personal belief exemptions are crucial, but ultimately they can't protect against the destruction of the human genome from the abominable concoctions of genetically modified organisms and synthetic monstrosities that make up modern vaccines. There is no middle ground. As long as the vaccine industry is run by sociopaths, people who are pro-vaccine are either knowingly or unknowingly anti-health, anti-freedom, and, for people of faith, anti-God.

The Unholy Trinity—industry, the medical establishment, and government—is really even worse than a metaphorical sinister religion. It's a cancerous cult on a conspiratorial mission to turn all of humanity into a compliant herd. When the corralling is done and the gate is locked, the cult overlords—those who stand outside of The Herd—will use their massive resources to conjure up increasingly absurd formulations to be added to mandatory schedules and that will further sicken and suck the life out of the human race.

Whether individuals have syphilis, gonorrhea, herpes, HIV, high blood pressure, acne, or tooth decay, jabs for those diseases and others may soon be included on the mandated schedule.[23] Next will come the vaccines to treat the effects of the vaccines caused by the previous vaccines.

Appealing to government, the pharmaceutical industry, and the medical establishment to rein itself in is like begging cancer to cure itself. For decades, investigations have been conducted, hearings have been held, and reports have been written, but, in the end, the government has betrayed the public by partnering with, profiting from, and protecting corporate criminals.

That is not to say that vaccine truth and safety advocacy is not important. It's crucial! The citizens of Leicester, England, and elsewhere were influential in repealing compulsory vaccination laws in the early 1900s, and vaccine-informed advocacy groups have successfully defeated repressive vaccination legislation. But the circumstances are more ominous today than ever before. Numerous citizens have appealed to Congress—most members of which are little more than tools for industry—to subpoena William Thompson, but to date, there's little evidence of progress. And that case is just a drop in the ocean of corruption. In the end, John W. Hodge's 1902 statement may prove prophetic:

> That reforms are not made by those who profit by them so the doctors or the government cannot be depended upon to abolish vaccination of their own volition; that the people, themselves, must rise up and make demands for freedom from this curse of greed, ignorance and destruction, for only then can we hope to see the light of a new day of health, progress and harmonious adjustment.[24]

Sheila Ealey, speaking as only the mother of a vaccine-injured child can speak, made similar pronouncements 114 years later:

> No one has the right to mandate and demand you inject known neurotoxins into your body! Everyone MUST Rise UP and put an end to forced medical procedures because THAT'S what a vaccination is, it's FORCED control over your body by this government [emphasis in original]![25]

As Ealey stated after a screening of *Vaxxed*,

> What we have is a holocaust. Our children are being maimed and they are being killed. And you've got a government sitting in Washington, DC that doesn't think enough to subpoena Dr. Thompson who came out and said what they were doing. So what we have to do today is take back our communities and take back our children. And how do we do that? We walk out of the doctors' offices, we decide no, we're not going to take that shot in the dark.[26]

The holocaust is here. It's now. It's real. At this very moment, somewhere a family is burying a low birth weight infant who stopped breathing following a vaccination. A mother is walking into her baby's room and discovering that her recently vaccinated child is dead. A father is asking a clueless doctor why his son stopped walking and talking after receiving the MMR vaccine. A grandmother is frantic from watching her two-month-old grandson scream out in pain from the pressure of his swollen brain against his skull. A physician tells her it's normal for babies to cry after their shots. Another doctor is pressuring his pregnant patient to roll up her sleeve. Teachers are meeting yet again to discuss the new normal: Billy messed his pants . . . again. Susan flew into a rage . . . again. Ted is still rocking in the corner. Ricardo's anti-anxiety meds are out. And someone call the police because John has wandered off and is missing . . . again. Eleven-year-old Helen hasn't been to school in a month since the nurse talked her into getting the HPV vaccine.

On a broader scale, thousands of school children in India are facing lives limited by paralysis following their polio vaccinations. Armed soldiers are going door to door in Uganda searching for vaccine holdouts. Countless mothers and fathers are spending money they don't have on treatments for their autistic teenage children—victims of the thimerosal and aluminum generations. Millions of vaccine-injured kids around the world are being bullied due to their behavioral, social, medical, or emotional difficulties. Tens of thousands are being prescribed psychotropic medications known to increase suicidal ideation, aggression, and rage. Some of those kids are bringing guns to school and using them. Couples, single parents, and grandparents are having hushed conversations about who will take care of a disabled adult child after they're gone, and, in many cases, it's no one.

Andrew Wakefield has told numerous audiences:

> . . . When a government subverts the rights of the individuals that it is sworn to serve, . . . when those are superseded by special interests, by serving corporations, particularly the pharmaceutical industry, over and above the well-being of the citizens who put them in place, then that republic has come to an end.[27]

Wakefield is right yet again. The American republic is dying. Corporations exert fascistic, oligarchical control over the once-great United States of America. With corporations at the helm, the American Academy of Pediatrics and other medical cartels continue to deny their role in the vaccine holocaust. Highly paid pimps like Richard Pan, Paul Offit, and Benard P. Dreyer continue to fabricate myths about herd immunity and the greater good, and the pharmaceutical industry exerts its power to pass ever more repressive legislation.

But, in the end, none of that will matter. The strength of the global vaccine-informed community is growing. Vaccine believers—those who are still locked in the paradigm—will eventually awaken, and, when they do, they'll be outraged. They'll hold accountable the likes of Dr. William Cosgrove for telling legislators to ignore "troubled parents." They'll be outraged at Richard Pan and his gang for being cowards and liars. They'll be furious at profiteer and false prophet Paul Offit for . . . for everything. And, for the Americans who become aware, there will be outrage when they realize that their republic has been stolen.

As soon as enough people have awakened, revolution will follow. Freedom emerges out of tyranny, and revolution is the path to freedom. That statement is not a call to arms; it's historical fact. The only question that remains is when will vaccine sociopaths have injured and killed enough of us to spark the revolution?

Dr. Andrew Wakefield gave the answer: "Now is the time to overthrow the corporate rule of this country and to bring the power back to the people."[28]

AFTERWORD
by Shawn Siegel

"Vaccine injury is a death, the death of the life my son could've had."

"Yes, I cannot die. I must continue to live long enough for my son to pass before me."

Reflecting the horror that is severe vaccine injury—the loss of neurological and immunological integrity, if not the very life of the child, the loss of a n y possibility of independence—those comments were made by two moms on social media. What they don't reflect are the ripple effects: the stress within the family, the enormous expense often involved in care and treatment, the toll taken on sibling relationships, the strain on the very vows that forged the marriage.

Ultimately they don't reflect how self-defeating is the very concept of injecting disease to prevent disease, how foolish the circumvention of the highly developed, intricate, successful natural process of self-cleanse and detox that is the phenomenon we call infectious illness—a process that requires the participation of the innate cellular response that takes place in the mucosal membranes of the respiratory and gastrointestinal tracts, where in the vast majority of cases the body expects to see potential pathogens after natural exposure. That response "plays a crucial part in the initiation and subsequent direction of adaptive immune responses," we're told in the journal *Immuobiology*. That is, the adaptive response, targeted by vaccination, is secondary. The innate cellular response is crucial to both successful recovery and productive immunity.

And it's bypassed by injection.

A relevant aside: the story posted by a woman who for years would get the flu, go to the doctor, get the Rx du jour, and recover, only to repeat the cycle the following year—until one year she decided to let the illness play out, sans doctor visit and prescriptions. That was years ago, and she hasn't had the flu since. The fundamental purpose of the symptoms of infectious illness, so dissed by the vaccine industry, so misrepresented, is to heal, not harm, and in a customized, unique, individual manner science can't hope to understand, let alone duplicate. Where that process fails is where we'd expect it to fail—in those individuals—or populations, in the case of developing nations—where due to malnutrition and other complicating factors, compromised immune systems are the norm. The obvious solution in those instances is to provide the needed nutrition and other support, not to impose vaccination, a fundamentally self-defeating paradigm. The consequences of vaccinating immunocompromised populations are evident in an African study addressed in the article, "DTP Vaccine Increases Mortality in Young Infants 5 to 10 Fold Compared to Unvaccinated Infants," published by *The Lancet* in *EBioMedicine*.

Also confounding the persistent industry portrait of the supposedly vaccine-preventable illnesses as fearsome and threatening are the various scientific studies telling us that febrile childhood infections are associated with protection against cancer and other chronic diseases later in life—benefits that go well beyond the typical gained lifetime of natural immunity.

It's dumbfounding when you then consider the known(!) neurotoxins in vaccines. The arrogance of the vaccine industry is boundless. There's no known way to reliably assess the susceptibility of any child to the aluminum and mercury—and other toxins—found in vaccines. Meanwhile, aluminum attacks the myelin which makes up the insulating sheath that surrounds our nerves, interfering with signals to, from, and within the brain. Thus the preponderance of related injuries "compensated" by the Vaccine Injury Compensation Program in the US, among them spinal cord myelitis and transverse myelitis, which can resemble polio in display. The movie Trace Amounts provides adequate evidence that even a single part per billion of injected mercury can cause neurological havoc in the susceptible child. Yet we're told, carte blanche, that vaccines are safe.

In the rather amazing compendium of valuable information that is *Jabbed*, we find the undeniable portrait of a paradigm rooted in statistical manipulation and outright lies, and of steadfast mainstream denial of the underbelly of the industry: the true nature and extent of vaccine injury. The pregnant question of motivation, posed by Brett in this encyclopedic work, remains: why the vaccination paradigm?

Since the initial publication of *Jabbed* both Maine and New York have joined the unhappy group of US states that have removed non-medical vaccine exemptions—New York, in draconian fashion, with a bill that had sat in committee for months suddenly and with no public notice being approved, sent to the floor for vote, passed, and signed by the Governor. This cloak-and-dagger approach smacks of disdain for the public, of the tight-fisted control exercised by the industry, of deception. Coupled with the ever-present alarmist mainstream articles, warning us of this or that fearsome—"vaccine-preventable"—disease, stoking the fire of fear, steering public opinion, and laying the groundwork for such sordid legislative business, it smacks of motivation far deeper and darker than mere monetary gain.

Recently yet another restrictive vaccine bill was passed in California—SB276, which in essence removed the authority to issue medical vaccine exemptions, currently the only exemption available in the state, from the family doctor—from the very medical professional most intimately involved with the child, thus obviously most qualified to assess the need for a medical exemption. Instead the final decisions will now be made by a state board. The day of its passage, hundreds of parents converged on the state Capitol, in protest. Many of them gathered in the Senate chamber, and were able with their strong chorus of voices to delay the vote for a little while, but ultimately to no avail.

Meanwhile, several moms were arrested outside the Capitol after refusing to move when ordered.

Based on our modern history of seemingly inexorable increase in the ferocity of vaccine laws, state by state, the road ahead, I fear, is filled with turmoil. Some families are having to find the means to home school their kids to avoid vaccinating, others are literally leaving for friendlier states, where the law allows vaccine refusal on either religious or personal grounds. Meanwhile, the vaccine myth, so divisive in the widespread irrational belief that unvaccinated children are a threat to everyone else's kids, so unquestioningly propelled by the mainstream media, becomes even more deeply entrenched. That tyrannical hold on public perception stretches from the vaccine manufacturers to the government to the medical establishment to state legislatures to the courts—seemingly insurmountable. Non-violent civil disobedience will undoubtedly increase as a result, as more and more parents, aware of the threat to the integrity of their children's well-being that are vaccines, nonetheless find themselves legally compelled to vaccinate.

The integrity of our children's lives is indeed at stake. Using whatever communication platforms are available, the vaccine awareness community must continue to alert family, friends and the general public to the pitfalls of vaccination—one vaccine refusal at a time, if necessary. Ultimately the paradigm must be stopped, a daunting task, one in which this book plays a poignant role. But Herculean works such as *Jabbed* will have to be matched by an even more Herculean outreach.

No parent who's seen enough honest information about vaccines and the illnesses they supposedly prevent would ever vaccinate, or continue vaccinating her kids.

NOTES

Introduction

1. Kevin Barry, Esq., Vaccine Whistleblower: Exposing Autism Research Fraud at the CDC, Skyhorse Publishing, 2015, Introduction, p. xxi, https://www.amazon.com/Vaccine-Whistleblower-Exposing-Autism-Research/dp/1634509951/.
2. Sharyl Attkisson, Stonewalled: My Fight for Truth Against the Forces of Obstruction, Intimidation, and Harassment in Obama's Washington. Harper, 2014, p. 71, https://www.amazon.com/Stonewalled-Obstruction-Intimidation-Harassment-Washington/dp/0062322842/.
3. Andrew Gavin Marshall, "Biased? Damn Right I Am," occupy.com, June 12, 2012, http://www.occupy.com/article/biased-damn-right-i-am.
4. Paul Thomas, MD, "Vaccines – Is Your Doctor Committed to First Doing No Harm?" Dr Thomas's Blog, May 20, 2013, http://paulthomasmd.com/category/vaccines/page/39/.
5. Kelly Brogan, MD, A Mind of Your Own: The Truth About Depression and How Women Can Heal Their Bodies to Reclaim Their Lives, Harper Wave, 2016, p. 138, http://www.amazon.com/Mind-Your-Own-Depression-Reclaim/dp/0062405578/.
6. http://www.dictionary.com/browse/sociopath.
7. Kevin Barry, Esq., Vaccine Whistleblower: Exposing Autism Research Fraud at the CDC, Skyhorse Publishing, 2015, p. 116, https://www.amazon.com/Vaccine-Whistleblower-Exposing-Autism-Research/dp/1634509951/.

Chapter 1. Pharma, Medicine, Government, and the Religion of Vaccinology

1. Robert S. Mendelsohn, MD, Confessions of a Medical Heretic, Contemporary Books, 1979, pp. xiii, xiv, https://www.amazon.com/Confessions-Medical-Heretic-Robert-Mendelsohn/dp/0809241315/.
2. Mendelsohn, p. iv.
3. Mendelsohn, pp. xiii, xiv.
4. Mendelsohn, p. 143.

5. Richard Moskowitz, MD, "The Case Against Immunizations," http://doctor-rmosk.com/Site/The_Case_Against_Immunizations.html.

6-8. Olivier Clerc, Modern Medicine: The New World Religion: How Beliefs Secretly Influence Medical Dogmas and Practices, Personhood Press, 2004, https://www.amazon.com/Modern-Medicine-Religion-Influence-Practices/dp/1932181148/.

9. Timothy Alexander Guzman, "Big Pharma and Big Profits: The Multibillion Dollar Vaccine Market," file://localhost/Silent Crow News, January 26, 2016, http/::silentcrownews.com:wordpress: %3Fp=4539.

10. Arthur Wollaston Hutton, MA, The Vaccination Question, Methuen & Co., London, 1895, http://www.whale.to/vaccine/hutton_b.html.

11. Brandy Vaughan, "Why I Do What I Do," LearnTheRisk.org, http://www.learntherisk.org/news/why-i-do-what-i-do/.

Chapter 2. The Vaccine Paradigm: Invisible and Omnipresent

1. "ANTI-COMPULSORY VACCINATION DEMONSTRATION AT LEICESTER," Hawera & Normanby Star, Volume VL, Issue 1016, 19 May 1885, Page 2, http://paperspast.natlib.govt.nz/cgi-bin/paperspast?a=d&d=HNS18850519.2.14.

2. "Dr Tenpenny, What the CDC documents say about vaccines," April 29, 2013, https://www.youtube.com/watch?v=M1VwVBmx0Ng.

3. Marco Cáceres, "The Toxic Logic of Water and Applesauce," The Vaccine Reaction, December 8, 2015, http://www.thevaccinereaction.org/2015/12/the-toxic-logic-of-water-and-applesauce/.

4. Claudia Kalb, "Dr. Paul Offit: Debunking the Vaccine-Autism Link," Newsweek, October 24, 2008, http://www.newsweek.com/dr-paul-offit-debunking-vaccine-autism-link-91933.

5. Carl Sagan, The Demon-Haunted World: Science as a Candle in the Dark, Ballantine Books, 1997, p. 241, https://www.amazon.com/Demon-Haunted-World-Science-Candle-Dark/dp/0345409469/.

Chapter 3. Banking on Fear

1. "You've Got to Be Carefully Taught," Rogers and Hammerstein, South Pacific, online at http://www.ageofautism.com/2016/08/houston-chronicle-reports-vaccine-exemptions-on-rise.html.

2. "Houston Chronicle Reports Vaccine Exemptions on Rise," Age of Autism, August 16, 2016, http://www.ageofautism.com/2016/08/houston-chronicle-reports-vaccine-exemptions-on-rise.html.

3. "Politicians vs Doctors on Vaccines, Quacks and Hippies on the Internet," Global Freedom Movement, February 23, 2016, http://globalfreedommovement.org/politicians-vs-doctors-vaccines-quacks-hippies-internet/.

4. "Crucifying the Vaccine Heretics." by Roman Bystrianyk (coauthor Dissolving Illusions: Disease, Vaccines, and the Forgotten History), International Medical Council on Vaccination, October 9, 2014, http://www.vaccinationcouncil.org/2014/10/09/crucifying-the-vaccine-heretics-by-roman-bystrianyk-co-author-dissolving-illusions-disease-vaccines-and-the-forgotten-history/.

5. "Acute Hepatitis B Among Children and Adolescents—United States, 1990–2002," cdc, November 5, 2004, http://www.cdc.gov/mmwr/preview/mmwrhtml/mm5343a4.htm - fig1.

6. "BEXSERO® (Meningococcal Group B Vaccine)," Package Insert, https://gsksource.com/pharma/content/dam/GlaxoSmithKline/US/en/Prescribing_Information/Bexsero/pdf/BEXSERO.PDF.

7. "Meningococcal Disease," CDC, http://www.cdc.gov/vaccines/pubs/pinkbook/mening.html.

8. Gardiner Harris, "Panel Reviews New Vaccine That Could Be Controversial," The New York Times, October 27, 2004, http://www.nytimes.com/2004/10/27/health/panel-reviews-new-vaccine-that-could-be-controversial.html.

9. Kelly Brogan, MD, "Immunity: The Emerging Truth," http://kellybroganmd.com/immunity-emerging-truth/.

10. Glen Nowak, PhD, "Increasing Awareness and Uptake of Influenza Immunization," CDC, http://nationalacademies.org/hmd/~/media/Files/Activity%20Files/PublicHealth/MicrobialThreats/Nowak.pdf.

11. P. Doshi, "Are U.S. flu-death figures more PR than science?" BMJ 2005 Dec 10; 331: 1412.

12. "H1N1 'false pandemic' biggest pharma-fraud of century?" RT, January 12, 2010, https://www.youtube.com/watch?v=t9HamW8sH8Q&feature=youtu.be.

13-14. "Strong lobbying behind WHO resolution on mass vaccination," Information, November 16, 2009, Danish version at https://www.information.dk/udland/2009/11/staerk-lobbyisme-bag-who-beslutning-massevaccination, English version at http://translate.google.com/translate?js=y&prev=_t&hl=en&ie=UTF-8&layout=1&eotf=1&u=http%3A%2F%2Fwww.information.dk%2F215355&sl=da&tl=en.

15. "The handling of the H1N1 pandemic: more transparency needed," Council of Europe, http://assembly.coe.int/committeedocs/2010/20100604_h1n1pandemic_e.pdf.

16. "H1N1 'false pandemic' biggest pharma-fraud of century?" RT, January 12, 2010, https://www.youtube.com/watch?v=t9HamW8sH8Q&feature=youtu.be.

17. Sarah Knapton, "Tamiflu: drugs given for swine flu 'were waste of £500m,'" The Telegraph, April 10, 2014, http://www.telegraph.co.uk/news/health/swine-flu/10756200/Tamiflu-drugs-given-for-swine-flu-were-waste-of-500m.html.

18. R. Hama et al., "Oseltamivir and early deterioration leading to death: a proportional mortality study for 2009A/H1N1 influenza," Int J Risk Saf Med., 2011, https://www.ncbi.nlm.nih.gov/m/pubmed/22156085/.

19. Tom Porter, "Brain-Damaged UK Victims of Swine Flu Vaccine to Get £60 Million Compensation," International Business Times, March 2, 2014, http://www.ibtimes.co.uk/brain-damaged-uk-victims-swine-flu-vaccine-get-60-million-compensation-1438572.

20. "Panikens Pris," February 12, 2012, http://www.kostdemokrati.se/nyheter/files/2012/02/SvD-sid-14-19.pdf.

21. file://localhost/"Massvaccinering räddade sex liv," Svenska Dagbladet, http/::www.svd.se:massvaccinering-raddade-sex-liv_6851143.

22. "Health Benefits of Measles Infection," GreenMedInfo.com, http:// www .greenmedinfo.com/keyword/health-benefits-measles-infection.

23. Dr. William Thompson, Vaccine Whistleblower: Exposing Autism Research Fraud at the CDC, Skyhorse Publishing, 2015, p. 11, https://www.amazon.com/Vaccine-Whistleblower-Exposing-Autism-Research/dp/1634509951/.

24. "The Problem With Mandatory Vaccination as Public Health Policy," Stop Mandatory Vaccination, http://www.stopmandatoryvaccination.com/public-health/.

25. Jeanne Bendick, Have a Happy Measle, a Merry Mumps, and a Cheery Chickenpox, Hardcover – 1958, https://www.amazon.com/happy-measle-merry-cheery-chickenpox/dp/B0007HQ528.

26. Peter J. Hotez, "How the Anti-Vaxxers Are Winning," New York Times, February 8, 2017 https://www.nytimes.com/2017/02/08/opinion/how-the-anti-vaxxers-are-winning.html.

27. Lou Conte and Wayne Rohde, "Paul Offit, Fear, Intimidation and Astroturf," Age of Autism, February 10, 2015, http://www.ageofautism.com/2015/02/paul-offit-fear-intimidation-and-astroturf.html.

28. "Richard Pan's Lies on SB277," https://www.youtube.com/watch?v=caiCn57RNFc.

29. "Thimerosal in Vaccines Questions and Answers," FDA, http://www.fda.gov/BiologicsBloodVaccines/Vaccines/QuestionsaboutVaccines/ucm070430.htm.

30. Marco Cáceres, "The Toxic Logic of Water and Applesauce," The Vaccine Reaction, December 8, 2015, http://www.thevaccinereaction.org/2015/12/the-toxic-logic-of-water-and-applesauce/.

31. Sayer Ji, "Hep B Vaccine Damages The Liver It Is Supposed To Protect," GreenMedInfo.com, February 29, 2012, http://www.greenmedinfo.com/blog/hep-b-vaccine-damages-liver-it-supposed-protect.

32. C. Pande et al., "Hepatitis B vaccination with or without hepatitis B immunoglobulin at birth to babies born of HBsAg-positive mothers prevents overt

HBV transmission but may not prevent occult HBV infection in babies: a randomized controlled trial," Journal of Viral Hepatitis, April 23, 2013, DOI: 10.1111/jvh.12102, http://onlinelibrary.wiley.com/doi/10.1111/jvh.12102/ abstract.

Chapter 4. Vaccines are Safe and Effective and Other Lies

1. Carla Emery, Secret, Don't Tell: The Encyclopedia of Hypnotism, Acorn Hill Pub., 1998, p. 238, by Carla Emery p. 238.
2. Claire Dwoskin, "Are aluminum adjuvants plus Gardasil a uniquely damaging neuroinflammatory cocktail?" The Driven Researcher, July 28, 2016, http://info.cmsri.org/the-driven-researcher-blog/are-aluminum-adjuvants-plus-gardasil-a-uniquely-damaging-neuroinflammatory-cocktail.
3. Robert Whitaker, Anatomy of an Epidemic: Magic Bullets, Psychiatric Drugs, and the Astonishing Rise of Mental Illness in America, Broadway Books, 2011, http://www.amazon.com/Anatomy-Epidemic-Bullets-Psychiatric-Astonishing/dp/0307452425/.
4. Claudia Kalb, "Dr. Paul Offit: Debunking the Vaccine-Autism Link," Newsweek, October 24, 2008, http://www.newsweek.com/dr-paul-offit-debunking-vaccine-autism-link-91933.
5. "Reasons to Immunize," BYUNursing, June 19, 2013, https://www.youtube.com/watch?v=dYDzOy36zk0.
6. Jane Orient, MD, "STATEMENT of the ASSOCIATION OF AMERICAN PHYSICIANS & SURGEONS to the Subcommittee on Criminal Justice, Drug Policy, and Human Resources of the Committee on Government Reform, U.S. House of Representatives," Association of American Physicians & Surgeons, June 14, 1999, http://www.aapsonline.org/testimony/hepbcom.htm.
7. "200 Evidence Based Reasons Not to Vaccinate," Sourced from the US National Library of Medicine, GreenMedInfo.com, http://www.greenmedinfo.com/anti-therapeutic-action/vaccination-all.
8. Mary Holland, Louis Conte, Robert Krakow, and Lisa Colin, "Unanswered Questions from the Vaccine Injury Compensation Program: A Review of Compensated Cases of Vaccine-Induced Brain Injury," 28 Pace Envtl. L. Rev. 480 (2011), online at: http://digitalcommons.pace.edu/pelr/vol28/iss2/6.
9. Singh/Lin/Newell/Nelson, J Biomed Sci 2002;9:359–364.
10. Dr. Brian Hooker, PhD, Dr. Andrew Wakefield, MB, BS, James Moody, JD, "Re: Alleged Research Misconduct," ORI Complaint_rev_1.pdf, http://www.autismmediachannel.com/-!cdcwhistleblower/cmmo.

11. "Dr. Paul Offit is admitted to Philadelphia hospital after taking 100,000 vaccines – Reuters Health," The Refusers, April 1, 2012, http://therefusers.com/refusers-newsroom/dr-paul-offit-is-admitted-to-philadelphia-hospital-after-taking-100000-vaccines-reuters-health/.

12-13. Neil Z. Miller, "Combining Childhood Vaccines at One Visit Is Not Safe," Journal of American Physicians and Surgeons, Volume 21 Number 2 Summer 2016 47, http://www.jpands.org/vol21no2/miller.pdf.

14-15. "W.H.O. Ensures Third World Child Vaccine Deaths Will Not Be Recorded – New Weakened W.H.O. Criteria For Third World Child Deaths From Vaccines," ChildHealthSafety, February 5, 2014, http://wp.me/pfSi7-235.

16. Tozzi A.E et al., "Assessment of causality of individual adverse events following immunization (AEFI): a WHO tool for global use," Vaccine. 2013 Oct 17;31(44):5041-6. doi: 10.1016/j.vaccine.2013.08.087. Epub 2013 Sep 8, http://www.ncbi.nlm.nih.gov/pubmed/24021304 - cm24021304_2587.

Chapter 5. Safe and Effective: Not What You Think It Means

1. Kelly Brogan, MD, A Mind of Your Own: The Truth About Depression and How Women Can Heal Their Bodies to Reclaim Their Lives, Harper Wave, 2016, p. 136, http://www.amazon.com/Mind-Your-Own-Depression-Reclaim/dp/0062405578/.

2. Mark Blaxill, "From the Roman to the Wakefield Inquisition," Age of Autism blog, January 27, 2010, http://www.ageofautism.com/2010/01/from-the-roman-to-the-wakefield-inquisition.html.

3. Executive Reorganization and Government Research of the Committee on Government Operations United States Senate, Ninety-Second Congress, Second Session. Pp. 499-505. April 20,21; and May 3,4, 1972.

4. Marco Cáceres, "Bernice Eddy Warned of Defective Salk Polio Vaccine," The Vaccine Reaction, June 23, 2016, http://www.thevaccinereaction.org/2016/06/bernice-eddy-warned-of-defective-salk-polio-vaccine/.

5-6. David M. Oshinsky, Polio: An American Story, Oxford University Press, 2005, p. 231, http://www.amazon.com/Polio-American-David-M-Oshinsky/dp/0195307143/.

7. Richard Carter, Breakthrough: The Saga of Jonas Salk, Trident Press, New York, 1965, pp. 318-319. (Dissolving Illusions, p. 273.)

8. Executive Reorganization and Government Research of the Committee on Government Operations United States Senate, Ninety-Second Congress, Second Session. Page 499-505. April 20,21; and May 3,4, 1972.

9. Elizabeth H. Oakes, Encyclopedia of World Scientists, Infobase Publishing, 2002, p. 199.

10. Executive Reorganization and Government Research of the Committee on Government Operations United States Senate, Ninety-Second Congress, Second Session. Page 499-505. April 20,21; and May 3,4, 1972.

11. "Additional Standards for Viral Vaccines; Poliovirus Vaccine, Live, Oral," DEPARTMENT OF HEALTH AND HUMAN SERVICES, Food and Drug Administration, Federal Register / Vol. 49, No. 107 / Friday, June 1, 1984, / Rules and Regulations, 21 CFR Part 630 [Docket No. 84N-0178], online at http://www.beyondconformity.co.nz/_literature_80498/Federal_ Register_1984.

12-13. Andrea Rock, "The Lethal Dangers of the Billion-Dollar Vaccine Business," Money Magazine, December 1996, Vol. 25, online at http://www.whale.to/vaccines/money_mag.html.

14. Kent Keckenlively, Judy Mikovits, Plague: One Scientist's Intrepid Search for the Truth about Human Retroviruses and Chronic Fatigue Syndrome (ME/CFS), Autism, and Other Diseases, Skyhorse Publishing, 2014, https://www.amazon.com/Plague-Scientists-Intrepid-Retroviruses-Syndrome/dp/1626365652/.

15. "XMRV (Xenotropic Murine Leukemia Virus-related Virus)," CDC, http://www.cdc.gov/xmrv/questions-answers.html.

16. Allene Edwards, "VACCINES, RETROVIRUSES, DNA, AND THE DISCOVERY THAT DESTROYED JUDY MIKOVITS' CAREER," Organic Lifestyle Magazine, December 1, 2015, http://www.organiclifestylemagazine.com/vaccines-retroviruses-dna-and-the-discovery-that-destroyed-judy-mikovits-career.

17. Kent Keckenlively, Judy Mikovits, Plague: One Scientist's Intrepid Search for the Truth about Human Retroviruses and Chronic Fatigue Syndrome (ME/CFS), Autism, and Other Diseases, Skyhorse Publishing, 2014, https://www.amazon.com/Plague-Scientists-Intrepid-Retroviruses-Syndrome/dp/1626365652/.

19. Brandy Vaughan, "Why I Do What I Do," LearnTheRisk.org, http://www.learntherisk.org/news/why-i-do-what-i-do/.

19. Message from Brandy Vaughan to the author, July 18, 2016.

20. John W. Oller, Jr. and Stephen D. Oller, Autism: The Diagnosis, Treatment, & Etiology Of The Undeniable Epidemic, Jones & Bartlett Learning, 2009, pp. http://www.amazon.com/Autism-Diagnosis-Treatment-Etiology-Undeniable/dp/0763752800/.

21. Robert F. Kennedy, Jr. "Deadly Immunity," Salon, June 16, 2005, online at http://www.robertfkennedyjr.com/articles/2005_june_16.html.

22. Robert F. Kennedy, Jr., "Tobacco Science and the Thimerosal Scandal," p. 7, http://www.robertfkennedyjr.com/docs/ThimerosalScandalFINAL.PDF.

23. Rep. Bill Posey, C-SPAN, July 29, 2015, min. 1:03:24, http://www.c-span
.org/video/?327309-1/us-house-morning-hour&live.

24. Robert F. Kennedy, Jr., "CDC Forced Researchers To Lie About Mercury
in Vaccines," Office of Medical and Scientific Justice, February 15, 2015,
http://www.omsj.org/corruption/cdcvaxlies/2.

25. Kevin Barry, Esq., Vaccine Whistleblower: Exposing Autism Research Fraud
at the CDC, Skyhorse Publishing, 2015, p. xv, xxi, https://www.amazon.
com/Vaccine-Whistleblower-Exposing-Autism-Research/dp/1634509951/.

26. "Text of the Vaccine Safety Study Act," govtrack.us, 113th Congress, 1st Session, H.R. 1757, April 25, 2013, Mr. Posey (for himself and Mrs. Carolyn B.
Maloney of New York) introduced the following bill; which was referred to
the Committee on Energy and Commerce, https://www.govtrack.us/congress/
bills/113/hr1757/text.

27. Quoting Carol Stott, PhD, MSc, CSci, CPsychol, and Andrew Wakefield,
MB, BS, FRCS, FRCPath, in Louise Kuo Habakus, MA, and Mary Hol-
land, JD, Vaccine Epidemic: How Corporate Greed, Biased Science, and
Coercive Government Threaten Our Human Rights, Our Health, and Our
Children, Skyhorse Publishing, 2011, p. 56, https://www.amazon.com/
Vaccine-Epidemic-Corporate-Coercive-Government/dp/1620872129/.

28. "Text of the Vaccine Safety Study Act," govtrack.us, 113th Congress, 1st Session, H.R. 1757, April 25, 2013, Mr. Posey (for himself and Mrs. Carolyn
B. Maloney of New York) introduced the following bill; which was referred
to the Committee on Energy and Commerce, https://www.govtrack.us/con-
gress/bills/113/hr1757/text.

29. "Less than 30% of Congress Admits to Vaccinating Their OWN KIDS!!!"
VaxTruth, February 7, 2015, http://vaxtruth.org/2015/02/nbc-congress-
poll/.

30-32. "Studies comparing vaccinated to unvaccinated populations," Vermont
Coalition for Vaccine Choice, 1/7/2016, http://www.vaxchoicevt.com/sci-
ence/studies-comparing-vaccinated-to-unvaccinated-populations/.

33. I. Kristensen, P. Aaby, H. Jensen, "Routine vaccinations and child survival:
follow up study in Guinea-Bissau, West Africa," BMJ 2000; 321: 1435–
1441. "The children of 15,000 mothers were observed from 1990 to 1996
for 5 years. Result: the death rate in vaccinated children against diphtheria,
tetanus and whooping cough is twice as high as the unvaccinated children
(10.5% versus 4.7%)" – from footnote "7.a.".

34. Dan Olmsted, UPI Senior Editor, "The Age of Autism: Study sees vaccine
risk," United Press International, Inc., June 26, 2007, http://www.upi.com/
Health_News/2007/06/26/The-Age-of-Autism-Study-sees-vaccine-risk/
UPI-93181182890397/.

35. "Why we don't vaccinate," vaccine-injury.info, http://vaccine-injury.info/introduction.cfm, original article here: http://www.quotidiano.net/vaccini-medici-contrari-1.1429559.

36. Celeste McGovern, "Vaccinated vs. Unvaccinated: Mawson Homeschooled Study Reveals Who is Sicker," November 20, 2017, http://info.cmsri.org/the-driven-researcher-blog/vaccinated-vs.-unvaccinated-guess-who-is-sicker.

37. Anthony R. Mawson et al., "Preterm birth, vaccination and neurodevelopmental disorders: a cross-sectional study of 6- to 12-year-old vaccinated and unvaccinated children," Open Access Text, April 24, 2017, http://www.oatext.com/Preterm-birth-vaccination-and-neurodevelopmental-disorders-a-cross-sectional-study-of-6-to-12-year-old-vaccinated-and-unvaccinated-children.php.

38. Douglas L. Leslie et al., "Temporal Association of Certain Neuropsychiatric Disorders Following Vaccination of Children and Adolescents: A Pilot Case–Control Study," Front. Psychiatry, 19 January 2017, https://doi.org/10.3389/fpsyt.2017.00003.

39-40. Norman W. Baylor, PhD, FDA, "FDA's Role in Protecting Your Child's Health Through Safe and Effective Vaccines," slide number, http://www.fda.gov/downloads/aboutfda/transparency/basics/ucm 268440.ppt.

41. Louise Kuo Habakus, "Do Vaccines Cause Cancer?" Fearless Parent, April 10, 2016, http://fearlessparent.org/do-vaccines-cause-cancer/.

42. Louise Kuo Habakus quoting the IOM, "Do Vaccines Cause Cancer?" Fearless Parent, April 10, 2016, http://fearlessparent.org/do-vaccines-cause-cancer/.

43. Dr. Brian Hooker, "Dr. Hooker: CDC whistle blower Dr. Thompson," Autism One, May 29, 2015, min. 16:45, https://www.youtube.com/watch?v=vy2aWHbQzuI.

44-46. Norman W. Baylor, PhD, FDA, "FDA's Role in Protecting Your Child's Health Through Safe and Effective Vaccines," slide number 9, http://www.fda.gov/downloads/aboutfda/transparency/basics/ucm268440.ppt.

47. Heather Fraser, The Peanut Epidemic, What's Causing It and How to Stop It, Skyhorse Publishing, 2011, https://www.amazon.com/Peanut-Allergy-Epidemic-Whats-Causing/dp/1616082739/.

48. Robyn Charron, "How to Cause a Peanut Allergy Epidemic in 4 Easy Steps," The Thinking Moms Revolution, August 18, 2015, http://thinkingmoms-revolution.com/whats-really-behind-peanut-allergy-epidemic/.

49. Janet Levatin, MD, Board Certified Pediatrician, Clinical Instructor in Pediatrics, Harvard Medical School, quoted in: The Peanut Allergy Epidemic by Heather Fraser, Skyhorse Publishing, August 18, 2015, from the foreword, https://www.amazon.com/Peanut-Allergy-Epidemic-Whats-Causing/dp/1616082739/.

50. Neil Z. Miller, Miller's Review of Critical Vaccine Studies, New Atlantean Press, 2016, https://www.amazon.com/Millers-Review-Critical-Vaccine-Studies/dp/188121740X/.

51. T. Verstraeten, R. Davies, et al., "Increased risk of developmental neurologic impairment after high exposure to thimerosal-containing vaccines in first month of life," Proceedings of the Epidemic Intelligence Service Annual Conference, vol. 49 (Centers for Disease Control and Prevention; Atlanta, GA, USA, April 2000).

52. C. Gallagher, M. Goodman, "Hepatitis B triple series vaccine and developmental disability in US children aged 1-9 years. Toxicol Environ Chem 2008 Sep-Oct; 90(5): 997-1008.

53. D.A. Geier, P.C. King, et al., "Thimerosal: clinical, epidemiologic and biochemical studies," Clin Chim Acta 2015 Apr 15, 444: 212-20.

54. C.A. Shaw, L. Tomljenovic, "Aluminum in the central nervous system (CNS): toxicity in humans and animals,vaccine adjuvants, and autoimmunity," Immunol Res 2013 Jul; 56(2-3): 304-16.

55. Gherardi RK, Coquet M, et al. "Macrophagic myofasciitis lesions assess long-term persistence of vaccine-derived aluminium hydroxide in muscle," Brain 2001 Sep; 124(Pt 9): 1821-31.

56. F.R. Mooi, I.H. van Loo, et al., "Bordetella pertussis strains with increased toxin production associated with pertussis resurgence," Emerg Infect Dis 2009 Aug; 15(8): 1206-13.

57. J. Lavine, H. Broutin, et al., "Imperfect vaccine-induced immunity and whooping cough transmission to infants," Vaccine 2010 Dec 10; 29(1): 11-16.

58. G.S. Ribeiro, J.N. Reis, et al., "Prevention of Haemophilus influenzae type b (Hib) meningitis and emergence of serotype replacement with type a strains after introduction of Hib immunization in brazil," J Infect Dis 2003 Jan 1; 187(1): 109-16.

59. L. Tomljenovic, C.A. Shaw, "Human papillomavirus (HPV) vaccine policy and evidence-based medicine: are they at odds? Ann Med 2013 Mar; 45(2): 182-93.

60. G.S. Goldman, "Cost-benefit analysis of universal varicella vaccination in the U.S. taking into account the closely related herpes-zoster epidemiology," Vaccine 2005 May 9; 23(25): 3349-55.

61. Y.C. Lai, Y.W. Yew, "Severe autoimmune adverse events post herpes zoster vaccine: a case-control study of adverse events in a national database.

62. M.A. Hernan, S.S. Jick, "Recombinant hepatitis B vaccine and the risk of multiple sclerosis: A prospective study," Neurology 2004 Sep 14; 63(5): 838-42.

63. Wyeth internal memo, August 27, 1979, http://www.ageofautism.com/files/wyeth79.pdf.

64. Erin Elizabeth, "Holistic Doctor Death Series: Nearly 50 Dead on 1 Year Anniversary, but what's being done?" Health Nut News, March 12, 2016, http://www.healthnutnews.com/recap-on-my-unintended-series-the-holistic-doctor-deaths/.

65. Jim Edwards, "Merck Created Hit List to 'Destroy,' 'Neutralize' or 'Discredit' Dissenting Doctors," CBS News, May 6, 2009, http://www.cbsnews.com/news/merck-created-hit-list-to-destroy-neutralize-or-discredit-dissenting-doctors/.

66. Norman W. Baylor, PhD, FDA, "FDA's Role in Protecting Your Child's Health Through Safe and Effective Vaccines," http://www.fda.gov/downloads/aboutfda/transparency/basics/ucm268440.ppt.

Chapter 6. Smallpox Vaccine: Legend and Lies

1. Frederick F. Cartwright, Disease and History, Rupert-Hart-David, London, 1972, p. 124.

2. "The Practice of Inoculation Truly Stated," The Gentleman's Magazine and Historical Chronicle, vol. 34, 1764, p. 333.

3. M. Beddow Bayly, MRCS, LRCP, "Inoculation Dangers to Travelers," a speech at the Caxton Hall Westminster, October 2, 1952. Published by the London and Provincial Anti-Vivisection Society.

4. "The Practice of Inoculation Truly Stated," The Gentleman's Magazine and Historical Chronicle, vol. 34, 1764, p. 333.

5. W.J. Collins, MD, BS, BSc, MRCS, "Twenty Years' Experience of a Public Vaccinator," 1866, quote online at http://globalfreedommovement.org/politicians-vs-doctors-vaccines-quacks-hippies-internet/.

6. Arthur Wollaston Hutton, MA, The Vaccination Question, Methuen & Co., London, 1895, http://www.whale.to/vaccine/hutton_b.html.

7-8. J.T. Biggs, J.P. Leicester: Sanitation Versus Vaccination, 1912, chapter 20, http://www.whale.to/a/biggs.html.

9. J.T. Biggs, J.P. Leicester: Sanitation Versus Vaccination, 1912, chapter 24, http://www.whale.to/a/biggs.html.

10. "ANTI-COMPULSORY VACCINATION DEMONSTRATION AT LEICESTER," The Hawera & Normanby Star, Volume VL, Issue 1016, 19 May 1885, p. 2, http://paperspast.natlib.govt.nz/cgi-bin/paperspast?a=d&d=HNS18850519.2.14.

11-14. J.T. Biggs, J.P. Leicester: Sanitation Versus Vaccination, 1912, chapter 25, http://www.whale.to/a/biggs.html.

15. Arthur Wollaston Hutton, MA, The Vaccination Question, Methuen & Co., London, 1895, http://www.whale.to/vaccine/hutton_b.html.

16. Eleanor McBean, The Poisoned Needle: Suppressed Facts About Vaccination, 1957, http://www.whale.to/a/mcbean.html.

17. Vernon Coleman, MD, "The Smallpox Myth," http://www.vernoncoleman. com/vaccines.htm.
18. "Sanitation Obliterated Smallpox," The Outliers, January 17, 2016, https:// vaccinesbytheoutliers.wordpress.com/2016/01/17/sanitation-obliterated-smallpox/.
19. Donald A. Henderson, "Eradication: Lessons From the Past," CDC, MMWR Supplements, December 31, 1999 / 48(SU01);16-22, http://www .cdc.gov/mmwr/preview/mmwrhtml/su48a6.htm.
20-21. Neil Z. Miller, Russell Blaylock, Vaccine Safety Manual for Concerned Families and Health Practitioners, New Atlantean Press, 2009, p. 32, http:// www.amazon.com/Vaccine-Safety-Concerned-Families-Practitioners/ dp/188121737X/.
22. Suzanne Humphries, MD, Roman Bystrianyk, *Dissolving Illusions: Disease, Vaccines, and the Forgotten History,* 2015, p. 92, https://www.amazon.com/ Dissolving-Illusions-Disease-Vaccines-Forgotten/dp/1480216895/.
23. Dr. Viera Scheibner, "Hepatitis B Vaccine: Helping or Hurting Public Health," The Subcommittee on Criminal Justice, Drug Policy, and Human Resources, May 18, 1999, http://www.thinktwice.com/Hep_Hear.pdf.

Chapter 7. Polio Vaccine: More Lore, More Lies

1. Howard B. Urnovitz, PhD, statement made to the Committee on Government Reform and Oversight, August 3, 1999, online at http://www.i-sis .org.uk/ERCD.php.
2. Neil Miller, "The polio vaccine: a critical assessment of its arcane history, efficacy, and long-term health-related consequences," Medical Veritas, 1 (2004) 239-251, http://www.thinktwice.com/Polio.pdf.
3. "Origin of AIDS (2004) Documentary," CBC Witness, https://www.youtube.com/watch?v=yRDsYqvrYgI.
4. "ACIP Vote Regarding Routine Childhood Polio Vaccination Recommendations," CDC, June 17, 1999, http://www.cdc.gov/media/pressrel/r990617.htm.
5-9. Kihura Nkuba, "The Polio Vaccination Agenda in Africa Blown Wide Open by Kihura Nkuba," Vaccination Safety, National Vaccine Information Center, C-SPAN Nov 7th 2002, https://www.youtube.com/ watch?v=JyVPTgfe2QA.
10. "Origin of AIDS (2004) Documentary," CDC Witness, https://www.youtube.com/watch?v=yRDsYqvrYgI.
11. Brian Martin, "Polio vaccines and the origin of AIDS: some key writings," http://www.uow.edu.au/~bmartin/dissent/documents/AIDS/.
12-13. Neil Miller, "The polio vaccine: a critical assessment of its arcane history, efficacy, and long-term health-related consequences," Medical Veritas, 1 (2004) 239-251, http://www.thinktwice.com/Polio.pdf.

14. "SV40 stands for Simian Virus 40," SV40 Cancer Foundation, http://www.sv40foundation.org/.

15. Andrea Rock, "The Lethal Dangers of the Billion-Dollar Vaccine Business," Money Magazine, December 1996, Vol. 25, online at http://www.whale.to/vaccines/money_mag.html.

16. S.G. Fisher, L. Weber, M. Carbone, "Cancer risk associated with simian virus 40 contaminated polio vaccine," Anticancer Research, 1999, May-Jun;19(3B):2173-80, http://www.ncbi.nlm.nih.gov/pubmed/10472327.

17. Michael E. Horwin, MA, JD, "Simian Virus 40 (SV40): A Cancer Causing Monkey Virus from FDA-Approved Vaccines," Albany Law Journal of Science & Technology, Volume 13, Number 3, 2003, online at http://www.sv40foundation.org/CPV-link.html - _edn1.

18-19. "Historical Vaccine Safety Concerns," CDC, http://www.cdc.gov/vaccinesafety/concerns/concerns-history.html.

20. Viera Scheibner, PhD, "Polio eradication: a complex end game," BMJ 2012;344:e2398, April 2, 2012, http://www.bmj.com/content/344/bmj.e2398/rr/599724.

21-22. Centers for Disease Control and Prevention. Recommendations of the Advisory Committee on Immunization Practices (ACIP): Use of vaccines and immune globulins in persons with altered immunocompetence, MMWR 1993; 42(No. RR-4), http://www.cdc.gov/mmwr/preview/mmwrhtml/00023141.htm.

23. "WHO vaccine-preventable diseases: monitoring system. 2015 global summary," World Health Organization, http://apps.who.int/immunization_monitoring/globalsummary/schedules.

24. Russell L. Blaylock, MD, "The Truth Behind the Vaccine Cover-Up," Vaccine Choice Canada, December 9, 2008, http://vaccinechoicecanada.com/health-risks/brain-neurological-injuries/the-truth-behind-the-vaccine-cover-up/.

25-26. Prasun Sonwalkar, "8 Indian states = 25 African nations: Oxford study on poverty," Hindustan Times, June 26, 2015, http://www.hindustantimes.com/india/8-indian-states-25-african-nations-oxford-study-on-poverty/story-ys7Oths8HIzK21WWdB8AnL.html.

27. Neetu Vashisht and Jacob Puliyel, "Polio programme: let us declare victory and move on," Indian Journal of Medical Ethics, Vol 9, No 2, 2012, http://www.issuesinmedicalethics.org/index.php/ijme/article/view/110/1065.

28. "Poliomyelitis," The Pink Book: Course Textbook - 13th Edition (2015) CDC, 2015, http://www.cdc.gov/vaccines/pubs/pinkbook/polio.html.

29-30. Jagannath Chatterjee, "India's Polio-Free Status a Cruel Joke," The Current Health Scenario, March 26, 2014, http://currenthealthscenario.blogspot.com/2014/03/indias-polio-free-status-cruel-joke.html.

31. Neetu Vashisht, Jacob Puliyel, Vishnubhatla Sreenivas, "Trends in Nonpolio Acute Flaccid Paralysis Incidence in India 2000 to 2013," Pediatrics, February 2015, VOLUME 135 / ISSUE Supplement 1, http://pediatrics.aappublications.org/content/135/Supplement_1/S16.2.

32. William Muraskin, Polio Eradication and Its Discontents: A Historian's Journey Through an International Public Health (Un)Civil War, Orient Blackswan, 2012, Introduction, http://www.amazon.com/Polio-Eradication-Its-Discontents-International-ebook/dp/B00BAWQFOW/.

33-34. Jagannath Chatterjee, "India's Polio-Free Status a Cruel Joke," The Current Health Scenario, March 26, 2014, http://currenthealthscenario.blogspot.com/2014/03/indias-polio-free-status-cruel-joke.html.

35. Neetu Vashisht and Jacob Puliyel, "Polio programme: let us declare victory and move on," Indian Journal of Medical Ethics, Vol 9, No 2, 2012, http://www.issuesinmedicalethics.org/index.php/ijme/article/view/110/1065.

36. William Muraskin, Polio Eradication and Its Discontents: A Historian's Journey Through an International Public Health (Un)Civil War, Orient Blackswan, 2012, Introduction, http://www.amazon.com/Polio-Eradication-Its-Discontents-International-ebook/dp/B00BAWQFOW/.

37. William Muraskin, Polio Eradication and Its Discontents: A Historian's Journey Through an International Public Health (Un)Civil War, Orient Blackswan, 2012, chapter 1, http://www.amazon.com/Polio-Eradication-Its-Discontents-International-ebook/dp/B00BAWQFOW/.

38. "Polio Endgame and Legacy," CDC, http://www.cdc.gov/polio/plan/.

39. Donald A. Henderson, "Eradication: Lessons From the Past," CDC, MMWR Supplements, December 31, 1999 / 48(SU01);16-22, http://www.cdc.gov/mmwr/preview/mmwrhtml/su48a6.htm.

40-41. Neetu Vashisht and Jacob Puliyel, "Polio programme: let us declare victory and move on," Indian Journal of Medical Ethics, Vol 9, No 2, 2012, http://www.issuesinmedicalethics.org/index.php/ijme/article/view/110/1065.

42-43. Jagannath Chatterjee, "India's Polio-Free Status a Cruel Joke," The Current Health Scenario, March 26, 2014, http://currenthealthscenario.blogspot.com/2014/03/indias-polio-free-status-cruel-joke.html.

44. "W.H.O. Ensures Third World Child Vaccine Deaths Will Not Be Recorded – New Weakened W.H.O. Criteria For Third World Child Deaths From Vaccines," ChildHealthSafety, February 5, 2014, http://wp.me/pfSi7-235.

45. Suzanne Humphries, MD, Roman Bystrianyk, "Dissolving Illusions: Disease, Vaccines, and the Forgotten History," 2015, pp. 230-231, https://www.amazon.com/Dissolving-Illusions-Disease-Vaccines-Forgotten/dp/1480216895/.

46. Dr. Viera Scheibner, "Hepatitis B Vaccine: Helping or Hurting Public Health," The Subcommittee on Criminal Justice, Drug Policy, and Human Resources, May 18, 1999, http://www.thinktwice.com/Hep_Hear.pdf.

47-49. Dan Olmsted, Mark Blaxill, "Pesticides and The Age of Polio," Age of Autism, February 28, 2014, http://www.ageofautism.com/2014/04/pesticides-and-the-age-of-polio.html.

50. Kihura Nkuba, "The Polio Vaccination Agenda in Africa Blown Wide Open by Kihura Nkuba," Vaccination Safety, National Vaccine Information Center, C-SPAN Nov 7th 2002, https://www.youtube.com/watch?v=JyVPTgfe2QA.

Chapter 8. Vaccine Safety: Yesterday and Today

1. Vernon Coleman, MD, "The Smallpox Myth," http://www.vernoncoleman.com/vaccines.htm.

2. Archie Kalokerinos, Every Second Child, Thomas Nelson (Australia) Limited, 1974, p. 102, online at https://soilandhealth.org/copyrighted-book/every-second-child/ - afterpost.

3-4. "Dr. Archie Kalokerinos," International Vaccine Newsletter, June, 1995, online at http://www.whale.to/v/kalokerinos.html.

5. Michael Gaeta DAc, MS, CDN, LAc, Dipl Ac & ABT (NCCAOM), "An Unearned Reputation of Goodness," michaelgaeta.com, April 14, 2014, https://michaelgaeta.com/vaccine-myth-7-vaccines-eliminated-many-epidemics-and-saved-millions-of-lives/.

6. Suzanne Humphries, MD, quoted online at https://michaelgaeta.com/vaccine-myth-7-vaccines-eliminated-many-epidemics-and-saved-millions-of-lives/.

7. Robert S. Mendelsohn, MD, How to Raise a Healthy Child in Spite of Your Doctor, Ballantine Books, 1987, p. 231, http://www.amazon.com/Raise-Healthy-Child-Spite-Doctor/dp/0345342763/.

8. E. Richard Brown, Rockefeller Medicine Men: Medicine and Capitalism in America, University of California Press, Berkeley, Los Angeles, London, 1979, pp. 220, 221, https://www.amazon.com/Rockefeller-Medicine-Men-Capitalism-America/dp/0520042697/.

9. "Doctors Against Vaccines: Hear From Those Who Have Done the Research," Organic Lifestyle Magazine, June 7, 2015, http://www.organiclifestylemagazine.com/doctors-against-vaccines-hear-from-those-who-have-done-the-research.

10. "John Anthony Morris, MD (1919–2014)," Alliance for Human Research Protection, http://ahrp.org/john-anthony-morris-md/.

11. James A. Howenstine, MD, A Physician's Guide to Natural Health Products, Penhurst Books, 2002, p. 268, http://www.amazon.com/Physicians-Guide-Natural-Health-Products/dp/0970568487/.

12. "The Truth About Vivisection," In Defense of Animals, http://www.vivisectioninfo.org/faq.html.

13. Vernon Coleman, MD, "The Smallpox Myth," http://www.vernoncoleman.com/vaccines.htm.
14-16. "Consumer Safety Act of 1972," Hearings before the Subcommittee on Executive Reorganization and Government Research of the Committee on Government Operations, United States Senate, Ninety-Second Congress, Second Session on Titles I and II of S. 3419, April 20, 21; and May 3, 4, 1972, online at http://www.vaccinationcouncil.org/wp-content/uploads/2012/06/SENATE-HEARING-S3419+1972.pdf.
17. Hilary Butler and Peter Butler, Just a Little Prick, Robert Reisinger Memorial Trust, 2015, pp. 214-215, http://www.amazon.com/Just-Little-Prick-Hilary-Butler/dp/0473108445/.
18. Matt Schudel, "David J. Sencer, CDC chief who resigned over swine-flu vaccine, dies at 86," The Washington Post, May 4, 2011, https://www.washingtonpost.com/local/obituaries/david-j-sencer-cdc-chief-who-resigned-over-swine-flu-vaccine-dies-at-86/2011/05/03/AFVwKirF_story.html.
19-20. A. COckburn et al., 1977, "Scientist J. Anthony Morris – He fought the flu shots and the US fired him," Washington Post, 13 March: 22. 215.
21. "Consumer Safety Act of 1972," Hearings before the Subcommittee on Executive Reorganization and Government Research of the Committee on Government Operations, United States Senate, Ninety-Second Congress, Second Session on Titles I and II of S. 3419, April 20, 21; and May 3, 4, 1972, online at http://www.vaccinationcouncil.org/wp-content/uploads/2012/06/SENATE-HEARING-S3419+1972.pdf.
22. "VIDEO: The 1976 Swine Flu Pandemic and Vaccine, Government Propaganda Causes Many Deaths. Transcript of CBS 60 minutes," http://www.globalresearch.ca/video-the-1976-swine-flu-pandemic-and-vaccine/14433.
23-24. Matt Schudel, "David J. Sencer, CDC chief who resigned over swine-flu vaccine, dies at 86," The Washington Post, May 4, 2011, https://www.washingtonpost.com/local/obituaries/david-j-sencer-cdc-chief-who-resigned-over-swine-flu-vaccine-dies-at-86/2011/05/03/AFVwKirF_story.html.
25. "Dr. Archie Kalokerinos," International Vaccine Newsletter, June, 1995, online at http://www.whale.to/v/kalokerinos.html.
26. Thomas Stone, MD, "Open Letter to Pediatricians on Flu Vaccines," Mercola.com, January 2, 2008, http://articles.mercola.com/sites/articles/archive/1998/11/22/tom-stone-letter.aspx.
27. "Dr Andrew Wakefield – Feast of Consequences – Whistleblowing in the Public Interest," Presentation delivered in Orem, Utah, in October, 2015, video and transcript online at http://www.runningthecountry.com/dr-andrew-wakefield-feast-of-consequences-whistleblowing-in-the-public-interest/.

28-29. "MMR: Conflict of Interest Zone," Private Eye, 8 June – 21 June 2007, online at http://www.jabs.org.uk/forum/topic.asp?TOPIC_ID=668&whichpage=5.

30. "Secret British MMR Vaccine Files Forced Open By Legal Action," Child Health Safety, January 13, 2009, https://childhealthsafety.wordpress.com/2009/01/13/secret-british-mmr-vaccine-files-forced-open-by-legal-action/#British_Government_Reckless.

31. Dan Burton, "Mercury in Medicine," Congressional Record (May 20, 2003): E1016.

32. Quoted by Supreme Court Justice S. Sotomayor, "BRUESEWITZ ET AL. v. WYETH LLC, FKA WYETH, INC., ET AL." SUPREME COURT OF THE UNITED STATES, February 22, 2011, p. 2 of Justice Sotomayor's and Justice Ginsburg's dissenting opinion, http://www.supremecourt.gov/opinions/10pdf/09-152.pdf.

33. "CONTRACT/WORK/STATEMENT, Immunization Safety Review Panel," 2000, p. 9,10, http://www.putchildrenfirst.org/media/ 6.3.pdf.

34. "Thimerosal in Vaccines," FDA, http://www.fda.gov/BiologicsBloodVaccines/SafetyAvailability/VaccineSafety/UCM096228.

35-37. Louise Kuo Habakus, "Do Vaccines Cause Cancer?" Fearless Parent, April 10, 2016, http://fearlessparent.org/do-vaccines-cause-cancer/.

38. "Dr. Archie Kalokerinos," International Vaccine Newsletter, June, 1995, online at http://www.whale.to/v/kalokerinos.html.

Chapter 9. Herd Immunity: Artifact, Contrivance, and Control

1. Suzanne Humphries, MD, "Smoke, Mirrors, and the 'Disappearance' Of Polio," International Medical Council On Vaccination Nov. 17, 2011, online at http://whale.to/a/smoke_mirrors.html.

2. W.W.C. Topley, G.S. Wilson, "The spread of bacterial infection: the problem of herd immunity," J Hyg 1923;21:243-9, http://www.ncbi.nlm.nih.gov/pmc/articles/PMC2167341/pdf/jhyg00291-0051.pdf.

3. Paul Fine, Ken Eames, and David L. Heymann, "'Herd Immunity': A Rough Guide," Clin Infect Dis. (2011) 52 (7): 911-916, http://cid.oxfordjournals.org/content/52/7/911.full.

4. C.E.G. Smith, Prospects of the control of disease, Proc Roy Soc Med 1970; 63:1181-90.

5. Dietz K. Transmission and control of arbovirus diseases, In: Ludwig D, Cooke KL, editors. Epidemiology. Philadelphia PA: Society for Industrial and Applied Mathematics; 1975, p. 104-21.

6. Paul Fine, Ken Eames, and David L. Heymann, "'Herd Immunity': A Rough Guide," Clin Infect Dis. (2011) 52 (7): 911-916, http://cid.oxfordjournals.org/content/52/7/911.full.

7. Jane Orient, MD, "STATEMENT of the ASSOCIATION OF AMERI-
    CAN PHYSICIANS & SURGEONS" to the Subcommittee on Criminal
    Justice, Drug Policy, and Human Resources of the Committee on Govern-
    ment Reform, U.S. House of Representatives, Association of American Phy-
    sicians & Surgeons, June 14, 1999, http://www.aapsonline.org/testimony/
    hepbcom.htm.
8. "Physicians for Informed Consent Finds MMR Vaccine Causes Seizures in 5,700
    U.S. Children Annually," Physicians for Informed Consent, December 20,
    2017, https://physiciansforinformedconsent.org/news/physicians-informed-
    consent-finds-mmr-vaccine-causes-seizures-5700-u-s-children-annually/.
9. Kelly Brogan, MD, A Mind of Your Own: The Truth About Depression
    and How Women Can Heal Their Bodies to Reclaim Their Lives, Harper
    Wave, 2016, p. 138, http://www.amazon.com/Mind-Your-Own-Depression-
    Reclaim/dp/0062405578/.
10. Kelly Brogan, MD, A Mind of Your Own: The Truth About Depression
    and How Women Can Heal Their Bodies to Reclaim Their Lives, Harper
    Wave, 2016, p. 135, http://www.amazon.com/Mind-Your-Own-Depression-
    Reclaim/dp/0062405578/.
11. Suzanne Humphries, MD, Roman Bystrianyk, Dissolving illusions: Disease,
    Vaccines, and the Forgotten History, 2015, p. 479, https://www.amazon
    .com/Dissolving-Illusions-Disease-Vaccines-Forgotten/dp/1480216895/.
12. "Resurgence of Whooping Cough May Owe to Vaccine's Inability to Pre-
    vent Infections," Boston University School of Public Health, September
    21, 2017, http://www.bu.edu/sph/2017/09/21/resurgence-of-whooping-
    cough-may-owe-to-vaccines-inability-to-prevent-infections/.
13. "An Interview With Research Immunologist Tetyana Obukhanych PhD, part
    1, by Catherine Frompovich," Vaccination Council, June 20, 2012, http://
    www.vaccinationcouncil.org/2012/06/13/interview-with-phd-immunolo-
    gist-dr-tetyana-obukhanych-by-catherine-frompovich/.
14. G.S. Goldman and P.G. King, "Review of the United States universal vari-
    cella vaccination program: Herpes zoster incidence rates, cost-effectiveness,
    and vaccine efficacy based primarily on the Antelope Valley Varicella Active
    Surveillance Project data," Vaccine, 2013 Mar 25; 31(13): 1680–1694,
    http://www.ncbi.nlm.nih.gov/pmc/articles/PMC3759842/.
15. "Suzanne Humphries, MD on the Anti-Inflammatory Effects of Breast
    Milk," The Vaccine Reaction, February 29, 2016, http://www.thevaccine-
    reaction.org/2016/02/suzanne-humphries-md-on-the-anti-inflammatory-
    effects-of-breast-milk/.
16. Suzanne Humphries, MD, "Herd Immunity: Flawed Science and Mass
    Vaccination Failures," GreenMedInfo.com, July 16, 2012, http://www.
    greenmedinfo.com/blog/herd-immunity-flawed-science-and-mass-vaccina-
    tion-failures.

17. "The Emerging Risks of Live Virus & Virus Vectored Vaccines: Vaccine Strain Virus Infection, Shedding & Transmission," National Vaccine Information Center, November 2014, http://www.nvic.org/CMSTemplates/NVIC/pdf/Live-Virus-Vaccines-and-Vaccine-Shedding.pdf.

18. "The Emerging Risks of Live Virus & Virus Vectored Vaccines: Vaccine Strain Virus Infection, Shedding & Transmission," National Vaccine Information Center, November 2014, p. 14, http://www.nvic.org/CMSTemplates/NVIC/pdf/Live-Virus-Vaccines-and-Vaccine-Shedding.pdf.

19-20. Jacob M.Puliyel, MD, note by Puliyel: "The Guardian published an edited version of this article. This is the fuller version that obviates the need to read in-between the lines." Online at http://www.vaccinationcouncil.org/wp-content/uploads/2012/07/Puliyel-counterpoint1.pdf.

21. "Meningococcal Disease," The Pink Book: Course Textbook - 13th Edition (2015) CDC, 2015, http://www.cdc.gov/vaccines/pubs/pinkbook/mening.html.

22. Jacob M.Puliyel, MD, note by Puliyel: "The Guardian published an edited version of this article. This is the fuller version that obviates the need to read in-between the lines." Online at http://www.vaccinationcouncil.org/wp-content/uploads/2012/07/Puliyel-counterpoint1.pdf.

23. "Dr. Shiv Chopra," DaveJanda.com, July 17, 2016, min 3:40, http://www.davejanda.com/guests/dr-shiv-chopra/sunday-july-17-2016.

24. Dr. Russell Blaylock, "The Deadly Impossibility Of Herd Immunity Through Vaccination, by Dr. Russell Blaylock," International Medical Council on Vaccination, February 12, 2012, http://www.vaccinationcouncil.org/2012/02/18/the-deadly-impossibility-of-herd-immunity-through-vaccination-by-dr-russell-blaylock/.

25. Michael Gaeta, "Herd Immunity: The Foundational Lie of the Forced Vaccination Agenda, Part One," October 27, 2015, https://michaelgaeta.com/category/vaccines/.

26. Marcella Piper-Terry, FB post, July 24, 2016, https://www.facebook.com/marcellaterry?fref=nf.

27. Janet Levatin, MD, Board Certified Pediatrician, Clinical Instructor in Pediatrics, Harvard Medical School, quoted in: The Peanut Allergy Epidemic by Heather Fraser, Skyhorse Publishing, August 18, 2015, from the foreword, https://www.amazon.com/Peanut-Allergy-Epidemic-Whats-Causing/dp/1616082739/.

Chapter 10. American Academy of Pediatrics: Parental Discretion Advised

1. Ken Stoller, MD, Pediatrician, International Hyperbaric Medical Association, "Ken Stoller's Letter to Pediatrics on the Verstraeten Study," Adventures in

Autism, June 21, 2008, http://adventuresinautism.blogspot.com/2008/06/ken-stollers-letter-to-pediatrics-on.html.

2. "AAP Policy on Conflict of Interest and Relationships with Industry and Other Organizations," 2010, https://www.aap.org/en-us/about-the-aap/aap-leadership/Documents/20-IndustryRelations.pdf.

3. Jessica Martucci and Anne Barnhill, "Unintended Consequences of Invoking the 'Natural' in Breastfeeding Promotion," Pediatrics, April, 2016, http://pediatrics.aappublications.org/content/early/2016/03/02/peds.2015-4154.

4. Naomi Baumslag, MD, MPH, Dia L. Michels, Milk, Money, and Madness: The Culture and Politics of Breastfeeding, Bergin and Garvey, 1995, p. 172.

5-8. Melody Petersen, "Pediatric Book on Breast-Feeding Stirs Controversy With Its Cover," The New York Times, September 18, 2002, http://www.nytimes.com/2002/09/18/business/media-business-advertising-pediatric-book-breast-feeding-stirs-controversy-with.html.

9. "SUPERFOOD FOR BABIES: How overcoming barriers to breastfeeding will save children's lives," Save the Children, 2013, http://www.savethechildren.org.uk/sites/default/files/images/Superfood_for_Babies_UK_version.pdf.

10-11. Kimberly Seals Allers, "Does the A.A.P. Logo Belong on Formula Gift Bags?" The New York Times, December 19, 2013, http://parenting.blogs.nytimes.com/2013/12/19/does-the-a-a-p-logo-belong-on-formula-gift-bags/.

12. Sheldon Rampton, John Stauber, Trust Us, We're Experts, TarcherPerigee, 2002, p. 15, http://www.amazon.com/Trust-Us-Were-Experts-Manipulates/dp/1585421391/.

13. Moon SS et al., "Inhibitory effect of breast milk on infectivity of live oral rotavirus vaccines," Pediatr Infect Dis J. 2010 Oct;29(10):919-23, http://www.ncbi.nlm.nih.gov/pubmed/20442687.

14. "'Friends of Children Fund' Annual Report," American Academy of Pediatrics, July 1, 1996 – June 30, 1997, http://www.cspinet.org/integrity/corp_funding.html.

15. "AAP Policy on Conflict of Interest and Relationships with Industry and Other Organizations," American Academy of Pediatrics, June 2010, https://www.aap.org/en-us/about-the-aap/aap-leadership/Documents/ 20-IndustryRelations.pdf.

16. Melody Petersen, "Pediatric Book on Breast-Feeding Stirs Controversy With Its Cover," The New York Times, September 18, 2002, http://www.nytimes.com/2002/09/18/business/media-business-advertising-pediatric-book-breast-feeding-stirs-controversy-with.html.

17. Richard Gale, "Why Does the American Academy of Pediatrics Put Corporate Profits Ahead of Children's Health?" CounterPunch, December 21,

2012, http://www.counterpunch.org/2012/12/21/why-does-the-american-academy-of-pediatrics-put-corporate-profits-ahead-of-childrens-health/.

18. Dan Olmsted, "Best of A of A: Autism Explosion Followed Big Change in MMR Shot," Age of Autism, January 29, 2009, http://www.ageofautism.com/2009/02/olmsted-on-autism-autism-explosion-followed-big-change-in-mmr-shot.html.

19-20. Richard Gale, "Why Does the American Academy of Pediatrics Put Corporate Profits Ahead of Children's Health?" CounterPunch, December 21, 2012, http://www.counterpunch.org/2012/12/21/why-does-the-american-academy-of-pediatrics-put-corporate-profits-ahead-of-childrens-health/.

21. Joel Forman, MD, Janet Silverstein, MD, "Organic Foods: Health and Environmental Advantages and Disadvantages," Pediatrics, October 22, 2012, http://pediatrics.aappublications.org/content/pediatrics/early/2012/10/15/peds.2012-2579.full.pdf.

22. Brett Wilcox, We're Monsanto: Feeding the World, Lie After Lie, Book Two, pp. 107-109, http://www.amazon.com/Were-Monsanto-Still-Feeding-World/dp/1511742690/.

23. Sharyl Attkisson, "How Independent Are Vaccine Defenders?" CBSNews.com, July 25, 2008, http://www.cbsnews.com/news/how-independent-are-vaccine-defenders/.

24-25. "Conflicts of Interest in Vaccine Policy Making," Majority Staff Report, Committee on Government Reform, U.S. House of Representatives, June 15, 2000, online at http://www.nvic.org/nvic-archives/conflicts-of-interest.aspx.

26-27. Douglas S. Diekema, MD, MPH; and the Committee on Bioethics, "Responding to Parental Refusals of Immunization of Children," Pediatrics, May 2005, VOLUME 115 / ISSUE 5, http://pediatrics.aappublications.org/content/115/5/1428.full.

28-29. A. Soriano, G. Nesher, Y. Shoenfeld, "Predicting post-vaccination autoimmunity: who might be at risk?" Pharmacol Res 2015 Feb; 92: 18-22.

30. Alex Jones interviewing Dr. Andrew Wakefield, "Dr. Andrew Wakefield, director of the new bombshell documentary 'Vaxxed: From Cover-up to Catastrophe,' joins the show to break down why the film was pulled from the Tribeca Film Festival," InfoWars, April 19, 2016, min 31:55, http://www.infowars.com/doctor-reveals-secrets-behind-the-vaccine-autism-cover-up/.

31. Kenneth P. Stoller, MD, "My Open Letter to The American Academy of Pediatrics, 'Why Are Doctors Silent?'" Vaccines Uncensored, http://www.vaccinesuncensored.org/doctors.php.

32. "Mental Illness," National Institute of Mental Health, Last Updated November 2017, https://www.nimh.nih.gov/health/statistics/mental-illness.shtml.

Chapter 11. Conflicts of Interest in Every Jab

1. "Why Are Doctors Silent?" *Vaccines Uncensored*, http://www.vaccinesuncensored.org/doctors.php.
2. Jon Rappoport, "Incredible pandemic hoax from the Ministry of Truth," Feb 19, 2018, https://jonrappoport.wordpress.com/2018/02/19/incredible-pandemic-hoax-from-the-ministry-of-truth/.
3-4. Joel Roberts, "The Man Behind The Vaccine Mystery," The New York Times, December 12, 2002, http://www.cbsnews.com/news/the-man-behind-the-vaccine-mystery/.
5. Robert F. Kennedy, Jr., "Deadly Immunity," Salon, June 16, 2005, online at http://www.robertfkennedyjr.com/articles/2005_june_16.html.
6. Bob Herbert, "Whose Hands Are Dirty?" The New York Times, November 25, 2002, http://www.nytimes.com/2002/11/25/opinion/whose-hands-are-dirty.html.
7-9. Ceci Connolly, "Bush Plan for Smallpox Vaccine Raises Medical, Fiscal Worries," Washington Post, December 15, 2002, online at http://www.ph.ucla.edu/epi/bioter/bushplansmallpoxvac.html.
10. Robert F. Kennedy, Jr., "Tobacco Science and the thimerosal Scandal," p. 60, http://www.robertfkennedyjr.com/docs/thimerosalScandalFINAL.PDF.
11. Marcia Angell, MD, The Truth About the Drug Companies: How They Deceive Us and What to Do About it, Random House, 2004, p. xx, https://www.amazon.com/Truth-About-Drug-Companies-Deceive/dp/0375760946/.
12. Laurie Powell, "THE DANGER OF BIG PHARMA'S SILENT HOLD OVER THE US GOVERNMENT," Collective Evolution," May 2, 2016, http://www.collective-evolution.com/2016/05/02/the-danger-of-undue-influence-big-pharmas-silent-hold-over-us-government/.
13. John Hrabe, "Resigning lawmaker Henry Perea takes job with pharmaceutical industry," CalWatchdog.com, December 26, 2015, http://calwatchdog.com/2015/12/26/resigning-lawmaker-henry-perea-takes-job-pharmaceutical-industry/.
14. Jim Miller, "Drug companies donated millions to California lawmakers before vaccine debate," The Sacramento Bee, June 18, 2015, http://www.sacbee.com/news/politics-government/capitol-alert/article24913978.html.
15. "#PanRan like the Pink Panther," Vax Facts, May 10, 2016, https://www.youtube.com/watch?v=2PcGxLdLgzI.
16. Kenneth Lovett, "Lovett: Health Committee pol raises eyebrows with investments in drug firms," New York Daily News, November 30, 2015, http://www.nydailynews.com/news/politics/lovett-heath-pol-big-money-drug-firms-article-1.2449907.

17. "Mandatory Meningitis Vaccine Bill Author, Kemp Hannon, Caught Taking $420k From Pharma!" vaxxter.com, December 2, 2015, http://vaxxter.com/mandatory-meningitis-vaccine-bill-author-kemp-hannon-caught-taking-420k-from-pharma/.

18. "No jab, no pay laws pass parliament," November 23, 2015, sbs.com.au, http://www.sbs.com.au/news/article/2015/11/23/no-jab-no-pay-laws-pass-parliament.

19. "Department of Health and Human Services," https://www.whitehouse.gov/sites/default/files/omb/budget/fy2014/assets/health.pdf.

20. "About the National Vaccine Program Office (NVPO)," http://www.hhs.gov/nvpo/about/index.html.

21-23. "Partners," HHS, http://www.hhs.gov/nvpo/about/partners/index.html.

24. "What's NACCHO got to do with Oregon's vaccine exemption fight?," NoOnSB442, March 6, 2015, https://medium.com/@sb442no/what-s-naccho-got-to-do-with-oregon-s-vaccine-exemption-fight-87b16c7c0c77.

25. "About Us," Association of State and Territorial Health Officials, http://astho.org/About/.

26. "About AIM," Association of Immunization Managers, http://www.immunizationmanagers.org/?page=AboutAIM.

27. "Partners/Funders," National Association of County & City Health Officials, http://archived.naccho.org/about/partners_funders.cfm.

28. "What's NACCHO got to do with Oregon's vaccine exemption fight?," NoOnSB442, March 6, 2015, https://medium.com/@sb442no/what-s-naccho-got-to-do-with-oregon-s-vaccine-exemption-fight-87b16c7c0c77.

29. "State Legislative Liaisons," Association of State and Territorial Health Officials, http://astho.org/Public-Policy/State-Health-Policy/Legislative-Liaisons/.

30. "Cooperative Agreement to the Association of Immunization Managers; Notice of Award of Funds," Federal Register, https://www.federalregister.gov/articles/2002/10/02/02-24986/cooperative-agreement-to-the-association-of-immunization-managers-notice-of-award-of-funds.

31. "Partners/Funders," National Association of County & City Health Officials, http://archived.naccho.org/about/partners_funders.cfm.

32. "ASTHO Corporate Alliance," Association of State and Territorial Health Officials, http://www.astho.org/about/corporate-alliance/.

33. "Corporate Alliance Program Benefits," Association of Immunization Managers, http://c.ymcdn.com/sites/www.immunizationmanagers.org/resource/resmgr/AIM_Corporate_Alliance_Benef.pdf.

34. "Corporate Alliance Program," Association of Immunization Managers, http://www.immunizationmanagers.org/?page=Alliance.

35. "Seqirus," CSL, http://www.csl.com.au/Seqirus.htm.

36. Miloud Kaddar, Senior Adviser, Health Economist, WHO, IVB, Geneva, "Global Vaccine Market Features and Trends," WHO, April, 2008, http://who.int/influenza_vaccines_plan/resources/session_10_kaddar.pdf.

37-38. "Jacob Puliyel, MD, MRCP, M Phil," Alliance for Human Research Protection, http://ahrp.org/jacob-puliyel-md/.

39. Mark Curtis, "Gated Development: Is the Gates Foundation always a force for good?" Global Justice Now, January 2016, http://www.globaljustice.org.uk/sites/default/files/files/resources/gated-development-global-justice-now.pdf.

40. "Member Companies," Phrma, http://www.phrma.org/about/member-companies.

41. "We Are BIO," *Biotechnology Innovation Organization*, http://www.bio.org/.

42. "BIO Members & Web Site Links," Biotechnology Innovation Organization, https://www.bio.org/articles/bio-members-web-site-links.

43. "Are You Concerned Over Genetically Modified Vaccines?" National Vaccine Information Center, October 2012, http://www.nvic.org/NVIC-Vaccine-News/October-2012/Are-You-Concerned-Over-Genetically-Modified-Vaccin.aspx.

44. John W. Oller, Jr., and Stephen D. Oller, Autism: The Diagnosis, Treatment, & Etiology Of The Undeniable Epidemic, Jones & Bartlett Learning, 2009, p. 119, http://www.amazon.com/Autism-Diagnosis-Treatment-Etiology-Undeniable/dp/0763752800/.

45. "The National Vaccine Advisory Committee (NVAC)," U.S. Department of Health & Human Services, http://www.hhs.gov/nvpo/nvac/adult4.html.

46. "National Vaccine Plan Implementation: Protecting the Nation's Health Through Immunization," HHS, http://www.hhs.gov/nvpo/vacc_plan/2010-2015-Plan/implementationplan.pdf.

47-48. "Members," National Vaccine Advisory Committee, U.S. Department of Health & Human Services, http://www.hhs.gov/nvpo/nvac/roster/index.html.

49. "NVAC Executive Secretary: Bruce G. Gellin, MD, MPH," hhs.gov, http://www.hhs.gov/nvpo/nvac/roster/gellin-bio.html.

50. "H1N1: The Report Card," Reader's Digest, March 2010, http://www.rd.com/health/wellness/h1n1-the-report-card/.

51. Jon Rappoport, "My interview with Sharyl Attkisson: vaccines, exposing the CDC," July 22, 2016, https://jonrappoport.wordpress.com/2016/07/22/my-interview-with-sharyl-attkisson-vaccines-exposing-the-cdc/.

52-53. Sharyl Attkisson, Stonewalled: My Fight for Truth Against the Forces of Obstruction, Intimidation, and Harassment in Obama's Washington, Harper, 2014, p. 72, https://www.amazon.com/Stonewalled-Obstruction-Intimidation-Harassment-Washington/dp/0062322842/.

54. Celia Farber, "BREAKING NEWS: HOUSTON FILM FEST HIT WITH 'VERY THREATENING CALLS' FROM GOVERNMENT OFFICIALS FORCING 'VAXXED' PULLED," The Truth Barrier, April 6, 2016, http://truthbarrier.com/2016/04/06/breaking-news-houston-government-officials-threaten-film-festival-vaxxed-pulled/.

55. Vera Sharav, "Blatant Censorship — Vaxxed Banned from Worldfest by 'High Gov Officials,'" Alliance for Human Research Protection, April 9, 2016, http://ahrp.org/heavy-handed-censorship-high-gov-officials-prevent-screening-of-vaxxed/.

56. Jean Clare Smith, "The structure, role, and procedures of the U.S. Advisory Committee on Immunization Practices (ACIP)," Vaccine, 28S (2010) A68–A75, http://www.cdc.gov/vaccines/acip/committee/downloads/article-2010-role-procedures-ACIP.pdf.

57. Linda A. Suydam, DPA, "FDA Advisory Committees," FDA, June 14, 2000, http://www.fda.gov/newsevents/testimony/ucm114932.htm.

58-60. "Conflicts of Interest in Vaccine Policy Making," Majority Staff Report, Committee on Government Reform, U.S. House of Representatives, June 15, 2000, online at http://www.nvic.org/nvic-archives/conflicts-of-interest.aspx.

61-62. Massimo Calabresi, "Candidate to Lead FDA Has Close Ties to Big Pharma," Time, February 19, 2015, http://time.com/3714242/candidate-to-lead-fda-has-close-ties-to-big-pharma/.

63-66. Martha Rosenberg, "Former FDA Reviewer Speaks Out About Intimidation, Retaliation and Marginalizing of Safety," Truthout, July 29, 2012, http://www.truth-out.org/news/item/10524-former-fda-reviewer-speaks-out-about-intimidation-retaliation-and-marginalizing-of-safety.

67. "Consumer Safety Act of 1972," Hearings before the Subcommittee on Executive Reorganization and Government Research of the Committee on Government Operations, United States Senate, Ninety-Second Congress, Second Session on Titles I and II of S. 3419, April 20, 21; and May 3, 4, 1972, online at http://www.vaccinationcouncil.org/wp-content/uploads/2012/06/SENATE-HEARING-S3419+1972.pdf.

68. "Our Story," CDC Foundation, http://www.cdcfoundation.org/who/story.

69. "Our Partners," CDC Foundation, http://www.cdcfoundation.org/what/partners.

70. Jeanne Lenzer, associate editor, "Why aren't the US Centers for Disease Control and Food and Drug Administration speaking with one voice on flu?" February 5, 2015, BMJ, 2015; 350 doi: http://dx.doi.org/10.1136/bmj.h658.

71. Rep. Dave Weldon, MD, Before The Institute of Medicine, February 9, 2004, online at http://www.putchildrenfirst.org/media/6.2.pdf.

72. Harold Buttram, MD, "Vaccine Scene 1999: Overview And Update," Originally posted in "Healthy News You Can Use" #112 - www.mercola.com, online at http://www.whale.to/vaccines/buttram1.html.

73. Gardiner Harris, "Advisers on Vaccines Often Have Conflicts, Report Says," The New York Times, December 17, 2009, http://www.nytimes.com/2009/12/18/health/policy/18cdc.html.

74. "Off The Grid: Robert F. Kennedy, Jr. Takes on Big Pharma & the Vaccine Industry," Jesse Ventura's Off The Grid, May 18, 2015, http://www.ora.tv/offthegrid/2015/5/18/grid-robert--kennedy-jr-takes-big-pharma--vaccine-industry-0_6ck7ne6j25bv.

75. Sarah Karlin-Smith, Brianna Ehley, "CDC Director Brenda Fitzgerald bought shares in a global tobacco giant even as her previous holdings were under review," Politico, January 30, 2018, https://www.politico.com/story/2018/01/30/cdc-director-tobacco-stocks-after-appointment-316245.

76. "Barbara Loe Fisher," http://www.whale.to/m/fisher9.html.

77. Barbara Loe Fisher, "Remove Vaccine Safety Oversight From DHHS," National Vaccine Information Center, September 1, 2014, http://www.nvic.org/NVIC-Vaccine-News/September-2014/Remove-Vaccine-Safety-Oversight-From-DHHS.aspx.

78. Kevin Barry, Vaccine Whistleblower: Exposing Autism Research Fraud at the CDC, Foreword, Skyhorse Publishing, 2015, p. xvii, https://www.amazon.com/Vaccine-Whistleblower-Exposing-Autism-Research/dp/1634509951/.

Chapter 12. Vaccines Cause Autism: The Words That Shall Not Be Spoken

1. Statement by Dr. William Thompson in Kevin Barry, Vaccine Whistleblower: Exposing Autism Research Fraud at the CDC, Skyhorse Publishing, 2015, p. 34, https://www.amazon.com/Vaccine-Whistleblower-Exposing-Autism-Research/dp/1634509951/.

2. Paul Offit, "Arthur Caplan And Cronies On The Vaccine Autism Link," Published May 18, 2017, 1:32, https://www.youtube.com/watch?v=_lnA9W2YgeE.

3. Dan Burton, "Mercury in Medicine," Congressional Record (May 20, 2003): E1016.

4. John W. Oller, Jr., and Stephen D. Oller, Autism: The Diagnosis, Treatment, & Etiology Of The Undeniable Epidemic, Jones & Bartlett Learning, 2009, p. 134, http://www.amazon.com/Autism-Diagnosis-Treatment-Etiology-Undeniable/dp/0763752800/.

5. Oller and Oller, p. 123, http://www.amazon.com/Autism-Diagnosis-Treatment-Etiology-Undeniable/dp/0763752800/.

6. Jon Mica, The Autistic Holocaust: The Reason Our Children Keep Getting Sick, Trine Day LLC, http://www.amazon.com/Autistic-Holocaust-Reason-Children-Getting/dp/1937584836/.

7-8. "Thimerosal in Vaccines," FDA, http://www.fda.gov/BiologicsBloodVaccines/SafetyAvailability/VaccineSafety/UCM096228.

9. Jon Mica, The Autistic Holocaust: The Reason Our Children Keep Getting Sick, Trine Day LLC, http://www.amazon.com/Autistic-Holocaust-Reason-Children-Getting/dp/1937584836/.

10. "Autism/thimerosal Timeline 2002," Autism Resource Foundation, http://autismgolf.org/info/info.2002.html.

11-15. Dan Burton, "Mercury in Medicine," Congressional Record (May 20, 2003): E1016.

16. Robert F. Kennedy, Jr., "Deadly Immunity," Salon, June 16, 2005, online at http://www.robertfkennedyjr.com/articles/2005_june_16.html.

17. Robert F. Kennedy, Jr., "Tobacco Science and the Thimerosal Scandal," http://www.robertfkennedyjr.com/docs/thimerosalScandalFINAL.PDF.

18. Dan Burton, "Mercury in Medicine," Congressional Record (May 20, 2003): E1016.

19. Brian Hooker et al., "Methodological Issues and Evidence of Malfeasance in Research Purporting to Show thimerosal in Vaccines Is Safe," Biomed Res Int. 2014; 2014: 247218, http://www.ncbi.nlm.nih.gov/pmc/articles/PMC4065774/.

20. Robert F. Kennedy, Jr., "Deadly Immunity," Salon, June 16, 2005, online at http://www.robertfkennedyjr.com/articles/2005_june_16.html.

21. "Dr. Frank B. Engley," Trace Amounts, http://traceamounts.com/dr-frank-b-engley/.

22. David Kirby, Evidence of Harm, Mercury in Vaccines and the Autism Epidemic: A Medical Controversy, St. Martin's Griffin, 2006, p. 81, http://www.amazon.com/Evidence-Harm-Vaccines-Epidemic-Controversy/dp/0312326459/.

23. "Thimerosal in Vaccines," FDA, http://www.fda.gov/BiologicsBloodVaccines/SafetyAvailability/VaccineSafety/UCM096228.

24. "Management Guidelines for Medicinals Containing Thimerosal," July 2010, https://denr.sd.gov/des/wm/hw/documents/Thimerosal.pdf.

25. Robert F. Kennedy, Jr., "Tobacco Science and the thimerosal Scandal," http://www.robertfkennedyjr.com/docs/thimerosalScandalFINAL.PDF.

26. "Protecting Children from Mercury-Containing Drugs," United Methodist Church, http://www.umc.org/what-we-believe/protecting-children-from-mercury-containing-drugs.

27. Dan Burton, "Mercury in Medicine," Congressional Record (May 20, 2003): E1016.

28. David Kirby, Evidence of Harm, Mercury in Vaccines and the Autism Epidemic: A Medical Controversy, St. Martin's Griffin, 2006, p. 81, http://www.amazon.com/Evidence-Harm-Vaccines-Epidemic-Controversy/dp/0312326459/.

29. Jon Christian Ryter, "Thimerosal . . . Autism's Daddy," http://www.jonchristianryter.com/2010/101016.html.

30. Dana Scott, "Is Your Dog's thimerosal-Free Vaccine Really Free Of Mercury?" Dogs Naturally Magazine, http://www.dogsnaturallymagazine.com/is-your-dogs-thimerosal-free-vaccine-really-free-of-mercury/.

31. David Kirby, Evidence of Harm, Mercury in Vaccines and the Autism Epidemic: A Medical Controversy, St. Martin's Griffin, 2006, p. 81, http://www.amazon.com/Evidence-Harm-Vaccines-Epidemic-Controversy/dp/0312326459/.

32. Andrew Wakefield, MD, "Response to Dr. Ari Brown and the Immunization Action Coalition," Medical Veritas, 6 (2009) 1907-1923, online at http://www.nvic.org/Downloads/manWakefield.aspx.

33-35. "Conflicts of Interest in Vaccine Policy Making," Majority Staff Report, Committee on Government Reform, U.S. House of Representatives, June 15, 2000, online at http://www.nvic.org/nvic-archives/conflicts-of-interest.aspx.

36. Robert F. Kennedy, Jr., Thimerosal: Let the Science Speak, Skyhorse Publishing, 2015, p. 267, https://www.amazon.com/Thimerosal-Supporting-Immediate-Mercury%C2%97-Neurotoxin%C2%97/dp/1634504429/.

37. David Kirby, Evidence of Harm, Mercury in Vaccines and the Autism Epidemic: A Medical Controversy, St. Martin's Griffin, 2006, p. 81, http://www.amazon.com/Evidence-Harm-Vaccines-Epidemic-Controversy/dp/0312326459/.

38. Arthur Allen, "The Not-So-Crackpot Autism Theory," The New York Times, November 10, 2002, http://www.nytimes.com/2002/11/10/magazine/the-not-so-crackpot-autism-theory.html.

39. "Neal Halsey Reaffirms Vaccines Do Not Cause Autism," Johns Hopkins Bloomberg School of Public Health," November 14, 2002, http://www.jhsph.edu/news/news-releases/2002/halsey-autism.html.

40. "Corrections," The New York Times, November 15, 2002, http://www.nytimes.com/2002/11/15/pageoneplus/corrections.html.

41. Dan Burton, "Mercury in Medicine," Congressional Record (May 20, 2003): E1016.

42. "Frequently Asked Questions about Thimerosal," CDC, http://www.cdc.gov/vaccinesafety/concerns/thimerosal/faqs.html.

43-44. Nicole Dube, "MERCURY-FREE VACCINE LEGISLATION IN OTHER STATES," OLR Research Report, October 26, 2010, https://www.cga.ct.gov/2010/rpt/2010-R-0352.htm.

45-46. Letter from Kris E. Calvin et al. to Diana Dooley, Secretary, Health and Human Services Agency, "Request for temporary exemption for use of thimerosal-containing vaccine," September 23, 2015, http://aap-ca.org/wp-content/uploads/2015/09/ExemptionRequest-InfluenzaVaccine09-252015cm.pdf.

47. Letter from Diana S. Dooley to the Honorable Kevin de Leon et al., State of California, Health and Human Services Agency, October 9, 2015, http://www.cdph.ca.gov/programs/immunize/Documents/Secretary Dooley Notification Letter to Legislature.pdf.

48. Paul Thomas, MD, spoken on camera after watching the movie Vaxxed, April 18, 2016, https://www.youtube.com/watch?v=yzMNxClUwNA&feature=youtu.be.

49. Remarks of Robert Krakow at American Rally for Personal Rights, Chicago, Il, May 26, 2010, http://www.americanpersonalrights.org.

50. Andrea Rock, "The Lethal Dangers of the Billion-Dollar Vaccine Business," Money Magazine, December 1996, Vol. 25, online at http://www.whale.to/vaccines/money_mag.html.

51. "Big Pharma Conspiracy: Health Epidemics & The Untold Story of Vaccines," min 1:23:45, https://www.youtube.com/watch?v=XLqSgrhQdq4.

52. Statement of Barbara Loe Fisher, President, National Vaccine Information Center, to California State Senate Committee on Health and Human Services, January 23, 2002, http://www.whale.to/v/fisher7.html.

53. "Unanswered Questions: A Review of Compensated Cases of Vaccine-Induced Brain Injury," Elizabeth Birt Center for Autism Law & Advocacy, 2011, http://www.ebcala.org/unanswered-questions.

54. Steven Novella, "MMR and Autism Rises from the Dead," Science-Based Medicine, September 4, 2013, https://www.sciencebasedmedicine.org/mmr-and-autism-rises-from-the-dead/.

55. Jon Rappoport, "A world waking up: damage after vaccination," April 25, 2016, https://jonrappoport.wordpress.com/2016/04/25/a-world-waking-up-damage-after-vaccination/.

56. Rev. Lisa K. Sykes, "'Ten Lies' Told About Mercury in Vaccines," Trace Amounts, http://traceamounts.com/ten-lies-told-about-mercury-in-vaccines/.

Chapter 13. Dr. Andrew Wakefield: The Vaccine Industry's Worst Nightmare

1. Statement by Václav Havel in Robert Andrews, The Columbia Dictionary of Quotations, Columbia University Press, 1993, p. 257, https://books.google.com/books?isbn=0231071949.

2. Journal of Medical Virology 39 (1993), p. 345-53.

3. The Lancet 345 (1995): 1071-74.
4. Andrew J. Wakefield, Callous Disregard: Autism and Vaccines—The Truth Behind a Tragedy, Skyhorse Publishing, 2010, p. 10, https://www.amazon.com/Callous-Disregard-Autism-Vaccines---Tragedy/dp/1616083239/.
5. Andrew J. Wakefield, Callous Disregard: Autism and Vaccines—The Truth Behind a Tragedy, Skyhorse Publishing, 2010, pp. 84-85, https://www.amazon.com/Callous-Disregard-Autism-Vaccines---Tragedy/dp/1616083239/.
6. "RETRACTED: Ileal-lymphoid-nodular hyperplasia, non-specific colitis, and pervasive developmental disorder in children," The Lancet, February 28, 1998, http://www.thelancet.com/journals/lancet/article/PIIS0140-6736(97)11096-0/fulltext.
7. Louise Kuo Habakus, MA, and Mary Holland, JD, Vaccine Epidemic: How Corporate Greed, Biased Science, and Coercive Government Threaten Our Human Rights, Our Health, and Our Children, Skyhorse Publishing, 2011, p. 225, https://www.amazon.com/Vaccine-Epidemic-Corporate-Coercive-Government/dp/1620872129/.
8. [2012] EWHC 503 (Admin), http://www.bailii.org/ew/cases/EWHC/Admin/2012/503.html.
9. "Retraction—Ileal-lymphoid-nodular hyperplasia, non-specific colitis, and pervasive developmental disorder in children," The Lancet, Volume 375, No. 9713, p445, 6 February 2010, http://www.thelancet.com/journals/lancet/article/PIIS0140-6736(10)60175-4/abstract.
10. Andrew J. Wakefield, Callous Disregard: Autism and Vaccines—The Truth Behind a Tragedy, Skyhorse Publishing, 2010, p. 3, https://www.amazon.com/Callous-Disregard-Autism-Vaccines---Tragedy/dp/1616083239/.
11. Andrew J. Wakefield, Callous Disregard: Autism and Vaccines—The Truth Behind a Tragedy, Skyhorse Publishing, 2010, p. 5, https://www.amazon.com/Callous-Disregard-Autism-Vaccines---Tragedy/dp/1616083239/.
12. Andrew J. Wakefield, Callous Disregard: Autism and Vaccines—The Truth Behind a Tragedy, Skyhorse Publishing, 2010, Afterword, cowritten with James Moody, Esq., p. 247,248. First appeared in The Autism File magazine in April 2010, https://www.amazon.com/Callous-Disregard-Autism-Vaccines---Tragedy/dp/1616083239/.
13. [2012] EWHC 503 (Admin), http://www.bailii.org/ew/cases/EWHC/Admin/2012/503.html.
14. "Unanswered Questions: A Review of Compensated Cases of Vaccine-Induced Brain Injury," Elizabeth Birt Center for Autism Law & Advocacy, 2011, http://www.ebcala.org/unanswered-questions.
15. "Doctor Andrew Wakefield: Hero or Quack?" VacTruth, April 23, 2016, https://vactruth.com/2016/04/23/doctor-andrew-wakefield/.

16. Andrew J. Wakefield, Callous Disregard: Autism and Vaccines—The Truth Behind a Tragedy, Skyhorse Publishing, 2010, Afterword, cowritten with James Moody, Esq. p. 245. First appeared in The Autism File magazine in April 2010, https://www.amazon.com/Callous-Disregard-Autism-Vaccines---Tragedy/dp/1616083239/.

17. Andrew J. Wakefield, Callous Disregard: Autism and Vaccines—The Truth Behind a Tragedy, Skyhorse Publishing, 2010, postscript by James Moody, Esq. p. 268, 269, https://www.amazon.com/Callous-Disregard-Autism-Vaccines---Tragedy/dp/1616083239/.

18. Who Killed Alex Spourdalakis? Autism Media Channel, http://www.autismmediachannel.com/#!film/cb30.

19-20. "Dr Andrew Wakefield – Feast of Consequences – Whistleblowing in the Public Interest," Running The Country, October 26, 2015, http://www.runningthecountry.com/dr-andrew-wakefield-feast-of-consequences-whistleblowing-in-the-public-interest/.

Chapter 14. Crisis and Damage Control

1. Arthur Allen quoting Representative Dan Burton, "The Not-So-Crackpot Autism Theory," The New York Times, November 10, 2002, http://www.nytimes.com/2002/11/10/magazine/the-not-so-crackpot-autism-theory.html.

2. "Unanswered Questions: A Review of Compensated Cases of Vaccine-Induced Brain Injury," Elizabeth Birt Center for Autism Law & Advocacy, 2011, http://www.ebcala.org/unanswered-questions.

3. Sarah C. Corriher, "The Inflammatory Topic of Vaccines During a Health Information War," The Health Wyze Report, June 9. 2009, http://healthwyze.org/reports/131-the-inflammatory-topic-of-vaccines-during-a-health-information-war.

4. "DTaP Side Effect: Autism. Now You See It. Now You Don't," Age of Autism, December 9, 2008, http://www.ageofautism.com/2008/12/dtap-side-effec.html.

5. "FDA Approved Vaccine with Autism and SIDS Listed as Adverse Events, Vaccine Safety Website Removes Information," Vactruth, September 9, 2008, https://vactruth.com/2012/09/18/fda-vaccine-autism-sids/.

6. J.B. Handley, "Rotavirus: The Vaccine Nobody Wants," Age of Autism, September 3, 2009, http://www.ageofautism.com/2009/09/rotavirus-the-vaccine-nobody-wants.html.

7-11. Dan Burton, "Mercury in Medicine," Congressional Record (May 20, 2003): E1016.

12-14. "Autism/thimerosal Timeline 1999," Autism Resource Foundation, http://autismgolf.org/info/info.1999.html.

15. Dan Burton, "Mercury in Medicine," Congressional Record (May 20, 2003): E1016.

16. Russell L. Blaylock, MD, "The Truth Behind the Vaccine Cover-Up," Vaccine Choice Canada, December 9, 2008, http://vaccinechoicecanada.com/health-risks/brain-neurological-injuries/the-truth-behind-the-vaccine-cover-up/.

17-18. "Recommendations Regarding the Use of Vaccines That Contain thimerosal as a Preservative," CDC, http://www.cdc.gov/mmwr/preview/mmwrhtml/mm4843a4.htm.

19. Russell L. Blaylock, MD, "The Truth Behind the Vaccine Cover-Up, Vaccine Choice Canada, December 9, 2008, http://vaccinechoicecanada.com/health-risks/brain-neurological-injuries/the-truth-behind-the-vaccine-cover-up/.

20. Dan Burton, "Mercury in Medicine," Congressional Record (May 20, 2003): E1016.

21-22. "Autism/thimerosal Timeline 1999," Autism Resource Foundation, http://autismgolf.org/info/info.1999.html.

23. "Conflicts of Interest in Vaccine Policy Making," Majority Staff Report, Committee on Government Reform, U.S. House of Representatives, June 15, 2000, online at http://www.nvic.org/nvic-archives/conflicts-of-interest.aspx.

24. "Vaccine Safety Datalink (VSD)," CDC, http://www.cdc.gov/vaccinesafety/ensuringsafety/monitoring/vsd/.

25. Barbara Lardy, "THE VACCINE SAFETY DATALINK (VSD) PROJECT: Annual Report for 2003," America's Health Insurance Plans, p. 12, online at http://www.putchildrenfirst.org/media/4.15.pdf.

26. Robert T. Chen et al., "Vaccine Safety Datalink Project: A New Tool for Improving Vaccine Safety Monitoring in the United States," Pediatrics, June 1997, VOLUME 99 / ISSUE 6, http://pediatrics.aappublications.org/content/99/6/765.

27. "A Brief Review of Verstraeten's 'Generation Zero' VSD Study Results," Safe Minds, http://www.safeminds.org/wp-content/uploads/2013/04/GenerationZeroNotes.pdf.

28-29. "Generation Zero: Thomas Verstraeten's First Analyses of the Link Between Vaccine Mercury Exposure and the Risk of Diagnosis of Selected Neuro-Developmental Disorders Based on Data from the Vaccine Safety Datalink: November-December 1999," Safe Minds, September, 2004, http://www.safeminds.org/wp-content/uploads/2014/04/GenerationZero-PowerPoint.pdf.

30. PDF of Verstraeten's December 17, 1999, email message is found at http://www.putchildrenfirst.org/media/2.7.pdf.

Chapter 15. Simpsonwood and Other Bull

1. Albert Einstein, "The NAS Building: The Einstein Memorial," National Academy of Sciences, http://www.nasonline.org/about-nas/visiting-nas/nas-building/the-einstein-memorial.html.
2. "Scientific Review of Vaccine Safety Datalink Information," Simpsonwood Retreat Center, Norcross, Georgia, June 7-8, 2000, http://www.putchildren-first.org/media/2.9.pdf.
3-4. "Chapter V: 2003, It's Rotten in Denmark," Put Children First, http://www.putchildrenfirst.org/chapter5.html.
5. David Kirby, Evidence of Harm, Mercury in Vaccines and the Autism Epidemic: A Medical Controversy, St. Martin's Griffin, 2006, p. 169-170, http://www.amazon.com/Evidence-Harm-Vaccines-Epidemic-Controversy/dp/0312326459/.
6. "Scientific Review of Vaccine Safety Datalink Information," Simpsonwood Retreat Center, Norcross, Georgia, June 7-8, 2000, http://www.putchildren-first.org/media/2.9.pdf.
7. Russell L. Blaylock, MD, "The Truth Behind the Vaccine Cover-Up," Vaccine Choice Canada, December 9, 2008, http://vaccinechoicecanada.com/health-risks/brain-neurological-injuries/the-truth-behind-the-vaccine-cover-up/.
8. Robert F. Kennedy, Jr., "Deadly Immunity," Salon, June 16, 2005, online at http://www.robertfkennedyjr.com/articles/2005_june_16.html.
9. "Chapter II: 1999-2000, Simpsonwood," Put Children First, http://www.putchildrenfirst.org/chapter2.html.
10. Russell L. Blaylock, MD, "The Truth Behind the Vaccine Cover-Up, Vaccine Choice Canada, December 9, 2008, http://vaccinechoicecanada.com/health-risks/brain-neurological-injuries/the-truth-behind-the-vaccine-cover-up/.
11. Robert F. Kennedy, Jr., "Tobacco Science and the Thimerosal Scandal," http://www.robertfkennedyjr.com/docs/thimerosalScandalFINAL.PDF.
12. "Less than 30% of Congress Admits to Vaccinating Their OWN KIDS!!!" VaxTruth, February 7, 2015, http://vaxtruth.org/2015/02/nbc-congress-poll/.
13. Mary Holland, Research Scholar, NYU School of Law, Vaccination Policies and Human Rights, 25th International Health and Environment Conference, United Nations, April 26, 2016, http://www.ageofautism.com/2016/04/professor-mary-holland-et-al-speaking-the-world-information-transfer-un-health-and-environment-confe.html.

14. Email message from Thomas Verstraeten to Philippe Grandjean et al., "Thimerosal and neurologic outcomes," July 14, 2000, online at http://www.putchildrenfirst.org/media/2.20.pdf.

15-17. "MERCURY IN MEDICINE—ARE WE TAKING UNNECESSARY RISKS?, HEARING before the COMMITTEE ON GOVERNMENT REFORM, HOUSE OF REPRESENTATIVES," JULY 18, 2000, https://bulk.resource.org/gpo.gov/hearings/106h/72722.txt.

18. William Egan, PhD, "Additives in Childhood Vaccines," FDA, June 18, 2000, http://www.fda.gov/newsevents/testimony/ucm114923.htm.

19. S. Bernard, A. Enayati, L. Redwood, H. Roger, T. Binstock, "Autism: a novel form of mercury poisoning," Medical Hypotheses (2001) 56(4), 462–471, online at http://www.putchildrenfirst.org/media/3.2.pdf.

20-21. "MERCURY IN MEDICINE—ARE WE TAKING UNNECESSARY RISKS?, HEARING before the COMMITTEE ON GOVERNMENT REFORM, HOUSE OF REPRESENTATIVES," JULY 18, 2000, https://bulk.resource.org/gpo.gov/hearings/106h/72722.txt.

Chapter 16. Vaccines Do Not Cause Autism: The Greatest Fraud in the History of Medical Science

1. David McCullough, American author, narrator, historian, and lecturer. He is a two-time winner of the Pulitzer Prize, "The Science," http://www.jabevalscalifornia.com/#!science/crdh.

2. Polly Tommey, "Portland #vaxxed Q&A," Autism Media Channel, June 19, 2016, min 30:55, https://www.periscope.tv/TeamVaxxed/1zqKVpodLzmJB.

3. Donald G. McNeil, Jr., "Court Says Vaccine Not to Blame for Autism," The New York Times, February 12, 2009, http://www.nytimes.com/2009/02/13/health/13vaccine.html.

4-5. "NATIONAL ACADEMY OF SCIENCES, INSTITUTE OF MEDICINE, Organizational Meeting of: IMMUNIZATION SAFETY REVIEW COMMITTEE, CLOSED SESSION," January 12, 2001, online at http://www.putchildrenfirst.org/media/6.4.pdf.

6. David Kirby, "EVIDENCE OF HARM—Presentation: SPRING 2006," slide #53, online at http://slideplayer.com/slide/264589/.

7-8. Immunization Safety Review: Vaccines and Autism, Institute of Medicine (US) Immunization Safety Review Committee, Washington (DC): National Academies Press (US); 2004, http://www.ncbi.nlm.nih.gov/books/NBK25349/box/a2000af8fbbb00004/?report=objectonly.

9. "IOM Slams the Door (Quickly)," putchildrenfirst.org, http://www.putchildrenfirst.org/chapter6.html.

10. Conflicts of Interest: Presentation for Senatorial Inquiry," November 15, 2005, http://www.putchildrenfirst.org/media/6.14.pdf.

11. Robert F. Kennedy, Jr., "Central Figure in CDC Vaccine Cover-Up Absconds With $2M," Huffington Post, November 17, 2011, http://www.huffington-post.com/robert-f-kennedy-jr/central-figure-in-cdc-vac_b_494303.html.

12. Kevin Barry, Esq., Vaccine Whistleblower: Exposing Autism Research Fraud at the CDC, Skyhorse Publishing, 2015, pp. 65-66, https://www.amazon.com/Vaccine-Whistleblower-Exposing-Autism-Research/dp/1634509951/.

13. James Ottar Grundvig, Master Manipulator: The Explosive True Story of Fraud, Embezzlement, and Government Betrayal at the CDC, Skyhorse Publishing, 2016, http://www.amazon.com/Master-Manipulator-Explosive-Embezzlement-Government/dp/151070843X/.

14. "Conflicts of Interest: Presentation for Senatorial Inquiry," November 15, 2005, http://www.putchildrenfirst.org/media/6.14.pdf.

15. Brian Hooker, PhD, Dr. Andrew Wakefield MB, BS, James Moody, JD, "Re: Alleged Research Misconduct," ORI Complaint_rev_1.pdf, pp. 1-2, http://www.autismmediachannel.com/#!cdcwhistleblower/cmmo.

16-17. Dr. Brian Hooker, PhD, Dr. Andrew Wakefield MB, BS, James Moody, JD, "Re: Alleged Research Misconduct," ORI Complaint_rev_1.pdf, p. 17, http://www.autismmediachannel.com/#!cdcwhistleblower/cmmo.

18. Dr. William Thompson in Kevin Barry, Vaccine Whistleblower: Exposing Autism Research Fraud at the CDC, Skyhorse Publishing, 2015, p. 34, https://www.amazon.com/Vaccine-Whistleblower-Exposing-Autism-Research/dp/1634509951/.

19. Rep. Bill Posey, C-SPAN, July 29, 2015, min. 1:30:24, http://www.c-span.org/video/?327309-1/us-house-morning-hour&live.

20. Rep. Dave Weldon, MD, Before The Institute of Medicine, February 9, 2004, http://www.putchildrenfirst.org/media/6.2.pdf.

21. David Kirby, Evidence of Harm, Mercury in Vaccines and the Autism Epidemic: A Medical Controversy, St. Martin's Griffin, 2006, p. 503, http://www.amazon.com/Evidence-Harm-Vaccines-Epidemic-Controversy/dp/0312326459/.

22. John W. Oller, Jr., and Stephen D. Oller, Autism: The Diagnosis, Treatment, & Etiology Of The Undeniable Epidemic, Jones & Bartlett Learning, 2009, p 119. http://www.amazon.com/Autism-Diagnosis-Treatment-Etiology-Undeniable/dp/0763752800/.

23. Frank DeStefano, MD, MPH, Cristofer S. Price, ScM, and Eric S. Weintraub, MPH, "Increasing Exposure to Antibody-Stimulating Proteins and Polysaccharides in Vaccines Is Not Associated with Risk of Autism," The Journal of Pediatrics, Vol. 163, No. 2. August 2013, http://www.jpeds.com/article/S0022-3476(13)00144-3/pdf?ext=.pdf.

24. Mayer Eisenstein MD, JD, MPH, "No Vaccine-Autism Link - April Fools!!!!!!" April 2, 2013, https://www.youtube.com/watch?v=V6Sk6yrZMOA.

25. Dr. Brian Hooker, "Can We Trust the CDC Claim that There is No Link Between Vaccines and Autism?," Health Impact News, March 31, 2013, http://healthimpactnews.com/2013/can-we-trust-the-cdc-claim-that-there-is-no-link-between-vaccines-and-autism/.

26. Donald G. McNeil, Jr., "Court Says Vaccine Not to Blame for Autism," The New York Times, February 12, 2009, http://www.nytimes.com/2009/02/13/health/13vaccine.html.

27. J.S. Poling, R.E. Frye, J. Shoffner, et al., Developmental regression and mitochondrial dysfunction in a child with autism. J Child Neurol. 2006;21:170-2.

28. J.S. Poling, R.E. R.E. Frye, J. Shoffner, A.W. Zimmernan, "Developmental regression and mitochondrial dysfunction in a child with autism," J Child Neurol. 2006 Feb;21(2):170-2.

29. Dr. Andrew Wakefield, "Response to Dr. Ari Brown and the Immunization Action Coalition," Medical Veritas 6 (2009) pp. 1915-1916, online at http://www.nvic.org/Downloads/manWakefield.aspx.

30. Donald G. McNeil, Jr., "Court Says Vaccine Not to Blame for Autism," The New York Times, February 12, 2009, http://www.nytimes.com/2009/02/13/health/13vaccine.html.

31. Dan Olmsted, "Weekly Wrap: Standing Up for Yates," Age of Autism, November 9, 2013, http://www.ageofautism.com/2013/11/standing-up-for-yates.html.

32. Rolf Hazelhurst, Congressional briefing on the status of the Vaccine Injury Compensation Program, November 7, 2013, min: 18:50, https://www.youtube.com/watch?v=qd5Y88ePhIg.

33. "Vaccine Awareness Presentation - Andrew Wakefield," YouTube Channel: Ashly Ochsner, August 14, 2014, min 1:01:30, https://www.youtube.com/watch?v=stUVpdgXmUo.

34. "The Vaccine Autism Link," Age of Autism, http://www.ageofautism.com/the-vaccine-autism-link.html.

35. "Vaccine History: Vaccine Availability Timeline," The Children's Hospital of Philadelphia, November 19, 2014, http://www.chop.edu/centers-programs/vaccine-education-center/vaccine-history/vaccine-availability-timeline.

36. "GARDASIL®9, Merck Sharp & Dohme Corp, 2015, https://www.merck.com/product/usa/pi_circulars/g/gardasil_9/gardasil_9_pi.pdf.

37. "Vaccine Timeline," http://www.immunize.org/timeline/.

38. Molly Walker, "ACIP Reinstates FluMist for 2018-2019 Flu Season," MedPage Today, February 21, 2018, https://www.medpagetoday.com/meeting-coverage/acip/71298.

Chapter 17. Flu Jabs, Preterm Jabs, and Other Atrocities

1. Robert S. Mendelsohn, MD, Confessions of a Medical Heretic, Contemporary Books, 1979, p. 145, https://www.amazon.com/Confessions-Medical-Heretic-Robert-Mendelsohn/dp/0809241315/.

2. "Top 5 Vaccine Companies by Revenue – 2012," FiercePharma, http://www.fiercepharma.com/special-report/top-5-vaccine-companies-by-revenue-2012.

3. "Influenza Vaccination Information for Health Care Workers," CDC, http://www.cdc.gov/flu/healthcareworkers.htm.

4. "Overview of Influenza Surveillance in the United States," CDC, http://www.cdc.gov/flu/weekly/overview.htm.

5. Jon Rappoport, "Bombshell: 18 people died of the flu, not 36,000," September 8, 2012, https://jonrappoport.wordpress.com/2012/09/08/bombshell-18-people-died-of-the-flu-not-36000/.

6. "Top 5 Vaccine Companies by Revenue – 2012," FiercePharma, http://www.fiercepharma.com/special-report/top-5-vaccine-companies-by-revenue-2012.

7-8. "Influenza Virus Vaccine, Fluvirin®, 2015-2016 FORMULA," http://flu.seqirus.com/assets/files/us package insert_fluvirin 2015-2016.pdf.

9. Vittorio Demicheli et al., "Vaccines for preventing influenza in healthy adults," Cochrane Database of Systematic Reviews, March 13, 2014, http://onlinelibrary.wiley.com/doi/10.1002/14651858.CD001269.pub5/full.

10. AAP News staff, "AAP backs new ACIP recommendation on influenza vaccine," AAP News, June 22, 2016, http://www.aappublications.org/news/2016/06/22/InfluenzaVaccine062216.

11. Daphne Chen, "Family searches for answers after daughter, 8, dies from flu," KSL.com, June 27, 2016, http://www.ksl.com/?nid=148& sid=40412210.

12. Molly Walker, "ACIP Reinstates FluMist for 2018-2019 Flu Season," MedPage Today, February 21, 2018, https://www.medpagetoday.com/meeting-coverage/acip/71298.

13. Vittorio Demicheli et al., "Vaccines for preventing influenza in healthy adults," Cochrane Database of Systematic Reviews, March 13, 2014, http://onlinelibrary.wiley.com/doi/10.1002/14651858.CD001269.pub5/full.

14. "Influenza Vaccination Information for Health Care Workers," CDC, http://www.cdc.gov/flu/healthcareworkers.htm.

15-16. "FLUARIX QUADRIVALENT (Influenza Vaccine)," GlaxoSmithKline, https://www.gsksource.com/pharma/content/dam/GlaxoSmithKline/US/en/Prescribing_Information/Fluarix_Quadrivalent/pdf/FLUARIX-QUADRIVALENT.PDF.

17. "Flu Symptoms & Complications," CDC, http://www.cdc.gov/flu/about/disease/symptoms.htm.

18. Author's conversation with anonymous pharmacist, 2016.

19. Rep. Bill Posey, Congressional Records, PROCEEDINGS AND DEBATES OF THE 113th, CONGRESS, FIRST SESSION, FRIDAY, APRIL 26, 2013, Vol. 159, No. 59, p. E576, https://www.gpo.gov/fdsys/pkg/CREC-2013-04-26/pdf/CREC-2013-04-26.pdf.

20. Dr. William Thompson in Kevin Barry, Vaccine Whistleblower: Exposing Autism Research Fraud at the CDC, Skyhorse Publishing, 2015, p. 23, https://www.amazon.com/Vaccine-Whistleblower-Exposing-Autism-Research/dp/1634509951/.

21. "Autism: Made in the USA," documentary, minute 57:00, https://www.youtube.com/watch?v=smywi4NjigU.

22. Russell Blaylock, MD, "How Vaccines Harm Child Brain Development - Dr Russell Blaylock MD," min: 10:40, https://www.youtube.com/watch?v=7QBcMYqlaDs.

23. T. Jefferson, S. Smith, et al. Assessment of the efficacy and effectiveness of influenza vaccines in healthy children: systematic review. Lancet 2005 Feb 26; 365(9461): 773-80.

24. A.Y. Joshi, V.N. Iyer, et al., Effectiveness of trivalent inactivated influenza vaccine in influenza-related hospitalization in children: a case-control study, Allergy Asthma Proc 2012 Mar-Apr; 33(2): e23-7.

25. D.M. Skowronski, G. DeSerres, et al., Association between the 2008-09 seasonal influenza vaccine and pandemic H1N1 illness during Spring-Summer 2009: four observational studies from Canada. PLoS Med 2010 April 6; 7(4): e1000258.

26. Rogier Bodewes et. al., "Annual Vaccination against Influenza Virus Hampers Development of Virus-Specific CD8+ T Cell Immunity in Children," Journal of Virology, 2011 Nov; 85(22): 11995–12000, https://www.ncbi.nlm.nih.gov/pmc/articles/PMC3209321/.

27. B.J. Cowling, V.J. Fang, et al., Increased risk of noninfluenza respiratory virus infections associated with receipt of inactivated influenza vaccine. Clin Infect Dis 2012 June 15; 54(12): 1778-83.

28. S.E. Ohmit, J.G. Petrie, et al., Influenza vaccine effectiveness in the community and the household. Clin Infect Dis 2013 May; 56(10): 1363-69.

29. T. Jefferson, C. DelMar, et al., Physical interventions to interrupt or reduce the spread of respiratory viruses: systematic review. BMJ 2009 Sep 21; 339: b3675.

30. L. Simonsen, T.A. Reichart, et al., Impact of influenza vaccination on seasonal mortality in the US elderly population. Arch Intern Med 2005 Feb 14; 165(3): 265:72.

31. L. Simonsen, C. Viboud, et al., Influenza vaccination and mortality benefits: new insights, new opportunities. Vaccine 2009; 27(45): 6300-4.

32. Neil Z. Miller, Miller's Review of Critical Vaccine Studies, New Atlantean Press, 2016, p. 78, http://www.amazon.com/Millers-Review-Critical-Vaccine-Studies/dp/188121740X/.

33. Z.H. Abramson, What, in fact, is the evidence that vaccinating healthcare workers against seasonal influenza protects their patients? A critical review. Int J Family Med 2012; 2012: 205464.

34. T. Jefferson, C. DiPietrantonj, et al., Relation of study quality, concordance, take home message, funding, and impact in studies of influenza vaccines: systematic review, BMJ 2009 Feb 12; 338: b354.

35. P. Doshi, Influenza vaccines: time for a rethink. JAMA Intern Med 2013 Jun 10; 173(11): 1014-16.

36. P. Doshi, Influenza: marketing vaccine by marketing disease. BMJ 2013 May 16; 346: f3037.

37. R.E. Thomas, T. Jefferson, T.J. Lasserson, Influenza vaccination for healthcare workers who care for people aged 60 or older living in long-term care institutions. Cochrane Database Syst Rev 2013; Issue 7: CD005187.

38. Vittorio Demicheli et al., "Vaccines for preventing influenza in healthy adults," Cochrane Database of Systematic Reviews, March 13, 2014, http://onlinelibrary.wiley.com/doi/10.1002/14651858.CD001269.pub5/full.

39. Gaston De Serres et. al., "Influenza Vaccination of Healthcare Workers: Critical Analysis of the Evidence for Patient Benefit Underpinning Policies of Enforcement," Published: January 27, 2017, https://doi.org/10.1371/journal.pone.0163586.

40. Vittorio Demicheli et al., "Vaccines for preventing influenza in the elderly," Cochrane Database of Systematic Reviews, February 1, 2018, http://onlinelibrary.wiley.com/doi/10.1002/14651858.CD004876.pub4/full.

41. Jing Yan, et. al., "Infectious virus in exhaled breath of symptomatic seasonal influenza cases from a college community," PNAS, January 18, 2018, https://doi.org/10.1073/pnas.1716561115.

42. "FLUARIX QUADRIVALENT (Influenza Vaccine)," GlaxoSmithKline, https://www.gsksource.com/pharma/content/dam/GlaxoSmithKline/US/en/Prescribing_Information/Fluarix_Quadrivalent/pdf/FLUARIX-QUADRIVALENT.PDF.

43. Kelly Brogan, MD, "Following Your Inner Compass: Rejecting Flu Vaccine in Pregnancy," http://kellybroganmd.com/rejecting-flu-vaccine-in-pregnancy/.

44. Frederick L. Ruben, Scientific and Medical Affairs, Aventis Pasteur, "Inactivated Influenza Virus Vaccines in Children," Clinical Infectious Diseases, 2004:38 (1 March), p. 678, http://cid.oxfordjournals.org/content/38/5/678.full.pdf.

45. Kelly Brogan, MD, "Following Your Inner Compass: Rejecting Flu Vaccine in Pregnancy," http://kellybroganmd.com/rejecting-flu-vaccine-in-pregnancy/.

46-49. Dan Burton, "Mercury in Medicine," Congressional Record (May 20, 2003): E1016.

50. Lynn R. Goldman, Michael W. Shannon, the Committee on Environmental Health, "Technical Report: Mercury in the Environment: Implications for Pediatricians," Pediatrics, July 2001, VOLUME 108 / ISSUE 1, http://pediatrics.aappublications.org/content/108/1/197.

51. Erin Elizabeth, "New Doubts On Zika As Cause Of Microcephaly," Health Nut News, July 5, 2016, http://www.healthnutnews.com/new-doubts-zika-cause-microcephaly/.

52-53. Institute of Medicine, Adverse Effects of Pertussis and Rubella Vaccines: A Report of the Committee to Review the Adverse Consequences of Pertussis and Rubella Vaccines, 1991, http://www.ncbi.nlm.nih.gov/books/NBK234367/.

54-55. Jagannath Chatterjee, "What is the Zika Virus Epidemic Covering Up?" GreenMedInfo.com, February 5, 2016, http://www.greenmedinfo.com/blog/what-zika-virus-epidemic-covering?.

56. Centro de Vigilância Epidemiológica, "Prof. Alexandre Vranjac" (CVE), INFORME TÉCNICO–VACINA DIFTERIA, TÉTANO E COQUE-LUCHE (dTpa). cve.saude.sp.gov.br October 2014, p. 8., https://web.archive.org/web/20160209181516/http://www.cve.saude.sp.gov.br/htm/imuni/pdf/IF14_VAC_DTpa.pdf, "Gestantes NÃO vacina das previamente. Administrar três doses de vacinas contendo toxoides tetânico e diftérico com intervalo de 60 dias entre as doses. Administrar as duas primeiras doses de dT e a última dose de dTpa entre 27ª e, preferencialmente até a 36ª semana de gestação." English Translation: "Pregnant women NOT previously vaccinated. Administer three doses of tetanus toxoids containing diphtheria with 60 days interval between doses. Administer the first two doses of dT and the last dose of dTpa between 27th and, preferably until the 36th week of gestation."

57. "Updated Recommendations for Use of Tetanus Toxoid, Reduced Diphtheria Toxoid, and Acellular Pertussis Vaccine (Tdap) in Pregnant Women — Advisory Committee on Immunization Practices (ACIP), 2012," CDC, February 22, 2013, http://www.cdc.gov/mmwr/preview/mmwrhtml/mm6207a4.htm.

58. Centro de Vigilância Epidemiológica "Prof. Alexandre Vranjac" (CVE), INFORME TÉCNICO–VACINA DIFTERIA, TÉTANO E COQUE-LUCHE (dTpa). cve.saude.sp.gov.br October 2014, https://web.archive.org/web/20160209181516/http://www.cve.saude.sp.gov.br/htm/imuni/pdf/IF14_VAC_DTpa.pdf.

59. Lise Alves, "Annual Flu Vaccination Campaign Starts in Brazil," The Rio Times, May 12, 2015, http://riotimesonline.com/brazil-news/rio-politics/flu-vaccination-campaign-starts-in-brazil/#.

60. Rafael Romo, "Brazil, world health officials deny link between pesticide and microcephaly," CNN, February 18, 2016, http://www.cnn.com/2016/02/17/health/brazil-who-pesticide-microcephaly-zika/.

61. Steven Mufson, Lena H. Sun, "$1.8 billion to fight Zika: CDC moves to highest alert level," The Washington Post, February 8, 2016, https://www.washingtonpost.com/news/post-politics/wp/2016/02/08/obama-to-ask-congress-for-1-8-billion-to-combat-zika-virus/.

62. Suzannah Gonzales, "Florida leads U.S. in ramping up mosquito programs over Zika virus," Reuters, February 2, 2016, https://www.reuters.com/article/us-health-zika-usa/florida-leads-u-s-in-ramping-up-mosquito-programs-over-zika-virus-idUSKCN0VB2HC.

63. "Takeda's Zika Vaccine Candidate Receives U.S. FDA Fast Track Designation," Takeda, January 29, 2018, https://www.takeda.com/newsroom/newsreleases/2018/takedas-zika-vaccine-candidate-receives-u.s.-fda-fast-track-designation/.

64. Stephanie Seneff, PhD, "Cutting Edge Information On Glyphosate Now In Flu Vaccine And Others, By Mistake!" Whole Healthy Living, interview hosted by Sharon Brenna, Lshc, Cnhc, Ntp, February 5, 2016, http://www.voiceamerica.com/episode/90143/cutting-edge-information-on-glyphosate-now-in-flu-vaccine-and-others-by-mistake#.VrVw_bGLZSE.facebook.

65. Erin Elizabeth quoting Dr. Suzanne Humphries, "This Holistic MD Says No Vaccine is Safe and She Won't Be Silenced!" Health Nut News, July 4, 2016, http://www.healthnutnews.com/holistic-md-fierce-anti-vaxer-wont-silenced/.

66. "Molecular and Supramolecular Bioinorganic Chemistry," chapter 3, p. 20, online at https://www.herbasale.eu/Exley.pdf.

67. "Molecular and Supramolecular Bioinorganic Chemistry," chapter 3, p. 21-22, online at https://www.herbasale.eu/Exley.pdf.

68. Matthew Mold, Dorcas Umar, Andrew King, Christopher Exley, "Aluminium in brain tissue in autism," Journal of Trace Elements in Medicine and Biology, Volume 46, March 2018, pp. 76-82, https://www.sciencedirect.com/science/article/pii/S0946672X17308763.

69. Professor Chris Exley, Professor in Bioinorganic Chemistry, Keele University, Honorary Professor, UHI Millennium Institute, Group Leader - Bioinorganic Chemistry Laboratory at Keele, "Autism and aluminium: The din of silence," January 14, 2018, https://www.hippocraticpost.com/ageing/autism-aluminium-din-silence/.

70. "Massive Recall of Mercury Containing Vaccines Requested," Vaccineinfo.net, http://www.vaccineinfo.net/issues/mercury/vaccine_with_mercury_recall.shtml.

71. Rep. Bill Posey, Congressional Records, PROCEEDINGS AND DEBATES OF THE 113th, CONGRESS, FIRST SESSION, FRIDAY, APRIL 26,

2013, Vol. 159, No. 59, p. E576, https://www.gpo.gov/fdsys/pkg/CREC-2013-04-26/pdf/CREC-2013-04-26.pdf.

72. "Epilogue: Present day, Better science, better kids, and a DJ," putchildren-first.org, http://www.putchildrenfirst.org/epilogue.html.

73. "Thimerosal," Eli Lilly and Company," December 22, 1999, http://www.putchildrenfirst.org/media/1.13.pdf.

74. "Recommendations of the Advisory Committee on Immunization Practices (ACIP) and the American Academy of Family Physicians (AAFP)," CDC, http://www.cdc.gov/mmwr/preview/mmwrhtml/rr5102a1.htm.

75. Barbara Loe Fisher, "FDA Prepares to Fast Track New Vaccines Targeting Pregnant Women," National Vaccine Information Center, November 17, 2015, http://www.nvic.org/NVIC-Vaccine-News/November-2015/fda-to-fasttrack-vaccines-targeting-pregnant-women.aspx.

76. "Un Amor Perdido: CDC Racist Propaganda," The Thinking Moms' Revolution, September 9, 2013, http://thinkingmomsrevolution.com/response-to-the-cdcs-racist-propaganda/.

77. "Petition to Suspend Vaccines with thimerosal," National Vaccine Information Center, http://www.nvic.org/vaccines-and-diseases/Autism/thimerosal-petition.aspx.

78. D.M. Ayoub, F.E. Yazbak, Influenza vaccination during pregnancy: a critical assessment of the recommendations of the Advisory Committee on Immunization Practices (ACIP). Journal of American Physicians and Surgeons 2006 Summer; 11(2): 41-47.

79. Dr. Brian Hooker, "Dr. Hooker: CDC whistle blower Dr.Thompson," Speech delivered at the AutismOne Conference, Published May 29, 2015, min 4:45, https://www.youtube.com/watch?v=vy2aWHbQzuI.

80-81. Kelly Brogan, MD, "Following Your Inner Compass: Rejecting Flu Vaccine in Pregnancy," http://kellybroganmd.com/rejecting-flu-vaccine-in-pregnancy/.

82. James G. Donahue, "Association of spontaneous abortion with receipt of inactivated influenza vaccine containing H1N1pdm09 in 2010–11 and 2011–12," Vaccine, Volume 35, Issue 40, 25 September 2017, Pages 5314-5322, https://www.sciencedirect.com/science/article/pii/S0264410X17308666.

83. "Flu Vaccination & Possible Safety Signal," CDC, https://www.cdc.gov/flu/professionals/vaccination/vaccination-possible-safety-signal.html.

84. Andrew Wakefield, MD, "Response to Dr. Ari Brown and the Immunization Action Coalition," Medical Veritas, 6 (2009) 1907-1923, online at http://www.nvic.org/Downloads/manWakefield.aspx.

85. David Kirby, Evidence of Harm, Mercury in Vaccines and the Autism Epidemic: A Medical Controversy, St. Martin's Griffin, 2006, p. 82, http://www.amazon.com/Evidence-Harm-Vaccines-Epidemic-Controversy/dp/0312326459/.

86. Eric Gladen, Shiloh Levine, Trace Amounts, 2015, http://www.TraceAmounts.com/.

87. M. Pourcyrous, S.B. Korones et al., Primary immunization of premature infants with gestational age less than 35 weeks: cardiorespiratory complications and C-reactive protein responses associated with administration of single and multiple separate vaccines simultaneously. J Pediatr 2007 Aug; 151(2): 167-72.

88. G. Faldella, S. Galletti et al., Safety of DTaP-IPV-Hib-HBV hexavalent vaccine in very premature infants. Vaccine 2007 Jan 22; 25(6): 1036-42.

89. Neil Z. Miller, Miller's Review of Critical Vaccine Studies, New Atlantean Press, 2016, p. 214, http://www.amazon.com/Millers-Review-Critical-Vaccine-Studies/dp/188121740X/.

90. A. Flatz-Jequier, K.M. Posfay-Barbe et al. Recurrence of cardiorespiratory events following repeat DTaP-based combined immunization in very low birth weight premature infants. J Pediatr 2008 Sep; 153(3): 429-31.

91. Neil Z. Miller, Miller's Review of Critical Vaccine Studies, New Atlantean Press, 2016, p. 213, http://www.amazon.com/Millers-Review-Critical-Vaccine-Studies/dp/188121740X/.

92. C. Meinus, G. Schmalisch et al., Adverse cardiorespiratory events following primary vaccination of very low birth weight infants. J Pediatr (Rio J) 2012 Mar-Apr; 88(2): 137-42.

93-94. S.C. Buijs, B. Boersma, Cardiorespiratory events after first immunization in premature infants: a prospective cohort study. Ned Tijdschr Geneeskd 2012; 156(3): A3797. [Dutch.]

95-96. Stephen D. DeMeo, DO, et al., "Adverse Events After Routine Immunization of Extremely Low-Birth-Weight Infants," JAMA Pediatrics, August 2015, Vol 169, No. 8, http://archpedi.jamanetwork.com/article.aspx?articleid=2300376.

97. "Nurses Against Mandatory Vaccines," NAMV, http://www.namv.org/.

98. Jefferey Jaxen, "DAILY ROUTINE INJURY IGNORED IN US HOSPITAL NICU UNITS," May 8, 2106, http://www.jeffereyjaxen.com/blog/daily-routine-injury-ignored-in-us-hospital-nicu-units.

99-100. Robert F. Kennedy, Jr., "Robert F. Kennedy, Jr.'s speech on the corruption surrounding the CDC's vaccine division," http://pathwaystofamilywellness.org/Informed-Choice/unchecked-power.html, watch it on YouTube here: "Robert F. Kennedy JR NO ON SB277 speech Sacramento at The Capitol on April 8, 2015," https://www.youtube.com/watch?v=U14TTEFqrlg.

101. Andrew J. Wakefield, Callous Disregard: Autism and Vaccines—The Truth Behind a Tragedy, Skyhorse Publishing, 2010, p. 6, https://www.amazon.com/Callous-Disregard-Autism-Vaccines---Tragedy/dp/1616083239/.

102. Frank B. Engley, PhD, at the 2008 Autism One Conference, "Part 1: thi-merosal -- 50+ years of known toxicity!" min 4:00, https://www.youtube.com/watch?v=2T0Qcbx48YM.

Chapter 18. HPV Vaccine: One More Con Job

1. Lucija Tomljenovic and Christopher A. Shaw, "Too Fast or Not Too Fast: The FDA's Approval of Merck's HPV Vaccine Gardasil," Journal of Law, Medicine & Ethics, 2012 Fall; 40(3): 673-81.

2. "What is HPV?" CDC, http://www.cdc.gov/hpv/parents/whatishpv.html.

3. Mark Blaxill, "A License to Kill? Part 2: Who Guards Gardasil's Guardians?" Age of Autism, May 12, 2010, http://www.ageofautism.com/2010/05/a-license-to-kill-part-2-who-guards-gardasils-guardians.html.

4. "Vaccine History: Vaccine Availability Timeline," The Children's Hospital of Philadelphia, November 19, 2014, http://www.chop.edu/centers-programs/vaccine-education-center/vaccine-history/vaccine-availability-timeline.

5. Lucija Tomljenovic, Christopher A. Shaw, "Too Fast or Not Too Fast: The FDA's Approval of Merck's HPV Vaccine Gardasil," Journal of Law, Medicine & Ethics, 2012 Fall; 40(3): 673-81, http://lme.sagepub.com/content/40/3/673.full.pdf+html.

6. Mary Holland, Research Scholar, NYU School of Law, Vaccination Policies and Human Rights, 25th International Health and Environment Conference, United Nations, April 26, 2016, http://www.ageofautism.com/2016/04/professor-mary-holland-et-al-speaking-the-world-information-transfer-un-health-and-environment-confe.html.

7. Mark Blaxill, "A License to Kill? Part 1: How A Public-Private Partnership Made the Government Merck's Gardasil Partner," Age of Autism, May 12, 2010, http://www.ageofautism.com/2010/05/a-license-to-kill-part-1-how-a-publicprivate-partnership-made-the-government-mercks-gardasil-partner.html.

8. B. Herskovits, 2007, Brand of the Year, Pharmaceutical Executive, 27 (2): 58-65, http://www.pharmexec.com/brand-year-0.

9. Mark Blaxill, "A License to Kill? Part 1: How A Public-Private Partnership Made the Government Merck's Gardasil Partner," Age of Autism, May 12, 2010, http://www.ageofautism.com/2010/05/a-license-to-kill-part-1-how-a-publicprivate-partnership-made-the-government-mercks-gardasil-partner.html.

10. Mark Blaxill, "A License to Kill? Part 2: Who Guards Gardasil's Guardians?" Age of Autism, May 12, 2010, http://www.ageofautism.com/2010/05/a-license-to-kill-part-2-who-guards-gardasils-guardians.html.

11. Mark Blaxill, "A License to Kill? Part 3: After Gardasil's Launch, More Victims, More Bad Safety Analysis and a Revolving Door Culture," Age of Autism, May 13, 2010, http://www.ageofautism.com/2010/05/a-license-

to-kill-part-3-after-gardasils-launch-more-victims-more-bad-safety-analysis-and-a-revolvin.html.

12. Mark Blaxill, "A License to Kill? Part 1: How A Public-Private Partnership Made the Government Merck's Gardasil Partner," Age of Autism, May 12, 2010, http://www.ageofautism.com/2010/05/a-license-to-kill-part-1-how-a-publicprivate-partnership-made-the-government-mercks-gardasil-partner.html.

13. National Archives and Records Administration Office of Government Information Services, email sent November 24, 2010, http://www.vietnamcervicalcancer.org/dmdocuments/ogis%20suba%2024%20november%202010.pdf.

14. Mark Blaxill, "A License to Kill? Part 1: How A Public-Private Partnership Made the Government Merck's Gardasil Partner," Age of Autism, May 12, 2010, http://www.ageofautism.com/2010/05/a-license-to-kill-part-1-how-a-publicprivate-partnership-made-the-government-mercks-gardasil-partner.html.

15-16. Mark Blaxill, "A License to Kill? Part 2: Who Guards Gardasil's Guardians?" Age of Autism, May 12, 2010, http://www.ageofautism.com/2010/05/a-license-to-kill-part-2-who-guards-gardasils-guardians.html.

17-18. Lucija Tomljenovic, Christopher A. Shaw, "Too Fast or Not Too Fast: The FDA's Approval of Merck's HPV Vaccine Gardasil," Journal of Law, Medicine & Ethics, 2012 Fall; 40(3): 673-81, http://lme.sagepub.com/content/40/3/673.full.pdf+html.

19. GARDASIL® Package Insert, Merck Sharp & Dohme Corp, 2011, http://www.merck.com/product/usa/pi_circulars/g/gardasil/gardasil_pi.pdf.

20. "The Greater Good," min: 23:00, https://www.youtube.com/watch?v=o_nWp6ZHA2Q.

21. Mark Blaxill, "A License to Kill? Part 3: After Gardasil's Launch, More Victims, More Bad Safety Analysis and a Revolving Door Culture," Age of Autism, May 13, 2010, http://www.ageofautism.com/2010/05/a-license-to-kill-part-3-after-gardasils-launch-more-victims-more-bad-safety-analysis-and-a-revolvin.html.

22. Lucija Tomljenovic, Christopher A. Shaw, "Too Fast or Not Too Fast: The FDA's Approval of Merck's HPV Vaccine Gardasil," Journal of Law, Medicine & Ethics, 2012 Fall; 40(3): 673-81, http://lme.sagepub.com/content/40/3/673.full.pdf+html.

23. Mark Blaxill, "A License to Kill? Part 2: Who Guards Gardasil's Guardians?" Age of Autism, May 12, 2010, http://www.ageofautism.com/2010/05/a-license-to-kill-part-2-who-guards-gardasils-guardians.html.

24. Andrew J. Wakefield, Callous Disregard: Autism and Vaccines—The Truth Behind a Tragedy, Skyhorse Publishing, 2010, postscript by James Moody, Esq. p. 268, 269, https://www.amazon.com/Callous-Disregard-Autism-Vaccines---Tragedy/dp/1616083239/.

25-26. J. Lenzer, "FDA Is Incapable of Protecting Us against Another Vioxx," BMJ 329, no. 7477 (2004): 1253.

27. Mary Holland, Research Scholar, NYU School of Law, Vaccination Policies and Human Rights, 25th International Health and Environment Conference, United Nations, April 26, 2016, http://www.ageofautism.com/2016/04/professor-mary-holland-et-al-speaking-the-world-information-transfer-un-health-and-environment-confe.html.

28. GARDASIL® Package Insert, Merck Sharp & Dohme Corp, 2011, http://www.merck.com/product/usa/pi_circulars/g/gardasil/gardasil_pi.pdf.

29. Nancy B Miller, MD, Medical Officer, Vaccines Clinical Trial Branch, Division of Vaccines and Related Products Applications, Office of Vaccines Research and Review, Center for Biologics Evaluation and Research, Food and Drug Administration, "Clinical Review of Biologics License Application Supplement for Human Papillomavirus Quadrivalent (Types 6, 11, 16, 18) Vaccine, Recombinant (Gardasil®) to extend indication for prevention of vaginal and vulvar cancers related to HPV types 16 and 18," FDA, September 11, 2008, pp. 137-139, online at http://holyhormones.com/wp-content/uploads/2013/03/gardasil091108-Closing-Statement.pdf.

30. X.C. Liu et al., "Adverse events following HPV vaccination, Alberta 2006-2014." Vaccine. 2016 Apr 4;34(15):1800-5, http://www.ncbi.nlm.nih.gov/pubmed/26921782.

31. Tom Blackwell, "Concordia professor condemns HPV vaccine after winning $270K federal grant to study it," National Post, Oct 8, 2015, http://news.nationalpost.com/news/canada/concordia-professor-condemns-hpv-vaccine-after-winning-270k-federal-grant-to-study-it.

32. "GARDASIL®9," Merck Sharp & Dohme Corp, 2015, https://www.merck.com/product/usa/pi_circulars/g/gardasil_9/gardasil_9_pi.pdf.

33. "Brochure," Vaccine Papers, http://vaccinepapers.org/brochure/.

34. P.L. Moro et al., "Safety of quadrivalent human papillomavirus vaccine (Gardasil) in pregnancy: adverse events among non-manufacturer reports in the Vaccine Adverse Event Reporting System, 2006-2013," Vaccine. 2015 Jan 15;33(4):519-22, http://www.ncbi.nlm.nih.gov/pubmed/25500173.

35. Masami Ito, "It's as if time has stopped since the vaccine," Japan Times, October 4, 2014, http://www.japantimes.co.jp/life/2014/10/04/lifestyle/time-stopped-since-vaccine/.

36. "'De vaccinerede piger' (with English Subs) for international viewing," TV2Danmark, May 8, 2015, online at https://www.youtube.com/watch?v=GO2i-r39hok.

37-38. Jefferey Jaxen, "Report: Ireland Fights HPV Vaccine Injury & Pharma Control," min 6:20, https://www.youtube.com/watch?v=5tmeshBn4EE.

39. Anubhuti Vishnoi, "Centre shuts health mission gate on Bill & Melinda Gates Foundation," The Economic Times, February 9, 2017, https://economictimes.

indiatimes.com/news/politics-and-nation/centre-shuts-gate-on-bill-melinda-gates-foundation/articleshow/57028697.cms.

40. K.P. Narayana Kumar, E.T. Bureau, "Controversial vaccine studies: Why is Bill & Melinda Gates Foundation under fire from critics in India?" The Economic Times, August 31, 2014, http://articles.economictimes.indiatimes.com/2014-08-31/news/53413161_1_hpv-vaccine-cervarix-human-papil-loma-virus.

41. "Not A Coincidence (Extended)," Canary Party, https://www.youtube.com/watch?v=Ijwlo_NnPQc.

42. "GARDASIL®9," Merck Sharp & Dohme Corp, 2015, https://www.merck.com/product/usa/pi_circulars/g/gardasil_9/gardasil_9_pi.pdf.

43. "Merck's Former Doctor Predicts that Gardasil will Become the Greatest Medical Scandal of All Time," Vaccine Impact, April 15, 2014, http://vaccineimpact.com/2014/mercks-former-doctor-predicts-that-gardasil-will-become-the-greatest-medical-scandal-of-all-time/, Original interview (French) online at http://ddata.over-blog.com/xxxyyy/3/27/09/71/2012-2013/Juin-2013/Dr-Dalbergue--Gardasil--plus-grand-scandale-de-tous-les-tem.pdf.

44. "Urgent Action Required: Stop Forced HPV Vaccines for Florida's Kids," GreenMedInfo.com, January 30, 2018, http://www.greenmedinfo.com/blog/urgent-action-required-stop-forced-hpv-vaccines-floridas-kids.

45. Sin Hang Lee, MD, "Allegations of Scientific Misconduct by GACVS/WHO/CDC Representatives et al," http://sanevax.org/wp-content/uploads/2016/01/Allegations-of-Scientific-Misconduct-by-GACVS.pdf.

46. "THE PROBLEMS WITH THE VACCINE," Uncensored, August 7, 2009, http://uncensored.co.nz/2009/08/07/the-problems-with-the-vaccine/.

47. Sin Hang Lee, MD, "Allegations of Scientific Misconduct by GACVS/WHO/CDC Representatives et al," http://sanevax.org/wp-content/uploads/2016/01/Allegations-of-Scientific-Misconduct-by-GACVS.pdf.

48. Dan Olmsted quoting Sin Hang Lee, MD, "Midweek Mashup: No, We Are Done With YOU Idiots!" Age of Autism, February 24, 2016, http://www.ageofautism.com/2016/02/midweek-mash-no-we-are-done-with-you-idiots.html.

49. B. Herskovits 2007, Brand of the Year, Pharmaceutical Executive, 27 (2): 58-65, http://www.pharmexec.com/brand-year-0.

Chapter 19. Racism and the Vaccine Program: It's a Black-and-White Issue

1. Harriet A. Washington, Medical Apartheid: The Dark History of Medical Experimentation on Black Americans from Colonial Times to the Present, Doubleday, 2006, pp. 2-3, https://www.amazon.com/Medical-Apartheid-Experimentation-Americans-Colonial/dp/076791547X/.

2. Harriet A. Washington, Medical Apartheid: The Dark History of Medical Experimentation on Black Americans from Colonial Times to the Present, Doubleday, 2006, https://www.amazon.com/Medical-Apartheid-Experimentation-Americans-Colonial/dp/076791547X/.

3. Allan M. Brandt, "Racism and Research: The Case of the Tuskegee Syphilis Study," p. 3, http://www.med.navy.mil/bumed/Documents/Healthcare Ethics/Racism-And-Research.pdf.

4. Harriet A. Washington, Medical Apartheid: The Dark History of Medical Experimentation on Black Americans from Colonial Times to the Present, Doubleday, 2006, pp. 5-6, https://www.amazon.com/Medical-Apartheid-Experimentation-Americans-Colonial/dp/076791547X/.

5. Quoting Vera Hassner Sharav, MLS, in Louise Kuo Habakus, MA, Mary Holland, JD, Vaccine Epidemic: How Corporate Greed, Biased Science, and Coercive Government Threaten Our Human Rights, Our Health, and Our Children, Skyhorse Publishing, 2011, pp 74-75, https://www.amazon.com/Vaccine-Epidemic-Corporate-Coercive-Government/dp/1620872129/.

6. Dr. Andrew Wakefield, https://www.facebook.com/OregoniansForVaccine-TruthAndHealthcareChoice/posts/927716207349441, https://www.youtube.com/watch?v=4QqkXIBTTro.

7-8. Allan M. Brandt, "Racism and Research: The Case of the Tuskegee Syphilis Study," p. 11, http://www.med.navy.mil/bumed/Documents/Healthcare Ethics/Racism-And-Research.pdf.

9. "Presidential Apology, CDC, May 16, 1997, http://www.cdc.gov/tuskegee/clintonp.htm.

10-11. "U.S. Public Health Service Syphilis Study at Tuskegee," CDC, http://www.cdc.gov/tuskegee/index.html.

12. "How Tuskegee Changed Research Practices," CDC, http://www.cdc.gov/tuskegee/after.htm.

13. Kihura Nkuba, "The Polio Vaccination Agenda in Africa Blown Wide Open by Kihura Nkuba,"Vaccination Safety, National Vaccine Information Center, C-SPAN Nov 7th 2002, https://www.youtube.com/watch?v=JyVPTgfe2QA.

14. "Thimerosal Should Not Be Banned From Vaccines Used Around The World, AAP Says," Huffington Post, 12/17/2012, http://www.huffingtonpost.com/2012/12/17/thimerosal-vaccines-aap-mercury_n_2316473.html.

15. Javier Cardenal Taján, "GSK fined over vaccine trials; 14 babies reported dead," Buenos Aires Herald, January 3, 2012, http://www.buenosairesherald.com/article/88922/gsk-fined-over-vaccine-trials-14--babies-reported-dead.

16. K.P. Narayana Kumar, E.T. Bureau, "Controversial vaccine studies: Why is Bill & Melinda Gates Foundation under fire from critics in India?" The Economic Times, August 31, 2014, http://articles.economictimes.indiatimes.

com/2014-08-31/news/53413161_1_hpv-vaccine-cervarix-human-papil-loma-virus.

17. "Presidential Apology," CDC, May 16, 1997, http://www.cdc.gov/tuskegee/clintonp.htm.

18. "Foster child drug trials," Source Watch, http://www.sourcewatch.org/index.php/Foster_child_drug_trials.

19. "Guinea Pig Kids: ARV-Babies in New York City," BBC, 2004, online at https://www.youtube.com/watch?v=is6Dtx8bXSU.

20. Liam Scheff, "The House That AIDS Built," altheal.org, January 2004, http://www.altheal.org/toxicity/house.htm.

21. "Guinea Pig Kids: How New York City is Using Children to Test Experimental AIDS Drugs," Democracy Now!, December 22, 2004, http://www.democracynow.org/2004/12/22/guinea_pig_kids_how_new_york.

22. "Foster child drug trials," Source Watch, http://www.sourcewatch.org/index.php/Foster_child_drug_trials.

23. Russell L. Blaylock, MD, "The Truth Behind the Vaccine Cover-Up," Vaccine Choice Canada, December 9, 2008, http://vaccinechoicecanada.com/health-risks/brain-neurological-injuries/the-truth-behind-the-vaccine-cover-up/.

24. Rep. Bill Posey, C-SPAN, July 29, 2015, min. 1:30:24, http://www.c-span.org/video/?327309-1/us-house-morning-hour&live.

25. Robert, F. Kennedy, Jr., in Kevin Barry, Vaccine Whistleblower: Exposing Autism Research Fraud at the CDC, Foreword, Skyhorse Publishing, 2015, p. xvii, https://www.amazon.com/Vaccine-Whistleblower-Exposing-Autism-Research/dp/1634509951/.

26. Sheila Ealey, "Vaxxed Q&A in Compton," Jefferey Jaxen Update, published May 20, 2016, https://www.youtube.com/watch?v=Jxl7xYiHgjg.

27. "Vaxxed movie makes women furious," https://www.youtube.com/watch?v=wTFKUBZTJeY&feature=share&app=desktop.

28. Anne Dachel, "Samsarah Morgan on CA Vaccine Mandates & African American Children," Age of Autism, October 12, 2105, http://www.ageofautism.com/2015/10/samsarah-morgan-on-ca-vaccine-mandates-african-american-children.html.

29. Cara Judea Alhadeff, PhD, "Is Vaccination a 'Public Good'? Fearless Parent, http://fearlessparent.org/is-vaccination-a-public-good/.

30. Anne Dachel, "Samsarah Morgan on CA Vaccine Mandates & African American Children," Age of Autism, October 12, 2105, http://www.ageofautism.com/2015/10/samsarah-morgan-on-ca-vaccine-mandates-african-american-children.html.

31. Betsy Hartmann, "Everyday Eugenics," ZNet, September 22, 2006, https://zcomm.org/znetarticle/everyday-eugenics-by-betsy-hartmann/.

32. Steve Weissman, "Why The Population Bomb Is a Rockefeller Baby," originally published in Ramparts in 1970, online at https://pulsemedia.org/2009/10/03/why-the-population-bomb-is-a-rockefeller-baby/.

33. John Sharpless, "World Population Growth, Family Planning, and American Foreign Policy," Journal of Policy History, / Volume 7 / Special Issue 01 / January 1995, pp 72-102, http://journals.cambridge.org/action/displayAbstract?fromPage=online&aid=7879093.

34. "The Human Laboratory," BBC Television, November 5, 1995, transcript at http://www.oldthinkernews.com/2010/12/09/human-laboratory-documentary-transcript/.

35. "About the Population Council," Population Council, http://www.pop-council.org/about.

36-37. "Norplant Information," Population Research Institute, November 30, 1999, https://www.pop.org/content/norplant-background-a-pri-petition-888.

38-39. "The Human Laboratory," BBC Television, November 5, 1995, transcript at http://www.oldthinkernews.com/2010/12/09/human-laboratory-documentary-transcript/.

40. Ute Sprenger, "The Development of Anti-Fertility Vaccines," Biotechnology and Development Monitor, No 25, December 1995, p. 2-5, http://home.snafu.de/usp/antifert.htm.

41. "A Vaccine Against Pregnancy," Women's Global Network for Reproductive Rights, http://www.fwhc.org/health/vaccine.htm.

42. R.K. Naz, "Contraceptive vaccines," Drugs. 2005;65(5):593-603, http://www.ncbi.nlm.nih.gov/pubmed/15748095.

43. M.A. Isahakia, C.S. Bambra, "Anti-sperm and anti-ovum vaccines: the selection of candidate antigens and the outcome of preclinical studies." Scand J Immunol Suppl. 1992;11:118-22. http://www.ncbi.nlm.nih.gov/pubmed/1514025.

44. R.K. Naz, "Contraceptive vaccines," Drugs. 2005;65(5):593-603, http://www.ncbi.nlm.nih.gov/pubmed/15748095.

45. G.P. Talwar, "A unique vaccine for control of fertility and therapy of advanced-stage terminal cancers ectopically expressing human chorionic gonadotropin." Ann N Y Acad Sci. 2013 Apr;1283:50-6. http://www.ncbi.nlm.nih.gov/pubmed/23302029.

46. G.P. Talwar et al., "A birth control vaccine is on the horizon for family planning." Ann Med. 1993 Apr;25(2):207-12. http://www.ncbi.nlm.nih.gov/pubmed/7683889.

47. Celeste McGovern, "Big Pharma's Dirty Little Secret: Vaccine-Induced Autoimmune Injury," Green Med Info, May 17, 2016, http://www.greenmedinfo.com/blog/pharma-s-dirty-little-secret-do-bleeding-calves-narcolepsy-and-infertility-have-sa.

48-49. Joan Robinson, "Blasted Ovaries: The Failure of Contraceptive Vaccines," Population Research Institute, January 1, 2010, https://www.pop.org/content/blasted-ovaries-failure-contraceptive-vaccines-0.

50. "Vision, Mission, Values," Women's Global Network for Reproductive Rights, http://wgnrr.org/who-we-are/vision-mission-values/.

51-53. Anita Hardon, "Negotiating safety and acceptability of new contraceptive technologies," MEDISCHE ANTROPOLOGIE 16 (1) 2004, http://tma.socsci.uva.nl/16_1/negotiating.pdf.

54. "A Vaccine Against Pregnancy," Women's Global Network for Reproductive Rights, http://www.fwhc.org/health/vaccine.htm.

55. Quoted in Judith Richter, "Research on antifertility vaccines—priority or problem?" Vena Journal, Volume 3, no. 2, Nov. 1991.

56. "The Human Laboratory," BBC Television, November 5, 1995, transcript at http://www.oldthinkernews.com/2010/12/09/human-laboratory-documentary-transcript/.

57. Celeste McGovern, "Vaccine Conspiracy or Racist Population Control Campaign: The Kenyan Tetanus Shot - Page 2," Green Med Info, November 7, 2014, http://www.greenmedinfo.com/blog/vaccine-conspiracy-or-racist-population-control-campaign-kenyan-tetanus-shot?page=2.

58. Anita Hardon, "Negotiating safety and acceptability of new contraceptive technologies," MEDISCHE ANTROPOLOGIE 16 (1) 2004, p. 119, http://tma.socsci.uva.nl/16_1/negotiating.pdf.

59. "The Human Laboratory," BBC Television, November 5, 1995, transcript at http://www.oldthinkernews.com/2010/12/09/human-laboratory-documentary-transcript/.

60. "CATHOLIC church WARNING: Neonatal tetanus Vaccine by WHO is DEADLY and bad for women reproductivity," Kenya Today, November 4, 2014, http://www.kenya-today.com/news/catholic-warning-neonatal-tetanus-vaccine-wto-deadly-bad-women-reproductivity.

61. Gregory Warner, "Catholic Bishops In Kenya Call For A Boycott Of Polio Vaccines," NPR News, August 9, 2015, http://www.npr.org/sections/goatsandsoda/2015/08/09/430347033/catholic-bishops-in-kenya-call-for-a-boycott-of-polio-vaccines.

62. Kenya NTV, "Doctors who blew the whistle over tetanus vaccine grilled by medical board," June 9, 2016, https://www.youtube.com/watch?v=K_KT7aqcJW8.

63. Dr. Stephen Kimotho Karanja, June 7, 2016, https://www.facebook.com/drstephen.kimothokaranja.

64. "The Problem With Mandatory Vaccination as Public Health Policy," Stop Mandatory Vaccination, http://www.stopmandatoryvaccination.com/public-health/.

65. "Infertility on the Rise: 1 in 6 are Infertile, Study Says," FertilityAuthor-ity.com, January 14, 2013, https://www.fertilityauthority.com/news/2013/jan/14/infertility-rise-1-6-are-infertile-study-says.

66. "New Concerns about the Human Papillomavirus Vaccine," American College of Pediatricians, January 2016, https://www.acpeds.org/the-col-lege-speaks/position-statements/health-issues/new-concerns-about-the-human-papillomavirus-vaccine.

67. Dr. Stephen Kimotho Karanja, June 2, 2016, https://www.facebook.com/drstephen.kimothokaranja.

Chapter 20. Indoctrinating The Herd

1. "Jefferey Jaxen HEALTH FREEDOM RALLY speech San Francisco City Hall on April, 22 2016," min 2:23, https://www.youtube.com/watch?v=9K_YTguXi5o.

2. Dr. Andrew Wakefield, Polly Tommey, "Update on the Sunday Lies," Autism Media Channel, July 5, 2016, min 18:15, https://www.periscope.tv/TeamVaxxed/1PlKQjNlaAvGE.

3. "Columbia University Press and Dr. Paul Offit Sued for Autism's False Prophets," Age of Autism, February 10, 2009, http://www.ageofautism.com/2009/02/columbia-university-press-and-dr-paul-offit-sued-for-au-tisms-false-prophets.html.

4. J.B. Handley, "Dr. Paul Offit, The Autism Expert. Doesn't See Patients with Autism?" Age of Autism, October 26, 2009, http://www.ageofautism.com/2009/10/dr-paul-offit-the-autism-expert-doesnt-see-patients-with-au-tism.html.

5. Rep. Bill Posey, C-SPAN, July 29, 2015, min. 1:30:24, http://www.c-span.org/video/?327309-1/us-house-morning-hour&live.

6. Tami Canal, "VAXXED: A Statement From The Producer Of Controversial Film Exposing CDC Corruption & MMR/Autism Link," March Against Monsanto, April 7, 2016, http://www.march-against-monsanto.com/vaxxed-a-statement-from-the-producer-of-controversial-film-exposing-cdc-corruption-mmrautism-link/.

7. Mollie Schreffler, "Vaxxed: The powerful new documentary the CDC wishes would just go away," The Autism File, March 26, 2016, http://www.autismfile.com/uncategorized/vaxxed-the-powerful-new-documentary-the-cdc-wishes-would-just-go-away.

8. Levi Quackenboss, "The top 3 things that #VAXXED is not: a movie review," April 12, 2016, https://leviquackenboss.wordpress.com/2016/04/12/the-top-3-things-that-vaxxed-is-not-a-movie-review/.

9. Robert F. Kennedy, Jr., "Tobacco Science and the thimerosal Scandal," p. 58, http://www.robertfkennedyjr.com/docs/thimerosalScandalFINAL.PDF.

10. Robert F. Kennedy, Jr., "Off The Grid: Robert F. Kennedy Jr. Takes on Big Pharma and the Vaccine Industry," Daily Motion, 2015, http://www.daily-motion.com/video/x2qmjj8.

11. Jon Rappoport, "How the media promote fake research on viruses," March 1, 2016, https://jonrappoport.wordpress.com/2016/03/01/how-the-media-promote-fake-research-on-viruses/.

12. Marcia Angell, MD, The Truth About the Drug Companies: How They Deceive Us and What to Do About it, Random House, 2004, p. 117, https://www.amazon.com/Truth-About-Drug-Companies-Deceive/dp/0375760946/.

13. Jerry Diamond, "U.S. slips again in press freedom ranking with blame on Obama administration," CNN, February 13, 2015, http://www.cnn.com/2015/02/13/politics/u-s-press-freedom-ranking-obama-administration-leaks/.

14. Sharyl Attkisson, "Astroturf and manipulation of media messages | Sharyl Attkisson | TEDxUniversityofNevada," TEDx Talks, February 6, 2015, https://www.youtube.com/watch?v=-bYAQ-ZZtEU.

15. Sharyl Attkisson, "Top 10 Astroturfers," Sharyl Attkisson.com, February 17, 2015, https://sharylattkisson.com/top-10-astroturfers/.

16. Lou Conte, Wayne Rohde, "Paul Offit, Fear, Intimidation and Astroturf," Age of Autism, February 10, 2015, http://www.ageofautism.com/2015/02/paul-offit-fear-intimidation-and-astroturf.html.

17. Sharyl Attkisson, "Top 10 Astroturfers," Sharyl Attkisson.com, February 17, 2015, https://sharylattkisson.com/top-10-astroturfers/.

18. Jake Crosby, "David Gorski's Financial Pharma Ties: What He Didn't Tell You," Age of Autism, June 21, 2010, http://www.ageofautism.com/2010/06/david-gorskis-financial-pharma-ties-what-he-didnt-tell-you.html.

19. "How The Refusers secretly infiltrated ORAC's Respectful Insolence science blog," The Refusers, July 15, 2012, http://therefusers.com/refusers-newsroom/how-the-refusers-secretly-infiltrated-oracs-respectful-insolence-science-blog/.

20. Sharyl Attkisson, Stonewalled: My Fight for Truth Against the Forces of Obstruction, Intimidation, and Harassment in Obama's Washington, Harper, 2014, pp. 63-64, https://www.amazon.com/Stonewalled-Obstruction-Intimidation-Harassment-Washington/dp/0062322842/.

21. "Wikipedia: Neutral point of view," https://en.wikipedia.org/wiki/Wikipedia:Neutral_point_of_view.

22. Julie Wilson, "EXCLUSIVE: Hijacked by pro-vaccine troll Dr. David Gorski, Wikipedia publishes deceitful entry on VAXXED documentary," Natural News, March 17, 2016, http://www.naturalnews.com/053719_David_Gorski_Wikipedia_VAXXED_documentary.html.

23-24. Professor TMR, "Changing Media Perception: 'Anti-Vaxxers Are [Fill in the Blank],'" Thinking Moms' Revolution, March 26, 2016, http://thinking-momsrevolution.com/changing-media-perception-anti-vaxxers-fill-blank/.

25. "About," Voices for Vaccines, http://www.voicesforvaccines.org/about/.

26-27. Jeffry John Aufderheide, "Voices for Vaccines: 11 Facts Show How it's a Propaganda Ploy for Emory University, CDC, and Big Pharma," Vac-Truth.com, February 19, 2014, https://vactruth.com/2014/02/19/cdc-and-emory-university/.

28. J.B. Handley, "Every Child By Two: Frozen Caveman Pharma Front Group," Age of Autism, November 10, 2012, http://www.ageofautism.com/2012/11/every-child-by-two-frozen-caveman-pharma-front-group.html.

29-30. Brandon Turbeville, "ALEC Behind Recent Push For Mandatory Vac-cination," NaturalBlaze.com, July 31, 2015, http://www.naturalblaze.com/2015/07/alec-behind-recent-push-for-mandatory.html.

Chapter 21. Indoctrinating Doctors

1. Quote attributed to George Merck, "The CDC's Fictional Flu Death Stats and Tamiflu's Lethal Side Effects," GreenMedinfo, February 14, 2018, http://www.greenmedinfo.com/blog/cdcs-fictional-flu-death-stats-and-tamiflus-lethal-side-effects.

2. Ben Swann, "Truth In Media: How Big Pharma Avoids Accountability With 'Off Label' Drugs," July 8, 2016, min: 5:45, http://truthinmedia.com/truth-media-big-pharma-evades-fda-off-label-drugs/.

3. Ron Chernow, Titan: The Life of John D. Rockefeller, Sr., Warner Books, 1998, https://www.amazon.com/Titan-Life-John-Rockefeller-Sr/dp/1400077303/.

4. "American Medical Association," SourceWatch, http://www.sourcewatch.org/index.php/American_Medical_Association.

5. Robert Scott Bell, "What is the hidden history of modern medicine in America? RSB reveals it," The Robert Scott Bell Show, http://www.robertscottbell.com/natural-remedies/what-is-the-hidden-history-of-modern-medicine-in-america-rsb-reveals-it/.

6. "Quackery: A Brief History of Quack Medicines & Peddlers," AuthenticHistory.com, http://www.authentichistory.com/1898-1913/2-progressivism/8-quackery/.

7. Robert Scott Bell, "What is the hidden history of modern medicine in America? RSB reveals it," The Robert Scott Bell Show, http://www.robertscottbell.com/natural-remedies/what-is-the-hidden-history-of-modern-medicine-in-america-rsb-reveals-it/.

8. "Pharmaceutical Industry," The Center for Media and Democracy, http://www.sourcewatch.org/index.php/Pharmaceutical_industry.

9. E. Richard Brown, Medicine Men: Medicine and Capitalism in America, University of California Press, Berkeley, Los Angeles, London, 1979, p. 14, https://www.amazon.com/Rockefeller-Medicine-Men-Capitalism-America/dp/0520042697/.

10-12. Eleanor McBean, The Poisoned Needle: Suppressed Facts About Vaccination, 1957, http://www.whale.to/a/mcbean.html#REGARDING THE MEDICAL MONOPOLY.

13. Dr. Richard Shulze, "Forbidden words, and diagnosis," http://whale.to/a/cure_word.html.

14. "American Medical Association," SourceWatch, http://www.sourcewatch.org/index.php/American_Medical_Association.

15. "U.S. Judge Finds Medical Group Conspired Against Chiropractors," The New York Times, August 29, 1987, http://www.nytimes.com/1987/08/29/us/us-judge-finds-medical-group-conspired-against-chiropractors.html.

16. Martin Gilens, Benjamin I. Page, "Testing Theories of American Politics: Elites, Interest Groups, and Average Citizens," Perspectives on Politics, September 2014 | Vol. 12/No. 3, p. 577, https://scholar.princeton.edu/sites/default/files/mgilens/files/gilens_and_page_2014_-testing_theories_of_american_politics.doc.pdf.

17. Jon Levine, "Jimmy Carter Tells Oprah America Is No Longer a Democracy, Now an Oligarchy," Policy. Mic, September 24, 2015, http://mic.com/articles/125813/jimmy-carter-tells-oprah-america-is-no-longer-a-democracy-now-an-oligarchy.

18. Duff Wilson, "For $520 Million, AstraZeneca Will Settle Case Over Marketing of a Drug," The New York Times, April 26, 2010, http://www.nytimes.com/2010/04/27/business/27drug.html.

19. Nicholas Kristof, "When Crime Pays: J&J's Drug Risperdal," The New York Times, September 17, 2015, http://www.nytimes.com/2015/09/17/opinion/nicholas-kristof-when-crime-pays-jjs-drug-risperdal.html.

20. "WARNER-LAMBERT TO PAY $430 MILLION TO RESOLVE CRIMINAL & CIVIL HEALTH CARE LIABILITY RELATING TO OFF-LABEL PROMOTION," Department of Justice, May 13, 2004, https://www.justice.gov/archive/opa/pr/2004/May/04_civ_322.htm.

21. "Merck to Pay More than $650 Million to Resolve Claims of Fraudulent Price Reporting and Kickbacks," Department of Justice, February 7, 2008, https://www.justice.gov/archive/opa/pr/2008/February/08_civ_094.html.

22. "GlaxoSmithKline to Plead Guilty & Pay $750 Million to Resolve Criminal and Civil Liability Regarding Manufacturing Deficiencies at Puerto Rico Plant," Department of Justice, October 26, 2010, https://www.justice.gov/

opa/pr/glaxosmithkline-plead-guilty-pay-750-million-resolve-criminal-and-civil-liability-regarding.

23. "Novartis Pharmaceuticals Corp. to Pay More Than $420 Million to Resolve Off-label Promotion and Kickback Allegations," Department of Justice, September 30, 2010, https://www.justice.gov/opa/pr/novartis-pharmaceuticals-corp-pay-more-420-million-resolve-label-promotion-and-kickback.

24. "U.S. Pharmaceutical Company Merck Sharp & Dohme to Pay Nearly One Billion Dollars Over Promotion of Vioxx®," Department of Justice, November 22, 2011, https://www.justice.gov/opa/pr/us-pharmaceutical-company-merck-sharp-dohme-pay-nearly-one-billion-dollars-over-promotion.

25. "Sanofi US Agrees to Pay $109 Million to Resolve False Claims Act Allegations of Free Product Kickbacks to Physicians," Department of Justice, December 19, 2012, https://www.justice.gov/opa/pr/sanofi-us-agrees-pay-109-million-resolve-false-claims-act-allegations-free-product-kickbacks.

26. "GlaxoSmithKline to Plead Guilty and Pay $3 Billion to Resolve Fraud Allegations and Failure to Report Safety Data," Department of Justice, July 2, 2012, https://www.justice.gov/opa/pr/glaxosmithkline-plead-guilty-and-pay-3-billion-resolve-fraud-allegations-and-failure-report.

27. "United States Sues Novartis Pharmaceuticals Corp. For Allegedly Paying Multi-Million Dollar Kickbacks To Doctors In Exchange For Prescribing Its Drugs," Department of Justice, April 26, 2013, https://www.justice.gov/usao-sdny/pr/united-states-sues-novartis-pharmaceuticals-corp-allegedly-paying-multi-million-dollar.

28. Malcolm Moore, "GlaxoSmithKline accused of 'criminal godfather' behaviour in China," The Telegraph, July 15, 2013, http://www.telegraph.co.uk/finance/newsbysector/pharmaceuticalsandchemicals/10179241/GlaxoSmithKline-accused-of-criminal-godfather-behaviour-in-China.html.

29. "China fines GlaxoSmithKline £300m and deports British boss in sex and bribery scandal," DailyMail, September 19, 2014, http://www.dailymail.co.uk/news/article-2762210/Briton-handed-suspended-jail-sentence-drug-company-GlaxoSmithKline-fined-record-300-million-China-massive-bribery-scandal.html.

30. Sammy Almashat, MD, MPH, et al., "Rapidly Increasing Criminal and Civil Monetary Penalties Against the Pharmaceutical Industry: 1991 to 2010," Public Citizen, December 16, 2010, http://www.citizen.org/hrg1924.

31. "Merck—Too Big to Prosecute?" Alliance for Natural Health USA, December 6, 2011, http://www.anh-usa.org/merck-too-big-to-prosecute/.

32. Jerome P. Kassirer, MD, On the Take: How Medicine's Complicity with Big Business Can Endanger Your Health, Oxford University Press, 2005, https://www.amazon.com/Take-Medicines-Complicity-Business-Endanger/dp/0195300041/.

33. "ON THE TAKE: How Big Business Is Corrupting American Medicine," Publishers Weekly, 2005, http://www.publishersweekly.com/978-0-19-517684-1.

34. Amy Goodman, "Narrator, Big Bucks, Big Pharma: Marketing Disease and Pushing Drugs," September, 2014, https://www.youtube.com/watch?v=lAzh28nEoWU.

35. "EXCLUSIVE: How Big Pharma greed is killing tens of thousands around the world: Patients are over-medicated and often given profitable drugs with 'little proven benefits,' leading doctors warn," Daily Mail, February 23, 2016, http://www.dailymail.co.uk/health/article-3460321/How-Big-Pharma-greed-killing-tens-thousands-world-Patients-medicated-given-profitable-drugs-little-proven-benefits-leading-doctors-warn.html.

36. Duff Wilson, "Harvard Medical School in Ethics Quandary," The New York Times, March 2, 2009, http://www.nytimes.com/2009/03/03/business/03medschool.html.

37. Marcia Angell, "Big Pharma, Bad Medicine," Boston Review, May 1, 2010, http://bostonreview.net/angell-big-pharma-bad-medicine.

38. Thomas J. Ruane, Letter to the editor, New England Journal of Medicine, August 17, 2000, p. 510.

39. Marcia Angell, MD, The Truth About the Drug Companies: How They Deceive Us and What to Do About it, Random House, 2004, p. 135, https://www.amazon.com/Truth-About-Drug-Companies-Deceive/dp/0375760946/.

40-41. Marcia Angell, MD, The Truth About the Drug Companies: How They Deceive Us and What to Do About it, Random House, 2004, p. 142, https://www.amazon.com/Truth-About-Drug-Companies-Deceive/dp/0375760946/.

42-44. Richard Smith, "Medical Journals Are an Extension of the Marketing Arm of Pharmaceutical Companies," PLOS Medicine, May 17, 2005, http://dx.doi.org/10.1371/journal.pmed.0020138.

45. Charlie Cooper, "Scientific peer reviews are a 'sacred cow' ready to be slaughtered, says former editor of BMJ," Independent, April 22, 2015, http://www.independent.co.uk/news/science/scientific-peer-reviews-are-a-sacred-cow-ready-to-be-slaughtered-says-former-editor-of-bmj-10196077.html.

46. Richard Smith, "Medical Journals Are an Extension of the Marketing Arm of Pharmaceutical Companies," PLOS Medicine, May 17, 2005, http://dx.doi.org/10.1371/journal.pmed.0020138.

47. "Retraction—Ileal-lymphoid-nodular hyperplasia, non-specific colitis, and pervasive developmental disorder in children," The Lancet, Volume 375, No. 9713, p445, 6 February 2010, http://www.thelancet.com/journals/lancet/article/PIIS0140-6736(10)60175-4/abstract.

48. Andrew J. Wakefield, Callous Disregard: Autism and Vaccines—The Truth Behind a Tragedy, Skyhorse Publishing, 2010, https://www.amazon.com/Callous-Disregard-Autism-Vaccines---Tragedy/dp/1616083239/.

49. John Stone, "The Official Stamp of the CDC: IGNORANCE IS STRENGTH," Age of Autism, September 12, 2014, http://www.ageofautism.com/2014/09/the-official-stamp-of-the-cdc-ignorance-is-strength.html.

50. "America's Healthcare System is the Third Leading Cause of Death," http://www.health-care-reform.net/causedeath.htm.

51. Pauline W. Chen, MD, "Teaching Doctors About Nutrition and Diet," The New York Times, September 16, 2010, http://www.nytimes.com/2010/09/16/health/16chen.html.

52. T. Colin Campbell, PhD, Thomas M. Campbell II, MD, The China Study: The Most Comprehensive Study of Nutrition Ever Conducted And the Startling Implications for Diet, Weight Loss, And Long-term Health, BenBella Books, 2006, pp. 328-329, https://www.amazon.com/China-Study-Comprehensive-Nutrition-Implications/dp/1932100660/.

53-54. "Mercury, Vaccines and the Global Population Control Agenda - PART 1," Uploaded August 12, 2010, https://www.youtube.com/watch?v=ONKF3CCCM1Q.

55. "AMA Supports Tighter Limitations on Immunization Opt Outs," AMA, June 8, 2015, http://www.ama-assn.org/ama/pub/news/news/2015/2015-06-08-tighter-limitations-immunization-opt-outs.page.

Chapter 22. Gods, Pawns, and Perpetrators

1. Leo Tolstoy, "DON'T BOTHER ME WITH THE FACTS," Pediatrics, May 1989, Volume 83/Issue 5, http://pediatrics.aappublications.org/content/83/5/A92.1.

2. "Midwives And Health Professionals Against Vaccination," VaccineRiskAwareness.com, http://www.vaccineriskawareness.com/Midwives-And-Health-Professionals-Against-Vaccination.

3. Suzanne Humphries, MD, "Vaccines-Honesty vs Policy - Part VI. The Business of Vaccination," April 19, 2015, min 16:15, https://www.youtube.com/watch?v=3chlvoTdnvo.

4. "How Vaccines Harm Child Brain Development - Dr Russell Blaylock MD," Vaccination Information Network, October, 2008, min: 6:40, https://www.youtube.com/watch?v=7QBcMYqlaDs.

5. Louise B Andrew, MD, JD, "Physician Suicide," Medscape, June 1, 2016, http://emedicine.medscape.com/article/806779-overview.

6. Suzanne Humphries, MD, "Smoke, Mirrors, and the 'Disappearance' Of Polio." International Medical Council On Vaccination Nov. 17, 2011, online at http://whale.to/a/smoke_mirrors.html.

7. Bob Sears, MD, The Vaccine Book: Making the Right Decision for Your Child. Oct. 26, 2011, https://idsent.wordpress.com/2015/11/22/doctors-are-no-experts-on-vaccines-get-over-it/.

8. "'The Doctors' Star Rachael Ross MD says she feels like an ASS misunderstanding vaccines," Erin Elizabeth at Health Nut News, May 30, 2016, https://www.youtube.com/watch?v=qqwPUpkuOIA.

9. Kathryn A Hale, MD, MPH, "I saw VAXXED and I was shattered!" Abundant Health Life, May 13, 2016, http://www.abundanthealthlife.com/vaxxed/.

10. "Requirements & Laws," CDC, http://www.cdc.gov/vaccines/imz-managers/laws/.

11. Del Bigtree, Vaxxed, Producer, "VAXXED: the ABC News interview that Big Pharma didn't want you to see," March 27, 2016, min: 9:50, https://www.youtube.com/watch?v=tvcdh7KlgPI.

12. Mollie Schreffler, "Vaxxed: The powerful new documentary the CDC wishes would just go away," The Autism File, March 26, 2016, http://www.autismfile.com/uncategorized/vaxxed-the-powerful-new-documentary-the-cdc-wishes-would-just-go-away.

13. Dr. Nick Delgado, "THE VACCINE PANEL: The Insider's Report," March 29, 2016, https://www.youtube.com/watch? v=F8uradn98Ls.

14. "Dr. Jack Wolfson Discusses the Anti-Vaccine Movement," NBC Channel 12 News in Phoenix, published on May 6, 2014, https://www.youtube.com/watch?v=9pw8ri_eIiI.

15. "Anti-vaccine doctor under investigation," CNN, published on February 4, 2015, https://www.youtube.com/watch?v=la82yIJLUvI.

16-17. Dr. Jack Wolfson, "Case Dismissed," Wolfson Integrative Cardiology, July 20, 2015, https://www.wolfsonintegrativecardiology.com/case-dismissed/.

18. Dr. Daniel Neides, Cleveland Clinic, "Make 2017 the year to avoid toxins (good luck) and master your domain: Words on Wellness," Updated Jan. 10, 2017; Posted Jan. 6, 2017, http://www.cleveland.com/lyndhurst-south-euclid/index.ssf/2017/01/make_2017_the_year_to_avoid_to.html.

19. Brian Shilhavy, "Former Medical Director of Cleveland Clinic Speaks Out After Being Fired for Questioning Flu Vaccine," Vaccine Impact, January 25, 2018, http://vaccineimpact.com/2018/former-medical-director-cleveland-clinic-speaks-out-after-being-fired-for-questioning-flu-vaccine/.

20. J.B. Handley, "Vaccines Don't Cause Autism, Pediatricians Do," Age of Autism, January 12, 2010, http://www.ageofautism.com/2010/01/vaccines-dont-cause-autism-pediatricians-do.html.

21. "How Can it be About the Money? Immunizations are Free! Right?" Vac-Truth, September 14, 2011, http://vaxtruth.org/2011/09/how-can-it-be-about-the-money-immunizations-are-free-right/.

22. We are Vaxxed, Posted November 3, 2016, https://www.facebook.com/wearevaxxed/videos/vb.272455363101747/358736384473644/?type=2&theater.

23. Jamie Loehr, MD, FAAFP, "Immunizations: How to Protect Patients and the Bottom Line," Fam Pract Manag. 2015 Mar-Apr;22(2):24-29, https://www.aafp.org/fpm/2015/0300/p24.html.

24. "2016 Performance Recognition Program," Blue Cross Blue Shield, p. 15, http://thephysicianalliance.org/wp-content/uploads/2016/03/2016-BCN-BCBSM-Incentive-Program-Booklet.pdf.

25. Dr. Suzanne Humphries, FB Post.

26. Douglas S. Diekema, MD, MPH, and the Committee on Bioethics, "Responding to Parental Refusals of Immunization of Children," Pediatrics, May 2005, VOLUME 115 / ISSUE 5, http://pediatrics.aappublications.org/content/115/5/1428.full.

27. "Reaffirmation: Responding to Parents Who Refuse Immunization for Their Children," http://pediatrics.aappublications.org/content/131/5/e1696.

28. "American Academy of Pediatrics Publishes New Policies to Boost Child Immunization Rates," American Academy of Pediatrics, August 29, 2016, https://www.aap.org/en-us/about-the-aap/aap-press-room/Pages/American-Academy-of-Pediatrics-Publishes-New-Policies-to-Boost-Child-Immunization-Rates.aspx.

29. W. Osler, The reserves of life. St. Mary's Hosp Gaz (London) 1907;13: 95-8. Quoted in "Fever, Famine, and War: William Osler as an Infectious Diseases Specialist" by Charles S. Bryan, online at http://cid.oxfordjournals.org/content/23/5/1139.full.pdf.

30. Jeffrey Benabio, MD, MBA, "Flu shots and persuasion," Dermatology News, October 17, 2017, https://www.mdedge.com/edermatologynews/article/149600/infectious-diseases/flu-shots-and-persuasion.

31. Neil Z. Miller, "Thinktwice Bulletin (July 2016)," email message, June 25, 2016.

32. Andrew Wakefield, MD, "Dr. Wakefield speaking at the 68th Annual Meeting of AAPS in 2011," Association of American Physicians and Surgeons, https://www.youtube.com/watch?t=2&v= l67fWVrw8xU.

33-34. Jane Orient, MD, "STATEMENT of the ASSOCIATION OF AMERICAN PHYSICIANS & SURGEONS" to the Subcommittee on Criminal Justice, Drug Policy, and Human Resources of the Committee on Government Reform, U.S. House of Representatives, Association of American Physicians & Surgeons, June 14, 1999, http://www.aapsonline.org/testimony/hepbcom.htm.

35. David A. Geier et al., "A Cross-Sectional Study of the Association between Infant Hepatitis B Vaccine Exposure in Boys and the Risk of Adverse Effects as Measured by Receipt of Special Education Services," Environmental Research and Public Health, January 12, 2018, Int. J. Environ. Res. Public Health 2018, 15(1), 123; doi:10.3390/ijerph15010123.

36. World Mercury Project Team, "The Vaccine Program's Unintended Consequences: A Tale of Two Hepatitis B Studies," World Mercury Project, January 23, 2018, https://worldmercuryproject.org/news/two-hepatitis-b-studies-illustrate-vaccine-programs-unintended-consequences/.

37. Anne Dachel, "Dachel Interview: Dr. Paul Thomas," Age of Autism, February 7, 2017, http://www.ageofautism.com/2017/02/dachel-interview-dr-paul-thomas.html.

38. "More Than 22,000 Brave Nurses Refusing to Submit to Mandatory Vaccinations," The Event Chronicle, April 14, 2015, http://www.theeventchronicle.com/health/more-than-22000-brave-nurses-refusing-to-submit-to-mandatory-vaccinations/.

39. "Parents Share Why They Will Never Vaccinate Again," Stop Mandatory Vaccination, http://www.stopmandatoryvaccination.com/personal-choice/parents-who-refuse-vaccination/.

40. "Midwives And Health Professionals Against Vaccination," VaccineRiskAwareness.com, http://www.vaccineriskawareness.com/Midwives-And-Health-Professionals-Against-Vaccination.

41-42. Patti White, RN, "Hepatitis B Vaccine: Helping or Hurting Public Health", The Subcommittee on Criminal Justice, Drug Policy, and Human Resources, May 18, 1999, http://www.thinktwice.com/Hep_Hear.pdf.

43. "Why do parents refuse to vaccinate their children?" SEggertsen, April 23, 2013, https://www.youtube.com/watch?v=8LB-3xkeDAE.

44. "Cry for Vaccine Freedom Wall," National Vaccine Information Center, http://www.nvic.org/Forms/Cry-For-Vaccine-Freedom-Wall.aspx.

45. "Dare Doctor's Think?" Verbatim Report of the Great Meeting held at Queen's Hall, London, Fri, Feb. 6, 1925, In connection with the Rex versus Hadwen manslaughter charge, http://soilandhealth.org/wp-content/uploads/02/0201hyglibcat/020119hadwin/020119hadwin.daredocsthink.html.

46. Victoria BidWell, "Timeline for the Life & Hard Times of Dr. Shelton," http://soilandhealth.org/wp-content/uploads/02/0201 hyglibcat/shelton.bio.bidwell.htm.

47. Eleanor McBean, The Poisoned Needle: Suppressed Facts About Vaccination, 1957, http://www.whale.to/a/mcbean.html#CHAPTER 9: MEDICAL INTERFERENCE.

48-49. Larry Husten, "The Big Dirty Secret Every Doctor Knows," MedPageToday, August 2, 2016, http://www.medpagetoday.com/Cardiology/CardioBrief/59481.

50. Suzanne Humphries, MD, "Smoke, Mirrors, and the 'Disappearance' Of Polio." International Medical Council On Vaccination Nov. 17, 2011, online at http://whale.to/a/smoke_mirrors.html.

51. Suzanne Humphries, MD, Rising from the Dead, 2016, https://www.amazon.com/Rising-Dead-Suzanne-Humphries-M-D/dp/0692648186/.

52. Russell Blaylock, MD, quoted from the foreword of the book, Vaccine Safety Manual: For Concerned Families and Health Practitioners, New Atlantean Press; 2nd edition, December 1, 2011, p. 8, http://www.amazon.com/Vaccine-Safety-Concerned-Families-Practitioners/dp/188121737X.

53. Jim Meehan, MD, "Medical Doctor: Blood of Every Vaccine Injured or Killed Child on Hands of Murder-by-Vaccine Pediatricians," Vaccine Impact, October 22, 2017, http://vaccineimpact.com/2017/medical-doctor-blood-of-every-vaccine-injured-or-killed-child-on-hands-of-murder-by-vaccine-pediatricians/.

54. Statement made by a doctor to a mother on the author's FB wall.

55. Yuexuan Chen quoting Peter Hotez, "'Part of this is our fault': Global Health expert talks anti-vaccine movement, preventable diseases," The Chronicle, February 20, 2018, http://www.dukechronicle.com/article/2018/02/part-of-this-is-our-fault-global-health-expert-talks-anti-vaccine-movement-preventable-diseases.

56. "Medical errors are third leading cause of death in US," Fox News, May 4, 2016, https://www.youtube.com/watch?v=1OmI2PikrcM.

57. Savage, "There's No Beauty in Disease," Thinking Moms' Revolution, February 29, 2016, http://thinkingmomsrevolution.com/theres-no-beauty-in-disease/.

58. Alicia Davis Boone, "Injured by Gardasil: Ignored, Denied, or Despised," The Thinking Moms' Revolution, Inc., January 7, 2016, http://thinkingmomsrevolution.com/injured-by-gardasil-ignored-denied-or-despised/.

59. J.B. Handley, "Dr. David Gorski, a medical moron," Unmaskingorac.blogspot.com, February 11, 2012, http://unmaskingorac.blogspot.com/2012/02/dr-david-gorski-medical-moron.html.

60. J.B. Handley, "Vaccines Don't Cause Autism, Pediatricians Do," Age of Autism, January 12, 2010, http://www.ageofautism.com/2010/01/vaccines-dont-cause-autism-pediatricians-do.html.

61. Audrey H. Reynolds, Howard A. Joos, "ECZEMA VACCINATUM," Pediatrics, August 1958, VOLUME 22 / ISSUE 2, http://pediatrics.aappublications.org/content/22/2/259.

62. Polly Tommey Interviews Marie Hansen, June 9, 2016, https://www.periscope.tv/TeamVaxxed/1DXxyMdYgwvxM.

63. "M-M-R® II (MEASLES, MUMPS, and RUBELLA VIRUS VACCINE LIVE)," Merck Sharp & Dohme Corp., p. 8., http://www.merck.com/product/usa/pi_circulars/m/mmr_ii/mmr_ii_pi.pdf.

64. Thomas Stone, MD, "Open Letter to Pediatricians on Flu Vaccines" Mercola.com, http://articles.mercola.com/sites/articles/archive/1998/11/22/tom-stone-letter.aspx.

65. Camille Hayes, Nurse, "Journey of an anti-vaxxer," May 14, 2016, min: 8:40, https://www.youtube.com/watch?v=mZ6IuwjG134&feature=youtu.be.

66. Dan Olmsted, "Vaxxed's Del Bigtree: You Have Been Heard! Video," Age of Autism, July 5, 2016, http://www.ageofautism.com/2016/07/vaxxeds-del-bigtree-you-have-been-heard-video.html.

67. Suzanne Humphries, MD, Roman Bystrianyk, Dissolving illusions: Disease, Vaccines, and the Forgotten History, 2015, p. 479, https://www.amazon.com/Dissolving-Illusions-Disease-Vaccines-Forgotten/dp/1480216895/.

Chapter 23. Thou Shalt Have No Other God Before the Gods of Vaccinology

1. Dr. Isaac Golden, Vaccination & Homoeoprophylaxis?: A Review of Risks and Alternatives, Isaac Golden Publications, 2010, p. 379, https://www.amazon.com/Vaccination-Homoeoprophylaxis-Review-Risks-Alternatives/dp/0957872674/.

2. Mahatma Gandhi, "A Guide to Health," 1921, p. 106, http://www.gutenberg.org/files/40373/40373-h/40373-h.htm.

3. Debi Vinnedge, "Forsaking God For the Sake of Science," Children of God for Life, June 13, 2012, https://cogforlife.org/2012/06/13/polioperversion/.

4. "Aborted Fetal Cell Line Vaccines And The Catholic Family," Children of God for Life, October 2005, https://cogforlife.org/vaccines-abortions/.

5. Mee Sook Park, "Original Antigenic Sin Response to RNA Viruses and Antiviral Immunity," Immune Netw. 2016 Oct; 16(5): 261–270, Published online October 5, 2016, https://www.ncbi.nlm.nih.gov/pmc/articles/PMC5086450/.

6. Gaetano Romano, "Development of Safer Gene Delivery Systems to Minimize the Risk of Insertional Mutagenesis-Related Malignancies: A Critical Issue for the Field of Gene Therapy," ISRN Oncology, November 22, 2012, https://www.ncbi.nlm.nih.gov/pmc/articles/PMC3512301/.

7. Gabriel RInaldi et al., "Germline Transgenesis and Insertional Mutagenesis in Schistosoma mansoni Mediated by Murine Leukemia Virus," PLoS Pathogens, July 26, 2012, https://www.ncbi.nlm.nih.gov/pmc/articles/PMC3406096/.

8. Jon Rappoport, "New vaccines will permanently alter human DNA May," May 17, 2016, https://jonrappoport.wordpress.com/2016/05/17/new-vaccines-will-permanently-alter-human-dna/.

9. Jane M. Orient, MD, "Mandatory Influenza Vaccination for Medical Workers: a Critique," Journal of American Physicians and Surgeons, Volume 17 Number 4 Winter 2012, http://www.jpands.org/vol17no4/orient.pdf.

10. Debi Vinnedge, "Forsaking God For the Sake of Science," Children of God for Life, June 13, 2012, https://cogforlife.org/2012/06/13/polioperversion/.

11. Jon Rappoport, "New vaccines will permanently alter human DNA May," May 17, 2016, https://jonrappoport.wordpress.com/2016/05/17/new-vaccines-will-permanently-alter-human-dna/.

12. Sayer Ji, "Vaccination Agenda: An Implicit Transhumanism / Dehumanism," GreenMedinfo, January 10, 2012, http://www.greenmedinfo.com/blog/vaccination-agenda-implicit-transhumanismdehumanism.

13. Bob Unruh, "Bureaucrats misquote pope on vaccines, teach parents 'religion,;" WND, July 15, 2016, http://www.wnd.com/2016/07/bureaucrats-misquote-pope-on-vaccines-teach-parents-religion/.

14. Mark Oppenheimer, "Review: 'Bad Faith,' a Dr. Paul A. Offit Book on Religion and Modern Medicine," The New York Times, March 11, 2015, http://mobile.nytimes.com/2015/03/11/books/review-bad-faith-a-dr-paul-a-offit-book-on-religion-and-modern-medicine.html.

15. Paul Offit, "MISSISSIPPI MIRACLE: The Unhealthiest State in America Has the Best Vaccination Rate," The Daily Beast, December 15, 2017, https://www.thedailybeast.com/the-unhealthiest-state-in-america-has-the-best-vaccination-rate.

16. Marjorie Ordene, MD, "A Doctor's Personal Vaccine Dilemma," Orthodox Union, June 26, 2008, https://www.ou.org/life/parenting/ordene_a_doctors_dilemma_original/.

17-18. Richard Moskowitz, MD, "The Case Against Immunizations," http://doctorrmosk.com/Site/The_Case_Against_Immunizations.html.

19. "NATIONAL ADULT IMMUNIZATION PLAN," THE NATIONAL VACCINE PROGRAM OFFICE, http://www.hhs.gov/sites/default/files/nvpo/national-adult-immunization-plan/naip.pdf.

20. Minister Tony Muhammad, "Vaxxed Q&A in Compton," jeffereyjaxen.com, May 19, 2016, min 39:50, http://www.jeffereyjaxen.com/blog/video-compton-mayor-offers-free-premiere-of-vaxxed-community-revolts-against-big-pharma-control.

21. Patrick McGreevy, "Nation of Islam opposes California vaccine mandate bill," Los Angeles Times, June 22, 2015, http://www.latimes.com/local/political/la-me-pc-nation-of-islam-california-vaccine-mandate-bill-20150622-story.html.

22. "Vaxxed Q&A in Compton," jeffereyjaxen.com, May 19, 2016, http://www.jeffereyjaxen.com/blog/video-compton-mayor-offers-free-premiere-of-vaxxed-community-revolts-against-big-pharma-control.

23-24. Del Bigtree, "Vaxxed Q&A in Compton," jeffereyjaxen.com, May 19, 2016, min 35:00, http://www.jeffereyjaxen.com/blog/video-compton-mayor-offers-free-premiere-of-vaxxed-community-revolts-against-big-pharma-control.

25. "Protecting Children from Mercury-Containing Drugs," United Methodist Church, 2008, http://www.umc.org/what-we-believe/protecting-children-from-mercury-containing-drugs.

26. "Exemption from Hospital Vaccine Mandate," Association of American Physicians & Surgeons, December 23, 2015, http://www.aapsonline.org/index.php/article/exemption_from_hospital_vaccine_mandate/.

27. "Example Religious Exemption Letter," http://vaxtruth.org/2012/ 07/example-religious-exemption-letter/.

28. Conversation with the author.

29. Megan Heimer, "God Does Not Support Vaccines," Living Whole, July 7, 2014, http://www.livingwhole.org/god-does-not-support-vaccines/.

30. Quoting William Wagner, JD, in Louise Kuo Habakus, MA, Mary Holland, JD, Vaccine Epidemic: How Corporate Greed, Biased Science, and Coercive Government Threaten Our Human Rights, Our Health, and Our Children, Skyhorse Publishing, 2011, p. 47, https://www.amazon.com/Vaccine-Epidemic-Corporate-Coercive-Government/dp/1620872129/.

31. Barbara Loe Fisher, "Knowledge is the Antidote for Vaccine Orthodoxy," National Vaccine Information Center, January 10, 2016, http://www.nvic.org/NVIC-Vaccine-News/January-2016/knowledge-is-the-antidote-for-vaccine-orthodoxy.aspx.

32. Dan Olmsted, "Dan Olmsted: The Amish All Over Again," Age of Autism, May 12, 2012, http://www.ageofautism.com/2012/05/dan-olmsted-the-amish-all-over-again.html.

33. Mayer Eisenstein, MD, JD, MPH, "Smoke and Mirrors vs. Real Science on Vaccines," AutismOne, May, 2012, http://www.autismone.org/sites/default/files/eisenstein.pdf.

34. Dr. William H. Gaunt, "Let's Go Find Unvaccinated Children with Autism," Age of Autism, April 14, 2016, http://www.ageofautism.com/2016/04/lets-go-find-unvaccinated-children-with-autism.html.

35. "Amish children living in northern Indiana have a very low prevalence of allergic sensitization," Journal of Allergy and Clinical Immunology, Volume 129, Issue 6, June 2012, Pages 1671-1673, https://www.sciencedirect.com/science/article/pii/S0091674912005192.

36. "Church Leaders on Child Immunization," LDS Living, February 7, 2015, http://ldsliving.com/story/78000-church-leaders-parents-have-an-obligation-to-protect-their-families-through-immunization.

37. "Immunize Children, Leaders Urge," Liahona, July 1978, https://www.lds.org/liahona/1978/07/immunize-children-leaders-urge?lang=eng.

38. Marjorie Cortez, "Utah shows highest rate of autism in new study," KSL.com, March 29, 2012, https://www.ksl.com/?sid=19785956.

39-40. James O. Grundvig, "Six Lethal Sins of CDC A Toxic Legacy of Lies: Part 3 Autism Numbers," Age of Autism, June 9, 2016, http://www.ageofautism.com/2016/06/six-lethal-sins-of-cdc-a-toxic-legacy-of-lies-autism-numbers.html.

41. "Vaccine conspiracies, a common ground for cults," March 5, 2015, https://atimetovax.wordpress.com/2015/03/05/vaccine-conspiracies-a-common-ground-for-cults/.

42. Matt Phinney, "Official: Sect kids are 'healthy, robust,'" San Angelo Standard-Times, April 15, 2008, online at http://www.childbrides.org/raid_SAST_YFZ_kids_healthy_robust.html.

Chapter 24. Sticking It to Your Future

1. "An Open Letter to Legislators Currently Considering Vaccine Legislation from Tetyana Obukhanych, PhD in Immunology," Thinking Moms' Revolution, April 17, 2015, http://thinkingmomsrevolution.com/an-open-letter-to-legislators-currently-considering-vaccine-legislation-from-tetyana-obukhanych-phd-in-immunology/.

2. Jane Orient, MD, "STATEMENT of the ASSOCIATION OF AMERICAN PHYSICIANS & SURGEONS" to the Subcommittee on Criminal Justice, Drug Policy, and Human Resources of the Committee on Government Reform, U.S. House of Representatives, Association of American Physicians & Surgeons, June 14, 1999, http://www.aapsonline.org/testimony/hepbcom.htm.

3. George Fatheree, Esq., "SB277 George Fatheree CA Assembly Health Committee June 9 2015," https://www.youtube.com/watch?v=VPgNgTGwIoE.

4. Barbara Loe Fisher, cofounder & president, National Vaccine Information Center (NVIC), "SB 277 Testimony," California State Assembly Committee on Health, National Vaccine Information Center, June 9, 2015, http://www.nvic.org/cmstemplates/nvic/pdf/blf-ca-sb-277-testimony-2015.pdf.

5. Joshua Coleman, "How do Californians feel about SB277?" April 15, 2015, https://www.youtube.com/watch?v=SjZPoPaOk0s.

6. "Is Santa Barbara PHD violating SB277? Will #BenAct?" Truth Tube, Published June 8, 2016, https://www.youtube.com/watch?v=FzZbOFzDktTg.

7. Marcella, "Dear Dr. Charity Dean: You're Wrong About SB277. You're Wrong About Everything," VaxTruth, June 7, 2016, http://vaxtruth.org/2016/06/charity-dean-sb277/.

8-9. Jefferey Jaxen, "SOLUTIONS TO SANTA BARBARA PUBLIC HEALTH OVERREACH - THE PEOPLE ACTIVATE," JeffereyJaxen.com, June 9, 2016, http://www.jeffereyjaxen.com/blog/june-09th-2016.

10. Cathy Jameson, "Yes, Virginia, Your Vaccine Exemptions Are Safe. . .for now," *Age of Autism*, January 31, 2016, http://www.ageofautism.com/2016/01/yes-virginia-your-vaccine-exemptions-are-safefor-now.html.

11. "Utah's Immunization Rule, Individual Vaccine Requirements," NUIC Northern Utah Immunization Coalition, http://nuic.org/sites/default/files/Utahs Immunization Rule - Claudia Streuper.pdf.

12-13. "NATIONAL ADULT IMMUNIZATION PLAN," THE NATIONAL VACCINE PROGRAM OFFICE, http://www.hhs.gov/sites/default/files/nvpo/national-adult-immunization-plan/naip.pdf.

14. "How the Affordable Care Act Increases Access to Influenza Vaccination for Health Care Personnel," CDC, http://www.cdc.gov/flu/toolkit/long-term-care/aca.htm.

15. "Immunization Services for Adults," HHS, http://www.hhs.gov/healthcare/facts-and-features/fact-sheets/aca-and-immunization/index.html.

16. "Are Mandatory Flu Vaccines for Healthcare Workers part of Obamacare and Linked to Financial Reimbursement to Healthcare Facilities?" Health Impact News, January 7, 2013, http://healthimpactnews.com/2013/are-mandatory-flu-vaccines-for-healthcare-workers-part-of-obamacare-and-linked-to-financial-reimbursement-to-healthcare-facilities/.

17. "Facing penalties, hospitals take hard line on employee flu shots," The Advisory Board Company, November 4, 2103, https://www.advisory.com/daily-briefing/2013/11/04/facing-penalties-hospitals-take-hard-line-on-employee-flu-shots.

18-19. "PHYSICIAN GROUP PRACTICE DEMONSTRATION," Influenza Vaccination Strategies, Virtual Breakout Session Summary, Centers for Medicare & Medicaid Services, November 30, 2007, https://innovation.cms.gov/Files/x/PGP-Flu-Vaccination.pdf.

20. Allie Malloy, "Pregnant nurse: I was fired for refusing flu vaccine," CNN, December 29, 2013, http://www.cnn.com/2013/12/29/health/pregnant-nurse-flu-vaccine-refusal/.

21. "NATIONAL ADULT IMMUNIZATION PLAN," THE NATIONAL VACCINE PROGRAM OFFICE, http://www.hhs.gov/sites/default/files/nvpo/national-adult-immunization-plan/naip.pdf.

22. "SB 792 Clears California Legislature: Parents Will Need Shots To Volunteer in Pre-Schools," September 10, 2015, http://www.themomstreetjournal.com/vaccine-laws-in-california/.

23. Alec Rosenberg, "UC plans to require vaccinations for incoming students," University of California, February 6, 2015, http://universityofcalifornia.edu/news/uc-plans-require-vaccinations-incoming-students.

24. Del Bigtree, "UC Board of Regents Meeting, June 14, 2016," https://www.facebook.com/del.bigtree/videos/10153515669175964/.

25. Robert F. Kennedy, Jr., "Readers sound off on coed classrooms, vaccines and 'Sesame Street,'" Daily News, Opinion, November 7, 2015, http://www.nydailynews.com/opinion/nov-7-coed-classrooms-vaccines-sesame-street-article-1.2426184.

26. Heather Fraser, The Peanut Epidemic, What's Causing It and How to Stop It, Skyhorse Publishing, 2011, https://www.amazon.com/Peanut-Allergy-Epidemic-Whats-Causing/dp/1616082739/.

27. "Refused Vaccination, Got 15 Years," New York Times, May 2, 1918.

28. Dr. William Osler, Influence of Vaccination Upon Other Diseases, quoted in The Poisoned Needle: Suppressed Facts About Vaccination by Eleanor McBean, 1957, http://www.whale.to/a/mcbean.html.

29-30. Dan Burton, "Mercury in Medicine," Congressional Record (May 20, 2003): E1016.

31. Scott Miller, director, Direct Order, 2003, http://www.imdb.com/title/tt0391928/.

32. Jeff Moore, Tech Sgt, Air Force Reserve, "Direct Order" Documentary (Full) - Soldiers Ordered To Take Anthrax Vaccine & Got Brain Damaged, 2013, min. 7:00, https://www.youtube.com/watch?v=wDDMsvErsQw&.

33. Lt. Doug Rokke, US Army, "Beyond Treason: Depleted Uranium & Anthrax Vaccines," min 1:12:15, https://www.youtube.com/watch?v=DDQi9uMUodk&ebc.

34. Lt. Richard Rovet, U.S. Air Force, "ANTHRAX VACCINE ADVERSE REACTIONS," HEARING BEFORE THE SUBCOMMITTEE ON NATIONAL SECURITY, VETERANS AFFAIRS, AND INTERNATIONAL RELATIONS OF THE COMMITTEE ON GOVERNMENT REFORM, HOUSE OF REPRESENTATIVES, ONE HUNDRED SIXTH CONGRESS, FIRST SESSION, JULY 21, 1999, Serial No. 106–131, p. 15, https://www.gpo.gov/fdsys/pkg/CHRG-106hhrg65673/pdf/CHRG-106hhrg65673.pdf.

35. Rep. Benjamin A. Gilman, "ANTHRAX VACCINE ADVERSE REACTIONS," p. 15.

36-38. "FDA Anthrax vaccine documents show pentagon lied," Delaware News Journal, October 11, 20014, http://ahrp.org/fda-anthrax-vaccine-documents-show-pentagon-lied/.

39. Gary Matsumoto, "Vaccine A: The Covert Government Experiment That's Killing Our Soldiers—and Why GI's Are Only the First Victims," Basic Books, 2010, pp. 45-46, https://www.amazon.com/Vaccine-Government-Experiment-Killing-Soldiers/dp/0465021824.

40. Rep. Benjamin A. Gilman, "ANTHRAX VACCINE ADVERSE REACTIONS," HEARING BEFORE THE SUBCOMMITTEE ON

NATIONAL SECURITY, VETERANS AFFAIRS, AND INTERNA-
TIONAL RELATIONS OF THE COMMITTEE ON GOVERNMENT
REFORM, HOUSE OF REPRESENTATIVES, ONE HUNDRED
SIXTH CONGRESS, FIRST SESSION, JULY 21, 1999, Serial No. 106–
131, p. 15, https://www.gpo.gov/fdsys/pkg/CHRG-106hhrg65673/pdf/
CHRG-106hhrg65673.pdf.

41-42. "Improving Health Protection of Military Personnel Participating in
Particular Military Operations," The White House, September 30, 1999,
https://www.gpo.gov/fdsys/pkg/CFR-2000-title3-vol1/html/CFR-2000-ti-
tle3-vol1-eo13139.htm.

43. "Vaccine Dangers Exposed Part 2 Of 3," https://www.youtube.com/
watch?v=MGWWw89a0Y0.

44. "Direct Order" Documentary (Full) - Soldiers Ordered To Take Anthrax
Vaccine & Got Brain Damaged, 2013, https://www.youtube.com/
watch?v=wDDMsvErsQw&.

45. Sheila Ealey, "Vaxxed Q&A in Compton," jeffereyjaxen.com, May 19, 2016,
min 53:25, http://www.jeffereyjaxen.com/blog/video-compton-mayor-
offers-free-premiere-of-vaxxed-community-revolts-against-big-pharma-con-
trol.

46. John W. Hodge, MD, The Vaccination Superstition, 1902, p. 47,
https://books.google.com/books/about/The_Vaccination_Superstition.
html?id=eWRCCZmWd90C.

47. "Myths and Facts," National Vaccine Information Center, http://www.nvic
.org/Myths-and-Facts.aspx.

48-49. "Bush signs vaccine stockpile legislation," Associated Press, July 21, 2004,
http://www.nbcnews.com/id/5472564/ns/health-bioterror_news/t/bush-
signs-vaccine-stockpile-legislation/.

50. Carl Franzen, "Killer cure: why is the US creating new viruses and stockpiling the vaccines?" The Verge, April 17, 2013, http://www.theverge
.com/2013/4/17/4227570/project-bioshield-vaccine-stockpiling-bird-flu-
avian-influenza.

51-53. Carl Franzen, "Killer cure: why is the US creating new viruses and
stockpiling the vaccines?" The Verge, April 17, 2013, http://www.theverge
.com/2013/4/17/4227570/project-bioshield-vaccine-stockpiling-bird-flu-
avian-influenza.

54. Tia Ghose, "DARPA Is Developing Human Bio-Factories to Brew Lifesav-
ing Vaccines," LifeScience, September 11, 2015, https://www.livescience
.com/52150-humans-become-vaccine-factories.html.

55. Jane Orient, MD, "STATEMENT of the ASSOCIATION OF AMERI-
CAN PHYSICIANS & SURGEONS to the Subcommittee on Criminal

Justice, Drug Policy, and Human Resources of the Committee on Government Reform, U.S. House of Representatives, Association of American Physicians & Surgeons," June 14, 1999, http://www.aapsonline.org/testimony/hepbcom.htm.

56. U.S. Rep. Ron Paul, MD, "Government Vaccines — Bad Policy, Bad Medicine," International Medical Council on Vaccination, October 19, 2011, http://www.vaccinationcouncil.org/2011/10/19/ron-paul-mdgovernment-vaccines-bad-policy-bad-medicine/.

57. Barbara Loe Fisher, "No Pharma Liability? No Vaccine Mandates," National Vaccine Information Center, March 2, 2011, http://www.nvic.org/NVIC-Vaccine-News/March-2011/No-Pharma-Liability--No-Vaccine-Mandates-.aspx.

58. Supreme Court Justice S. Sotomayor joined by Justice Ginsburg, "BRUESEWITZ ET AL. v. WYETH LLC, FKA WYETH, INC., ET AL.," SUPREME COURT OF THE UNITED STATES, February 22, 2011, pp. 26-27 of Justice Sotomayor's and Justice Ginsburg's dissenting opinion, http://www.supremecourt.gov/opinions/10pdf/09-152.pdf.

59. "Control of Communicable Diseases," Federal Register, August 15, 2016, https://www.federalregister.gov/articles/2016/08/15/2016-18103/control-of-communicable-diseases.

60. Barack Obama, The White House, November 4, 2016, https://www.white-house.gov/the-press-office/2016/11/04/executive-order-advancing-global-health-security-agenda-achieve-world.

61. (https://www.facebook.com/shawn.siegel.7/posts/ 1931042850256506.)

Chapter 25. William Thompson, *Vaxxed,* and the Great Awakening

1. Glen Nowak, PhD, "Increasing Awareness and Uptake of Influenza Immunization," CDC, http://nationalacademies.org/hmd/~/media/Files/Activity%20Files/PublicHealth/MicrobialThreats/Nowak.pdf.

2. William W. Thompson, PhD, August 27, 2014 Press Release, "Statement of William W. Thompson, PhD, Regarding the 2004 Article Examining the Possibility of a Relationship Between MMR Vaccine and Autism," http://morganverkamp.com/statement-of-william-w-thompson-ph-d-regarding-the-2004-article-examining-the-possibility-of-a-relationship-between-mmr-vaccine-and-autism/.

3-4. Celia Farber, "BREAKING NEWS: CDC WHISTLEBLOWER TEXT MESSAGES TO ANDY WAKEFIELD: STUDY WOULD HAVE 'SUPPORTED HIS SCIENTIFIC OPINION'," The Truth Barrier, September 2, 2014, http://truthbarrier.com/2014/09/02/breaking-news-cdc-whistleblower-text-messages-to-andy-wakefield-study-would-have-supported-his-scientific-opinion/.

5. Andrew Wakefield, "I do not believe that any vaccines currently on the market meet the criteria for safety and efficacy," https://www.facebook.com/groups/1557208007861048/?multi_permalinks=1773742436207603&notif_t=group_highlights&notif_id=1470144013442113.

6. Amy Sherman, "Ben Carson says pediatricians realize need to cut down number and proximity of vaccines," Politifact, September 17, 2016, http://www.politifact.com/florida/statements/2015/sep/17/ben-carson/ben-carson-says-pediatricians-realize-need-cut-dow/.

7. Karen Remley, MD, MBA, MPH, FAAP, executive director, American Academy of Pediatrics, "American Academy of Pediatrics Reiterates Safety and Importance of Vaccines," American Academy of Pediatrics, September 17, 2015, https://www.aap.org/en-us/about-the-aap/aap-press-room/pages/American-Academy-of-Pediatrics-Reiterates-Safety-and-Importance-of-Vaccines.aspx.

8. Linda Williams, "Harkins pulls controversial Vaxxed film," Fox 10, April 27, 2016, http://www.fox10phoenix.com/news/arizona-news/133671199-story.

9. "InDOCtrination," Truth Tube, published June 28, 2016, min 1:18, https://www.youtube.com/watch?v=K6Xx0han0G8.

10. Carl Sagan, The Demon-Haunted World: Science as a Candle in the Dark, Ballantine Books, 1997, p. 241, https://www.amazon.com/Demon-Haunted-World-Science-Candle-Dark/dp/0345409469/.

11. Email from Dr. William E. Cosgrove, MD, FAAP, to Utah political leaders. June 14, 2016, copy in author's possession.

12. Harris L. Coulter, Vaccination, Social Violence, and Criminality: The Medical Assault on the American Brain, North Atlantic Books, 1993, p. 259, https://www.amazon.com/Vaccination-Social-Violence-Criminality-American/dp/1556430841.

13. Email from Dr. William E. Cosgrove, MD, FAAP, to Utah political leaders. June 14, 2016, copy in author's possession.

14. Shawn Siegel, FB post, August 12, 2016.

15. Paul Sisson, "Judge denies injunction against vaccine law," The San Diego Union Tribune, August 26, 2016, http://www.sandiegouniontribune.com/news/2016/aug/26/vaccination-order-judge-sabraw/.

16. "American Academy of Pediatrics Publishes New Policies to Boost Child Immunization Rates," American Academy of Pediatrics, August 29, 2016, https://www.aap.org/en-us/about-the-aap/aap-press-room/Pages/American-Academy-of-Pediatrics-Publishes-New-Policies-to-Boost-Child-Immunization-Rates.aspx.

17. "How Much Money Do Pediatricians Really Make From Vaccines?" WELLNESS AND EQUALITY, June 20, 2016, https://wellnessandequality.com/2016/06/20/how-much-money-do-pediatricians-really-make-from-vaccines/.

18. From the American Academy of Pediatrics Policy Statement, "Medical Versus Nonmedical Immunization Exemptions for Child Care and School Attendance," August 2016, http://pediatrics.aappublications.org/content/early/2016/08/25/peds.2016-2145.

19. "American Academy of Pediatrics Publishes New Policies to Boost Child Immunization Rates," American Academy of Pediatrics, August 29, 2016, https://www.aap.org/en-us/about-the-aap/aap-press-room/Pages/American-Academy-of-Pediatrics-Publishes-New-Policies-to-Boost-Child-Immunization-Rates.aspx.

20. D. Bennett, et al., "Project TENDR: Targeting Environmental Neuro-Developmental Risks. The TENDR Consensus Statement," Environ Health Perspect; DOI:10.1289/EHP358, Volume 124, Issue 7, July 2016, http://ehp.niehs.nih.gov/EHP358/#tab1.

21. Kelly Brogan, MD, A Mind of Your Own: The Truth About Depression and How Women Can Heal Their Bodies to Reclaim Their Lives, Harper Wave, 2016, p. 198, http://www.amazon.com/Mind-Your-Own-Depression-Reclaim/dp/0062405578/.

22. Stephanie Seneff, CSAIL, MIT, "Impact of Glyphosate: Possible Modes of Action," slide #7, March 6, 2016, SeneffSanDiego.pptx.

23. Anne Dachel, "NVIC's Barbara Loe Fisher on Vaccine Debate," Age of Autism, February 6, 2015, http://www.ageofautism.com/2015/02/nvics-barbara-loe-fisher-on-vaccine-debate.html.

24. John W. Hodge, MD, The Vaccination Superstition, 1902, p. 41, quoted in The Poisoned Needle: Suppressed Facts About Vaccination by Eleanor McBean, online at http://www.whale.to/a/mcbean.html.

25. https://www.facebook.com/sheila.ealey/posts/10208546971445994.

26. "Vaxxed Q&A in Compton," jeffereyjaxen.com, May 19, 2016, http://www.jeffereyjaxen.com/blog/video-compton-mayor-offers-free-premiere-of-vaxxed-community-revolts-against-big-pharma-control.

27. "Leadership & Longevity 2015 - Dr. Andrew Wakefield," Age of Autism, December 31, 2015, http://www.ageofautism.com/2015/12/leadership-longevity-2015-dr-andrew-wakefield.html.

28. "Andy Wakefield, Santa Monica," United for VaxXed, July 1, 2016, https://www.facebook.com/VaxXed/videos/vb.669084493234593/713749518768090/?type=2&theater.

INDEX

ABOUT THE AUTHOR

B rett Wilcox is a Licensed Professional Counselor and agnotologist (one who studies culturally induced ignorance or doubt). Through Brett's work and research, he realized that abusers at home, in industry, and in the government use the same tactics to gain and maintain control over others.

In 2013, Brett authored *We're Monsanto: Feeding the World, Lie After Lie, Book I*. In 2014, he and his 15-year-old son, David, ran across the United States advocating for a GMO-free USA and world. In 2015, Brett published his second book, *We're Monsanto: Still Feeding the World, Lie After Lie, Book II*.

While running across the country, Brett and his family met parents of autistic children. Some stated that their healthy children suffered severe vaccine reactions leading to their regression into autism. Shortly after finishing their run, Dr. William Thompson—the scientist now known as the CDC whistle-blower—acknowledged that he and his colleagues had buried the link between vaccines and autism.

These events compelled Brett to investigate the vaccine industry, which led to the conclusion that "the world's greatest scientific achievement" is built upon fraud, greed, corruption, racism, elitism, and tyranny. Brett is pleased to present his findings in his latest book, *Jabbed: How the Vaccine Industry, Medical Establishment, and Government Stick It to You and Your Family*.

Brett resides with his family in the island community of Sitka, Alaska, where he enjoys running the trails with Jenna, the dog they adopted from a Texas shelter while running across the USA.

Brett blogs at RunningTheCountry.com.